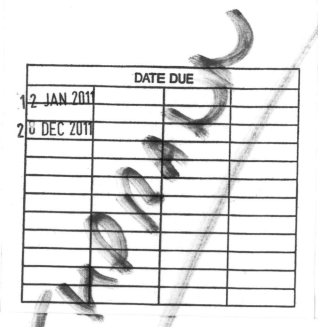

Psychotherapy Indications and Outcomes

Psychotherapy Indications and Outcomes

EDITED BY
David S. Janowsky, M.D.

American Psychopathological Association

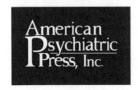

WASHINGTON, DC
LONDON, ENGLAND

Copyright © 1999 American Psychiatric Press, Inc.
ALL RIGHTS RESERVED
Manufactured in the United States of America on acid-free paper
02 01 00 99   4 3 2 1
First Edition

American Psychiatric Press, Inc.
1400 K Street, N.W., Washington, DC   20005
www.appi.org

Library of Congress Cataloging-in-Publication Data
Psychotherapy indications and outcomes / edited by David S. Janowsky. — 1st ed.
        p.   cm. — (American Psychopathological Association series)
    "Papers presented at the 86th Annual Meeting of the American Psychopathological Association" — Pref.
    Includes bibliographical references and index.
    ISBN 0-88048-761-5 (alk. paper)
    1. Psychodynamic psychotherapy—Congresses. 2. Mental illness—Congresses. 3. Psychology, Pathological—Congresses.
4. Psychotherapy—Congresses. I. Janowsky, David S. (David Steffan), 1939–   . II. American Psychopathological Association. Meeting (86th : 1996 : New York, N.Y.) III. Series.
    [DNLM: 1. Mental Disorders—therapy congresses.
2. Psychotherapy congresses. 3. Treatment Outcome congresses. 4. Mental Disorders—diagnosis congresses.
WM 420 P97435 1999]
RC489.P72P83   1999
616.89'14—dc21
DNLM/DLC
for Library of Congress   98-43413
                                                                                        CIP

British Library Cataloguing in Publication Data
A CIP record is available from the British Library.

Contents

Part II Dialectical Behavioral Therapy

Part III Cognitive-Behavioral Therapy

Part IV Interpersonal Therapy: Mechanisms and Efficacy

Part V Psychotherapy With the Medically Ill

Contributors

W. Stewart Agras, M.D.
Professor of Psychiatry and Behavioral Sciences, Stanford University School of Medicine, Stanford, California

Melanie M. Biggs, Ph.D.
Assistant Professor of Psychiatry, Department of Psychiatry, University of Texas Southwest Medical Center, Dallas, Texas

Sidney J. Blatt, Ph.D.
Professor of Psychiatry, Yale University, New Haven, Connecticut

Katherine A. Comtois, Ph.D.
Researcher, University of Washington, Seattle, Washington

Louis Diguer, Ph.D.
Laval University, Quebec, Canada

Irene Elkin, Ph.D.
Professor, School of Social Service Administration, University of Chicago, Chicago, Illinois

Ellen Frank, Ph.D.
Professor of Psychiatry and Psychology, University of Pittsburgh School of Medicine, Western Psychiatric Institute and Clinic, Pittsburgh, Pennsylvania

Ira D. Glick, M.D.
Professor of Psychiatry and Behavioral Sciences, Stanford University School of Medicine, Stanford, California

Michael J. Goldstein, Ph.D.
Professor of Psychology and Psychiatry, University of California, Los Angeles, California

Victoria J. Grochocinski, Ph.D.
University of Pittsburgh School of Medicine, Western Psychiatric Institute and Clinic, Pittsburgh, Pennsylvania

Steven D. Hollon, Ph.D.
Professor of Psychology, Vanderbilt University, Nashville, Tennessee

David S. Janowsky, M.D.
Professor of Psychiatry, University of North Carolina Chapel Hill, Chapel Hill, North Carolina

Jonathan W. Kanter, M.A.
Research Assistant, Department of Psychology, University of Washington, Seattle, Washington

Donald F. Klein, M.D.
Professor of Psychiatry, College of Physicians and Surgeons of Columbia University, New York, New York

David J. Kupfer, M.D.
Professor and Chair of Psychiatry, University of Pittsburgh School of Medicine, Western Psychiatric Institute and Clinic, Pittsburgh, Pennsylvania

Marsha M. Linehan, Ph.D.
Professor of Psychology, University of Washington, Seattle, Washington

Ellen Luborsky, Ph.D.
Senior Psychologist, Riverdale Mental Health Center, Philadelphia, Pennsylvania

Lester Luborsky, Ph.D.
Professor Emeritus of Psychology in Psychiatry, University of Pennsylvania Health System, Philadelphia, Pennsylvania

John C. Markowitz, M.D.
Associate Professor of Psychiatry and Director, Psychotherapy Clinic, Payne Whitney Clinic, The New York Hospital–Cornell Medical Center, New York, New York

Ann B. McEachran, M.A.
Department of Psychiatry, University of Pittsburgh School of Medicine, Western Psychiatric Institute and Clinic, Pittsburgh, Pennsylvania

A. John Rush, M.D.
Professor and Vice-Chairman for Research in Psychiatry, University of Texas Southwestern Medical Center, Dallas, Texas

Kelly A. Schmidt, B.A.
Department of Psychology, George Washington University, Washington, D.C.

Zindel V. Segal, Ph.D., C.Psych.
Associate Professor of Psychiatry and Psychology, University of Toronto, Head of Psychotherapy Research, Clarke Institute, Toronto, Canada

Stephen S. Sharfstein, M.D.
President, Medical Director and Chief Executive Officer, Sheppard
Pratt Health System, Baltimore, Maryland, Clinical Professor of
Psychiatry, University of Maryland

Brian F. Shaw, Ph.D., C.Psych.
Professor, Department of Psychiatry and Behavioral Science, University
of Toronto, Toronto, Canada

M. Tracie Shea, Ph.D.
Associate Professor of Psychiatry, Brown University, Providence, Rhode
Island

Stuart M. Sotsky, M.D., M.P.H.
Professor of Psychiatry, George Washington University Medical Center,
Washington, D.C.

Cynthia A. Spanier, Ph.D.
Department of Psychiatry, University of Pittsburgh School of Medicine,
Western Psychiatric Institute and Clinic, Pittsburgh, Pennsylvania

David Spiegel, M.D.
Professor of Psychiatry and Behavioral Sciences, Stanford University
School of Medicine, Stanford, California

Myrna M. Weissman, Ph.D.
Chief, Division of Clinical–Genetic Epidemiology, Professor of
Epidemiology in Psychiatry, College of Physicians and Surgeons of
Columbia University, New York, New York

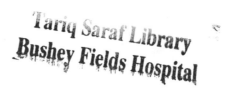

Preface

The practice of psychotherapy remains at the intellectual and philosophic heart of the work of those who treat emotional disorders. As a combination of scientifically driven techniques and an art requiring considerable creativity, intuitiveness, and empathy, psychotherapy is a phenomenon well worth celebrating, refining, and expanding. Nevertheless, obviously to retain its viability, the usefulness of psychotherapy needs to be objectively demonstrated. Over the last several decades considerable progress has been made toward understanding how truly useful various psychotherapies are, how they compare with pharmacotherapy, how psychotherapy and pharmacotherapy influence each other, and what general factors influence outcome. At the same time, since the 1980s and during the 1990s, the practice of psychotherapy has become very much altered by the economics and principles of managed care. The ability to offer medium-term to long-term psychotherapy has decreased considerably as managed care influences have pervaded the marketplace. Often, treatment is now restricted to attention to the acute crisis and may be limited to the briefest of psychotherapeutic interventions given in conjunction with pharmacotherapy. Thus, paradoxically, we are at a time when economic, political, and social pressures are undercutting our ability to offer effective psychotherapy at just the time when the scientific study of psychotherapy is helping us to understand how it works and demonstrating that it is very effective.

The purpose of this volume, a compendium of papers first presented at the 86th Annual Meeting of the American Psychopathological Association, held 29 February to 2 March 1996, in New York City, is to review the status of psychotherapy in the 1990s, paying special attention to existing evidence of its efficacy and effectiveness and to those underlying mechanisms that appear related to positive and negative outcomes. Another major theme of this volume is a consideration of the relative effectiveness of psychotherapy, as compared with pharmacotherapy, and to a combination of psychotherapy and pharmacotherapy.

At the American Psychopathological Association Annual Meeting and in the subsequent chapters created for this book, the principal authors, all esteemed researchers in the field of psychotherapy investigation, were asked to focus, from the perspective of their own work, on the theory and mechanisms, techniques, evidence of effectiveness, and indications for the psychotherapy or psychotherapies that they have devoted their research careers to understanding.

The chapters in this volume are divided into eight sections. The first of these focuses on those general mechanisms underlying psychotherapeutic efficacy. Chapters in this section begin with the Paul Hoch Award address by psychotherapy research pioneer Dr. Lester Luborsky and colleagues. This chapter explores the relative efficacy of dynamic and other therapies and those general therapist and patient characteristics that determine outcome. Other chapters, first-authored by Drs. Sidney Blatt, M. Tracie Shea, and David Janowsky, explore the interpersonal, patient, therapist, underlying personality, and general patient characteristics that determine psychotherapeutic outcome. In the second section, Dr. Marsha Linehan and colleagues describe the nature, theory, and efficacy of dialectical behavioral therapy. The third section offers an in-depth exploration of the mechanisms of action, therapeutic effects, and efficacy of cognitive-behavioral therapies, as provided in reviews by Drs. Melanie Biggs and A. John Rush, and by Drs. Brian Shaw and Zindel Segal. In addition, Dr. Stewart Agras here explores the usefulness of cognitive-behavioral therapy in the eating disorders. The fourth section similarly explores interpersonal therapy. This section leads off with a chapter by Dr. Myrna M. Weissman, the American Psychopathological Association's Zubin Award winner, in which she outlines how she and her late husband, Dr. Gerald Klerman, developed interpersonal therapy, as well as describing interpersonal therapy's nature, effectiveness, and future. This presentation is followed by an exploration of the interaction of interpersonal therapy and medications by Dr. John Markowitz and a chapter by Dr. Cynthia Spanier and colleagues exploring the use of interpersonal therapy in depression. The fifth section, authored by Dr. David Spiegel, elaborates a highly effective group therapy model for patients with cancer and other medical illnesses, a treatment method shown to increase life span and quality of life in those who participate. The sixth section contains reviews by Dr. Ira Glick, evaluating family therapy in general, and by the late Dr. Michael Goldstein, considering its use in the treatment of psychotic patients. The seventh section is largely focused on methodological considerations in psychotherapy and psychotherapy-psychopharmacological research. In this section, Drs. Steven Hollon and Donald Klein discuss, from varying perspectives, the types of methodological problems, difficulties, and challenges inherent in psychotherapy research. Finally, Dr. Steven Sharfstein presents an illuminating chapter on the relationship of psychotherapy to managed care, offering us important perspectives about how psychotherapy might best survive in these current difficult times.

It is hoped that from the chapters contained in this volume the reader can understand more about the current status of psychotherapy research as it relates to psychotherapeutic efficacy and can come to know more of those common underlying mechanisms that determine psychotherapeutic effectiveness. By bringing together the learned opinions of many leaders in the field of psychotherapy research, it is hoped that a usable volume of information will be presented that will allow the reader to have a clear view of the scientific basis underlying the practice of psychotherapy.

PART I

Individual and Interpersonal Determinants of Psychotherapeutic Effects

CHAPTER 1

The Efficacy of Dynamic Versus Other Psychotherapies

Is It True That "Everyone Has Won and All Must Have Prizes"?—An Update

Lester Luborsky, Ph.D.

Louis Diguer, Ph.D.

Ellen Luborsky, Ph.D.

Kelly A. Schmidt, B.A.

It is the fond wish of the practitioners of each form of psychotherapy that theirs be the most effective in treating patients, and this wish frequently becomes a conviction. Our wish here is to guard against any such tendency. By surveying evidence for the efficacy of each of the main forms of psychotherapy, we now focus on the dynamic therapies versus other therapies, a comparison omitted from our earliest version of the review of comparative treatment studies (Luborsky et al. 1975). We also update our previous review of a variety of psychotherapies compared with each other and with nontherapy control conditions.

Our current review only includes studies in which attention was paid to the main requisites of controlled comparative treatment re-

---

This chapter is an updated and revised version of Luborsky L, Diguer L, Luborsky E, et al.: "The Efficacy of Dynamic Psychotherapies: Is It True That Everyone Has Won So All Shall Have Prizes?" in Psychodynamic Treatment Research: A Handbook for Clinical Practice. *Edited by Miller N, Luborsky L, Barber JP, et al. New York, Basic Books, 1993, pp. 447–514. Copyright © 1993 by Basic Books, Inc. Reprinted by permission of Basic Books, a member of Perseus Books, L.L.C.*

search. These requisites were judged according to 12 criteria (given in more detail in Luborsky et al. 1975, the first review to evaluate each study according to detailed quality criteria). The main criteria for judging a study's adequacy of design are as follows:

1. Patients were assigned randomly (or stratified on prognostic variables) to each group.
2. Real patients, not actors or student volunteers, were used.
3. Therapists for each group were equally competent.
4. Therapists were experienced and knowledgeable about the form of therapy they were to conduct.
5. Treatments were equally valued by the patients and therapists in each group.
6. The outcome measures represented the target goals of the treatment (weight ½).
7. Treatment outcome was evaluated by independent measures.
8. Information was obtained about the patients' concurrent use of treatments other than that intended, both formal and informal (weight ½).
9. Samples of all compared treatments were independently evaluated for the extent to which the therapists adhered to the manual-designated form of treatment (weight ½).
10. Each of the compared treatments was given in equal amounts in terms of length and/or frequency.
11. Each treatment was given in a reasonable and appropriate amount.
12. Sample size was adequate.

Each criterion contributed a weight of 1, ½, or 0. But the primary purpose of our grading system was to weed out the worst studies rather than to provide highly reliable subdivisions of grading. Nevertheless, in the first agreement study (Luborsky et al. 1975) it was reassuring to find that the independent grading judgments of two of the authors (L.L. and B.S.) on 16 randomly selected studies yielded a reliability correlation of .84 ($P < .001$). In the present study, agreement of two judges (L.L. and L.D.) on 12 dynamic versus other studies was again highly satisfactory ($r = .90$, $P = .0001$).

The studies of dynamic psychotherapy in this review had to meet several other inclusion and exclusion criteria as well:

1. The studies had to be of young adults or adults.
2. The patients had to be nonpsychotic, although a few were patients with borderline personality disorder or psychosis.
3. The treatments needed to be bona fide treatments. (Thus we excluded role-playing studies, which makes our results more relevant to practitioners.)
4. Studies of patients who had only specific habit disturbances, such as smoking or overeating, were excluded.
5. We included mainly individual psychotherapy studies (except in comparisons with other forms of psychotherapy, such as group psychotherapy). The various forms of individual psychotherapy were all included, although some were merely designated verbal psychotherapy. We did not include studies of marital or family therapy.

Two main types of outcome measures were used: a general adjustment measure and a specific symptom outcome measure. When results differed on these two types of measures, we noted the trend of the difference. We counted each outcome measure's results at both termination of treatment and follow-up. Finally, to prevent distortion by the results of a few studies that contain many outcome measures, an upper limit of four outcome comparisons was set at termination and follow-up, a limit that affected only a few studies, such as those by Pierloot and Vinck (1978) and Cross et al. (1982).

Our review builds on studies collected in other reviews, including those of Crits-Christoph (1992), Elliott et al. (1993), Lambert et al. (1986), Meltzoff and Kornreich (1970), Shapiro and Shapiro (1982), Smith et al. (1980), and Svartberg and Stiles (1991).

Our results are expressed in Table 1–1 as box scores and effect sizes. Box scores give results in only three categories: significantly better (+), significantly worse (−), and not significantly different (0). Effect sizes give scores in terms of exact measures of the association of the variables, such as in Cohen's r in Table 1–1. The box score method

TABLE 1–1

Significance of differences in effect sizes: dynamic versus other psychotherapies

Study	Dynamic versus	Quality ratings	Termination Cohen's r	Z	N	1-year follow-up Cohen's r	Z	N	Box score Termination	Follow-up
Beutler and Mitchell 1981	Experiential	10.5	–.41	–2.59[a]	40				–	0
Brodaty and Andrews 1983	Family doctor	6	.03	.18	36	–.20	–1.13	32	0	0
Brom et al. 1989	Desensitization	9.5	.12	.93	60				0	0
	Hypnotherapy		.19	1.45	58				0	0
Cross et al. 1982	Behavior	7	.08	.44	30	–.40	–1.65	17	0	0
Elkin et al. 1989	Cognitive[b]	11	.08	.73	84				0	
Gallagher and Thompson 1982	Cognitive-behavioral	8	–.33	–1.92	20	–.39	–1.64	18	0	–
	Behavior		–.18	–.80	20	–.46	–1.95[a]	18	0	–
Marmar et al. 1988	Group	7	.20	1.56	61	.17	1.33	61	0	0
Patterson et al. 1971	Behavior	6.5	–.25	–1.82	53	0	0	20	–[a]	0
									0	
Pierloot and Vinck 1978	Desensitization	8	.12	.56	22				0	
Sloane et al. 1975	Behavior	10	.07	.54	60	0	0	60	0	0
Thompson et al. 1987	Cognitive-behavioral	10	–.01	–.08	61				0	
	Behavior		–.07	–.54	60				0	

Continued on next page

TABLE 1–1 (continued)

Study	Dynamic versus	Quality ratings	Termination Cohen's r	Termination Z	Termination N	1-year follow-up Cohen's r	1-year follow-up Z	1-year follow-up N	Box score Termination	Box score Follow-up
Woody et al. 1983	Cognitive-behavioral	10	.24	2.02[a]	71				0	
	Drug counseling		.26	2.19[a]	71				+	+
Zitrin et al. 1978	Behavior	9.5	.13	1.37	111				0	
Overall results										
Termination	Uncorrected	r = .008	Z = .80	P = .40						
	Corrected	r = .01	Z = 1.17	P = .24						
Follow-up	Uncorrected	r = −.19	Z = −1.90	P = .06						
	Corrected	r = −.19	Z = −1.85	P = .07						

Box score: dynamic better, +; nonsignificant difference, 0.

[a] Z was significant at P < .05.
[b] Interpersonal rather than dynamic therapy was used.

is not as precise as the effect size method, but our experience has shown that when the sample of studies is large, box scores adequately convey the general trend. For example, the box scores in the 1975 version of this chapter were in line with the effect-size-based results described by Smith et al. (1980).

Dynamic Versus Other Psychotherapies

The effectiveness of dynamic psychotherapy versus other psychotherapies is the only category of comparison that we review in detail. Dynamic psychotherapy is an early derivative of psychoanalytic treatment. It mimics the parent treatment, psychoanalysis, in its principles but is shorter in duration (Luborsky 1984). Dynamic psychotherapy itself has evolved into two forms: the time-limited type (Luborsky 1984; Luborsky and Mark 1991) and the time-unlimited type (Luborsky 1984). The earliest short versions of psychoanalysis (i.e., of dynamic psychotherapies) were those of Ferenczi (1920), Rank (1936), and Grinker and Spiegel (1944). The trend toward shortening treatment time was continued by Alexander and French (1946) to make treatment with psychoanalytic techniques more affordable than classical psychoanalysis.

With respect to the results of specific studies, the review by Svartberg and Stiles (1991) is a meta-analysis that found effect sizes to be smaller for dynamic therapy. However, shortly afterward Crits-Christoph (1992) undertook an even more controlled review of 11 studies. These studies were all manual guided, used therapists trained to provide the therapies, and fulfilled other criteria as well. Four studies in the Crits-Christoph review (1992) compared dynamic therapy with other therapies and found that effect sizes were about equal for dynamic versus other therapies. Dynamic therapy was more effective than minimal or no therapy.

In this review, when multiple measures were included in a given study, we calculated a mean Cohen's r by averaging the Fisher's Z transformation of these measures' r. (Statistics were calculated following Rosenthal [1991] and Rosenthal and Rubin [1986].) For combining results from different studies, we averaged Z and Z(r). Averaged corrected (i.e., weighted by quality ratings) Z and r across studies were computed. When researchers said only that a result was nonsignificant, we assumed that Z equaled zero.

For outcome measures we used three well-known domain measures: 1) general mental health and symptom indexes (i.e., the Health-Sickness Rating Scale (HSRS; Luborsky 1962) Global Assessment Scale [Endicott et al. 1976], and Symptom Check-list — 90 [Derogatis 1983]), 2) depression scales (i.e., the Beck Depression Inventory [Beck 1978] and Hamilton Rating Scale for Depression [Hamilton 1967]), and 3) social adjustment scales (i.e., the Social Adjustment Scales [SAS; Weissman and Bothwell 1976]). We included original measures devised for specific studies only where well-known measures were not available.

Our quality controls required that a study meet the set of 12 criteria listed earlier (i.e., attain a score of 6.5 or higher on our quality scale). An important criterion was the presence of evidence that the treatment was psychodynamic. For some studies we accepted less than the current high standard for adherence measures in that we relied on experienced therapists' stated *intention* to conduct insight-oriented psychotherapy. Nevertheless, the most fitting studies followed the example of Woody et al. (1983), with careful guidance offered by a treatment manual for psychoanalytic or psychodynamic psychotherapy.

Our report is of the results of the meta-analysis of the 13 psychodynamic treatment studies, using the easy-to-understand box score method and the effect size method shown in Table 1–1. At study termination, 14 of the 17 study comparisons had nonsignificant differences. In one, psychodynamic therapy was found to be more effective, and in two, the other treatment was found to be more effective. For seven studies of comparisons after a 1-year follow-up evaluation, eight of the comparisons showed nonsignificant differences. In one the dynamic therapy was more effective, and in two the other treatment was significantly more effective.

The overall effect sizes noted in Table 1–1 are based on the mean difference in the outcome measures between the treated and control groups, divided by the standard deviation of the control groups (Cohen 1969). This analysis reveals that there is no significant difference in terms of efficacy at the end of treatment between dynamic therapy and other forms of psychotherapy when results are corrected for the studies' quality. At 1-year follow-up, there is also no significant difference between dynamic and control therapies, which is consistent with our hypothesis that apparent differences between therapies are nonsignificant.

The comparison of our sample of studies with the meta-analyses by Svartberg and Stiles (1991) is illuminating. Our sample of 13 studies overlapped with only 7 of Svartberg and Stiles's studies. We focused only on comparing dynamic therapies with other therapies, whereas Svartberg and Stiles (1991) included comparisons of dynamic therapies and control therapies.

Our effect sizes sometimes differed from those found by Svartberg and Stiles (1991). When dynamic therapy was compared with more than one other type of therapy in a study, Svartberg and Stiles (1991) averaged their results and we did not. A few of the other bases for differences between our observations and those of Svartberg and Stiles are due to errors we found in their study. We believe it was an error for Svartberg and Stiles to take Strupp and Hadley's (1979) studies as wholly dynamic, because some experiential therapists were included. We also believe it was an error to include the work of Brockman et al. (1987) because the treatment in that study was not dynamic but something else—perhaps spontaneous and interactive. Another error is that Woody et al. (1983) were listed as having no termination evaluation, yet their 7-month evaluation *is* a termination assessment: it comes within the month following termination.

Comparisons Among Other Psychotherapies

Our first review (Luborsky et al. 1975) included about 100 selected studies. In contrast, the later review by Smith et al. (1980) of 475 studies accepted all studies, regardless of the quality of the research methods used. For example, the latter investigators included analogue studies with simulated treatments and simulated patients. Their decision to be all-inclusive reflected their desire to avoid any selection bias, and this all-inclusiveness was also an extrapolation from the observation of Luborsky et al. (1975) that trends in results were similar for studies with different ratings of quality. As it turned out, Smith et al. (1980) found a slight advantage in effect size for more rigorous studies. But their main conclusion was that the difference among the outcomes of different psychotherapies is nonsignificant, a conclusion with which we wholly agree. In addition, their use of an effect size measure enabled them to provide estimates of benefit from psychotherapy. For example, they could say that "a typical therapy client is better off than 75% of untreated individuals" (p. 60).

Briefly, our updated results considered five categories of comparisons among a variety of psychotherapies, including 1) group versus individual psychotherapy, 2) time-limited versus time-unlimited psychotherapy, 3) client-centered versus other psychotherapy, 4) behavior therapy versus other therapies, and 5) dynamic therapy versus other therapies. The main finding of these five treatment comparisons is that the nonsignificant difference effect is the most impressive result (Luborsky et al. 1975), and this main trend shows up about equally in all five comparisons.

Even with updated results that involve additional studies, the main trend has not changed since 1975: comparisons of outcomes of psychotherapies tend to show nonsignificant differences in efficacy. For example, the comparison of behavior therapies with other therapies was completely updated for this review, with a box score of 45 comparisons of outcome measures coming from 16 studies. The preparatory box score, which demonstrates that behavior therapy was more effective in 9 comparisons, showed a nonsignificant difference in 35 comparisons and showed that behavior therapy was less effective in 1 comparison. For studies in which effect size translations could be done, the results strongly showed the main nonsignificant difference trend. Furthermore, with a correction for the reactivity (i.e., the responsivity) of the outcome measures (as done by Smith et al. [1980]) the main trend for nonsignificance was even clearer.

By contrast, other types of comparisons, such as comparisons of psychotherapies with other nonpsychological forms of therapy (Luborsky et al. 1975), do show significant difference effects. Thus, combinations of psychotherapy with psychotropic medications tend to produce more benefit than the individual therapies alone. The combination of psychotherapy with a medical regimen for psychosomatic conditions shows superiority for the combination over the medication-only regimen. Finally, the comparison of psychotherapy alone with control (nonpsychotherapy) treatments shows an overwhelming superiority for psychotherapy.

Conclusions and Implications

The information we have reviewed so far leads to several conclusions:

Conclusion 1: The comparisons of treatments (Table 1–1) clearly show that dynamic psychotherapy seems no better or worse in its benefits than other psychotherapies.

Three meta-analyses have been devoted to comparing dynamic therapies with other therapies: those by Svartberg and Stiles (1991), Crits-Christoph (1992), and Luborsky et al. (1993). The first of these meta-analyses concluded that the outcomes for dynamic psychotherapy were less positive than for the other psychotherapies. However, several flaws in Svartberg and Stiles's method may explain their result, and we thus favor the results of the two meta-analyses that showed nonsignificant differences.

Conclusion 2. The main trend of the comparative studies among all other forms of psychotherapy is for nonsignificant differences to exist with respect to patients' benefits.

Because of the trend for nondynamic therapies not to differ in efficacy, and because these psychotherapies produce a high percentage of benefit, we can once again reach a "dodo bird" verdict — "Everyone has won and all must have prizes" — which means that nonsignificance predominates when different forms of psychotherapy are compared. (The dodo bird in *Alice in Wonderland* handed down this happy verdict after judging the race, and this also was the subtitle of the classic and prescient article by Rosenzweig [1936] entitled "Some Implicit Common Factors in Diverse Methods of Psychotherapy" that inspired our first paper.)

Specifically, comparisons between psychotherapies in our studies

(Luborsky et al. 1975), which involve group versus individual psychotherapy, time-limited versus time-unlimited psychotherapy, client-centered versus other traditional psychotherapies, behavior therapy versus other psychotherapies, and dynamic psychotherapies versus other psychotherapies, tend not to show differences in treatment outcomes. In addition, the few studies we reviewed that also reported results at follow-up show results that are consistent with the findings in non–follow-up studies in that patients who show improvement at study termination are generally able to maintain their gains (Garfield and Bergin 1986).

An ongoing large-scale review of all meta-analyses performed between 1975 and the present (Luborsky et al. 1997) was based on 1) the main psychotherapies common in practice, including dynamic psychotherapy, cognitive-behavioral psychotherapy, and behavioral psychotherapy, and 2) the main diagnostic categories, including anxiety disorders, depressive disorders, obsessive-compulsive disorders, and addictive disorders. Of 13 meta-analyses, all but 2 show the nonsignificant difference effect. These 2 are by Svartberg and Stiles (1991) and Shapiro and Shapiro (1982). The overwhelming result, therefore, is that when meta-analyses of comparative psychotherapy studies are examined, the nonsignificant difference effect is the most common.

The finding of nonsignificant differences among treatments should gain in impressiveness when one considers that 1) researchers as well as editors of journals probably have hesitated to publish results of studies with nonsignificant differences and 2) many of these comparisons are studied by partisans of one treatment or the other and are therefore vulnerable to allegiance effects (Luborsky et al., in press). Whatever the causes, a very close association (.85!) was found between the researcher allegiances and the outcomes of treatment comparisons. With such evidence the field cannot rule out the possibility that the researcher's allegiances have a role in treatment outcomes.

Conclusion 3. A high percentage of patients who go through each of the different psychotherapies improve.

One early review, that of Meltzoff and Kornreich (1970), estimated that for both individual and group therapy, about 80% of patients show mainly positive results. Similar high levels of treatment benefits were found for the other treatments in this review, such as in the Penn Psychotherapy Project (Luborsky et al. 1988) and the studies reviewed by Lambert et al. (1986) and Smith et al. (1980). This generally reported high level of benefit may contribute to the nonsignificant difference effect. Thus, the higher the percentage of patients who benefit from therapy, the harder it is to find significant differences among different forms of psychotherapy.

The effectiveness of psychotherapy expressed in terms of effect sizes has been stimulated by several meta-analyses. Smith et al. (1980) reported an effect size of .32, which accounts for only 10% of the variance. However, it is important to point out, as Rosenthal (1990) noted, that the benefits of psychotherapy versus a control condition are even more dramatic when shown in a binomial effect size display. Thus, labeling the .32 effect size as modest is incorrect, because an effect size that reflects increases in the success rate from 34% to 60% is impressive.

The practice of using minimal treatments as control conditions affects estimates of the benefits of psychotherapy. Even with minimal "treatments," such as a wait-list control, a moderate percentage of patients seem to make gains, as pointed out by Sloane et al. (1975). Thus, many control groups are actually minimal treatment groups. This fact may have contributed to a slight reduction in the true effect sizes and may also have contributed to our otherwise surprising finding that approximately one-third of the comparisons of psychotherapy groups with control groups did not show significant differences (Luborsky et al. 1975).

A fleeting furor was set off by the Prioleau et al. (1983) selection of 32 studies from Smith et al. (1980) of comparisons of treated groups with placebo control groups, in which the differences in outcome between them were nonsignificant. The most cogent explanations for this apparently paradoxical finding are consistent with the existence of treatment benefits coming from minimal treatment groups (i.e., that some of these placebo treatments are not justifiably considered placebos, as pointed out by Garfield and Bergin [1986] and Rosenthal [1991]). Rosenthal (1991) demonstrated from reanalysis of subgroups within the 32 studies described by Prioleau et al. (1983) that much depends on the particular kind of placebo control group. For the subgroup of college students and patients who were given *psychological* placebo controls (described as psychological controls), differences were significant at $P < .001$.

Another major limitation in studies of effectiveness is that most of the studies reviewed so far have been about brief therapy and do not include long-term therapy. Improvement might be greater for long-term therapy, such as psychoanalysis. A review by Bachrach et al. (1991) summarized the results from six clinical quantitative studies of psychoanalysis with a total of more than 500 patients. Improvement rates in these studies were in the 60%–90% range, which suggests some comparability of results between psychoanalysis and the other treatments. It should be noted, however, that the studies in the review are not comparative treatment studies but large single-sample studies.

Conclusion 4. Only a few special matches of type of treatment with type of patient show special efficacy for some forms of psychotherapy.

The difficulty of finding special matches is a logical consequence of the trend stated in conclusions 1 and 2. Even in the huge database in Smith et al. (1980), little convincing evidence for special matches appeared, although a few possible special matches could be identified.

Note that the authoritative review by Chambless et al. (1996) is not included here because that listing is explicitly only for forms of psychotherapy which have shown positive results from treatment comparisons, not to summarize the studies that have the most evidence for positive outcomes in treatment–patient matches.

Reasons for the Dodo Bird Verdict

The main reasons for the dodo bird verdict as it applies to the comparative efficacy of psychotherapies follow. They are ordered from most to least important, and some have been noted at various other places in this chapter and elsewhere (Stiles et al. 1986).

Common Components of Different Psychotherapies Exist

The different forms of psychotherapy have major components in common. The common components may be so large and so much more effective than the specific ingredients of the therapies that they obscure differences between them. Therefore, lumping horse-sized common components and canary-sized specific ones together is obviously wrong because they should not be given equal weight.

Common components include the support of a helping relationship with the therapist, the opportunity to express one's thoughts (sometimes called abreaction), and the opportunity to gain better self-understanding. This explanation of common components was put forward by Rosenzweig (1936), Frank and Frank (1991), and Strupp and Hadley (1979). Another common component, supportiveness, was also found to be virtually the same in amount in three differently designed treatments, as judged by two independent judges (Luborsky et al. 1982). One other generally applicable aspect of psychotherapeutic treatment that deserves further research was suggested by Rosenzweig (1936). It is the inclusion in all psychotherapies of a plausible system of explanation of the patient's problems. Such an organized explanatory and guidance system may facilitate realization of benefits from all forms of psychotherapy.

Extratherapeutic Conditions Vary

Extratherapeutic conditions vary for each study, and these conditions may differ between treatment groups despite researcher attempts to equate the groups. Extratherapeutic conditions may be crucial in explaining the dodo bird verdict. Such conditions reflect prognostic factors that are likely to be influential, including psychiatric severity, differences between patients in their capacity to form an alliance, differences in the adherence of therapists to treatment manuals, differences in patients' capacities to internalize the gains of treatment, and differences in therapists' capacities to effect change in their patients. These main prognostic factors are separate from the intrinsic quality of the treatment itself. Furthermore, to complete this argument, these differences in prognostic factors may almost randomly favor one group or the other in different studies, and therefore a large set of studies reveal a preponderance of nonsignificant difference effects.

Researcher's Allegiances to Each Therapy Are Consistent With the Outcome of the Treatment Comparison

A researcher's allegiance to each therapy might affect the amount of benefit that results from a given treatment, as first tallied by Luborsky et al. (1975) and more extensively demonstrated by Smith et al. (1980). Because therapist allegiance can vary for one treatment or another, the net effect in a set of studies might be to cause nonsignificant differences among treatments. These and other studies of the researcher's allegiance have been summarized by Luborsky et al. (in press).

Therapist Competence May Play a Part

Variations in therapists' competence may make for differences in outcomes of treatments compared. Such variations may be another extratherapy factor, because therapists are assigned to treatment comparisons by the luck of the draw or by meeting minimal standards of experience. Because therapists' previous success rates are not considered, and because these rates appear to differ considerably (Luborsky et al. 1985), the usual mode of distributing therapists may make for nonsignificant differences among treatments.

Outcome Measures May Be Insensitive

Some curative components in therapies may not be strong enough to influence outcome measures because of the insensitivity of these measures. One example may serve to illustrate this phenomenon: Auerbach and Johnson's (1977) review of the impact of the therapist's capacity to generate the patient's level of experiencing found 12 studies in which experienced therapists had established better relationships with their patients than had inexperienced therapists. Nevertheless, the outcome measures did not show a significant difference between the two groups.

Choice of Outcome Measures May Be Unrepresentative

The outcome measures used in a given study may not represent a treatment's intended outcomes. The most typical example is dynamic psychotherapy. Here, the therapy emphasizes the development of insight, yet its outcomes are typically measured by global ratings of improvement that may neglect changes in insight. The usual outcome measures used in studies do not adequately distinguish between short-term and long-lasting improvement or between the parallel related changes called nonstructural and structural changes. (A structural change is one that makes a long-lasting change in a central component of the transference.)

High Percentage of Benefits Limits Comparisons of Outcomes

Because all forms of psychotherapy tend to achieve high percentages of improvement in patients, it is difficult for any form of psychotherapy to show a statistically significant advantage over any other form: the higher the percentages of benefit in the compared treatments, the less room there is at the top for the existence of significant differences among treatments.

Small Samples and Small Effects May Limit Discovery of Therapy Effects

The nonsignificant differences among various treatments may often come about because the studies are not adequately designed to register meaningful differences. As explained by Kasdin and Bass (1989), in most of the comparisons of psychotherapies, statistical power may be weak because in small sample sizes it is difficult to detect the small effect sizes that may appear. Statistical power reflects the probability that a test will find differences when the treatments are truly different in their outcome.

The Hope for the Future

The dodo bird verdict may not be upheld forever, although there is still much evidence for it, as portrayed in this chapter and elsewhere (Luborsky et al. 1997). We can best point out the hoped-for direction of future research by engaging in an imaginary dialogue about these findings that paraphrases the responses of many psychotherapy researchers and practitioners and our responses to them.

QUESTION: I hadn't realized until I heard your papers that the dodo bird trends you found emerge so clearly within studies in which the quality of the research is considered. I also had the impression that there were certain most effective psychotherapies. Finally, wouldn't we learn more in future studies if we constructed studies to investigate specific treatments for specific types of patients?

ANSWER: Yes. Not enough of these studies have been undertaken, yet the outlook is good. Persistence, aided by our design recommendations, will bit by bit add more about the results of specific matches.

QUESTION: Don't you feel, despite all the evidence for the nonsignificant difference effect, that dynamic therapies have some special virtues to offer that are still not sufficiently recognized?

ANSWER: I'm glad you asked that. The answer is "definitely" yes. The studies have not yet dealt with their possible long-term benefits. Nor have they dealt adequately with the distinction between changes in symptoms and changes in general adjustment. The benefits of a treatment tend to reflect the focus of the treatment; thus, dynamic treatment tends to be focused less on symptom improvement and more on general adjustment changes, which are harder to accomplish. And, of course, the concept of insight has not yet been adequately operationalized and therefore has not been used as an outcome measure in any form of psychotherapy. All such mediators and moderators may not yet be sufficiently reflected in the results of meta-analyses, as Shadish and Sweeney (1991) point out.

References

Alexander F, French T: Psychoanalytic Therapy: Principles and Applications. New York, Ronald Press, 1946

Auerbach A, Johnson M: Research on the therapist's level of experience, in Effective Psychotherapy. Edited by Gurman A, Razin A. New York, Pergamon, 1977, pp 84–102

Bachrach H, Galatzer-Levy R, Skolnikoff A, et al: On the efficacy of psychoanalysis. J Am Psychoanal Assoc 39:871–916, 1991

Beck AT: Depression Inventory. Philadelphia, PA, Philadelphia Center for Cognitive Therapy, 1978

Brockman B, Ponton A, Ryle A, et al: Effectiveness of time-limited therapy carried out by trainees: comparison of two methods. Br J Psychiatry 151:602–610, 1987

Chambless D, Sanderson W, Shoham V, et al: An update on empirically validated therapies. The Clinical Psychologist 49:5–18, 1996

Cohen J: Statistical Power Analysis in the Behavioral Sciences. New York, Academic Press, 1969

Crits-Christoph P: The efficacy of brief dynamic psychotherapy: a meta-analysis. Am J Psychiatry 149:151–158, 1992

Cross D, Sheehan P, Kahn J: Short- and long-term follow-up of clients receiving insight-oriented therapy and behavior therapy. J Consult Clin Psychol 30:103–112, 1982

Derogatis L: SCL-90-R Manual II. Towson, MD, Clinical Psychometric Research, 1983

Elliott R, Stiles W, Shapiro D: Are some psychotherapies more equivalent than others? in Handbook of Effective Psychotherapy. New York, Plenum, 1993, 455–479

Endicott J, Spitzer RL, Fleiss JL, Cohen J: The global assessment scale: a procedure for measuring overall severity of psychiatric disturbance. Arch Gen Psychiatry 33:766–771, 1976

Ferenczi S: Further Contributions to the Theory and Technique of Psychoanalysis. London, Hogarth Press, 1920

Frank JD, Frank J: Persuasion and Healing: A Comparative Study of Psychotherapy, 3rd Edition. Baltimore, MD, Johns Hopkins University Press, 1991

Garfield S, Bergin A (eds): Handbook of Psychotherapy and Behavior Change: An Empirical Analysis, 3rd Edition. New York, Wiley, 1986

Grinker R, Spiegel J: Brief psychotherapy in war neuroses. Psychosom Med 6:123–131, 1944

Hamilton M: Development of a rating scale for primary depressive illness. British Journal of Social and Clinical Psychology 6:278–296, 1967

Kasdin A, Bass D: Power to detect differences between alternate treatments in comparative psychotherapy outcome research. J Consult Clin Psychol 57:138–147, 1989

Lambert M, Shapiro D, Bergin A: The effectiveness of psychotherapy, in Handbook of Psychotherapy and Behavior Change: An Empirical Analysis. Edited by Garfield S, Bergin A. New York, Wiley, 1986, pp 157–212

Luborsky L: The patient's personality and psychotherapeutic change, in Research in Psychotherapy, Vol 2. Edited by Strupp H, Luborsky L. Washington, DC, American Psychological Association, 1962, 115–133

Luborsky L: Principles of Psychoanalytic Psychotherapy: A Manual for Supportive-Expressive Treatment. New York, Basic Books, 1984

Luborsky L, Mark D: Short-term supportive expressive psychoanalytic psychotherapy, in Handbook of Brief Dynamic Therapies. Edited by Crits-Christoph P, Barber J. New York, Basic Books, 1991

Luborsky L, Singer B, Luborsky E: Comparative studies of psychotherapies: is it true that "everybody has won and all must have prizes?" Arch Gen Psychiatry 32:995–1008, 1975

Luborsky L, Woody GE, McLellan AT, et al: Can independent judges recognize different psychotherapies? an experience with manual-guided therapies. J Consult Clin Psychol 50:49–62, 1982

Luborsky L, McLellan AT, Woody GE, et al: Therapeutic success and its determinants. Arch Gen Psychiatry 42:602–611, 1985

Luborsky L, Crits-Christoph P, Mintz J, et al: Who Will Benefit From Psychotherapy? Predicting Therapeutic Outcomes. New York, Basic Books, 1988

Luborsky L, Diguer L, Luborsky E, et al: The efficacy of dynamic psychotherapies: is it true that "everyone has won so all shall have prizes?" in Psychodynamic Treatment Research: A Handbook for Clinical Practice. Edited by Miller N, Luborsky L, Barber JP, et al. New York, Basic Books, 1993, pp 447–514

Luborsky L, Diguer L, Seligman DA, et al: The researcher's own therapy allegiances: a "wild card" in comparisons of treatment efficacy. Clinical Psychology: Science and Practice, in press

Luborsky L, Seligman DA, Levine J, et al: The dodo bird is alive and well but so are the winners (abstract). Paper presented at the Society for Psychotherapy Research International Meeting, Geilo, Norway, June 1997

Meltzoff J, Kornreich M: Research in Psychotherapy. New York, Atherton, 1970

Pierloot R, Vinck J: Differential outcome of short-term dynamic psychotherapy and systematic desensitization in the treatment of anxious outpatients: a preliminary report. Psychology Belgium 18:87–98, 1978

Prioleau L, Murdock M, Brody N: An analysis of psychotherapy versus placebo studies. Behavioral and Brain Sciences 6:275–310, 1983

Rank O: Will Therapy. New York, Knopf, 1936

Rosenzweig S: Some implicit common factors in diverse methods of psychotherapy. Am J Orthopsychiatry 6:412–415, 1936

Rosenthal R: Meta-Analytic Procedures for Social Research. Newbury Park, CA, Sage, 1991

Rosenthal R: How are we doing in soft-psychology? Am Psychol 58:775–777, 1990

Rosenthal R, Rubin DB: Meta-analytic procedures for combining studies with multiple effect sizes. Psychol Bull 99:400–406, 1986

Shadish W, Sweeney R: Mediators and moderators and meta-analysis: there's a reason we don't let dodo birds tell us which psychotherapies should have prizes. J Consult Clin Psychol 59:883–893, 1991

Shapiro DA, Shapiro D: Meta-analysis of comparative therapy outcome studies: a replication and refinement. Psychol Bull 92:581–604, 1982

Sloane R, Staples F, Cristol A, et al: Psychotherapy Versus Behavior Therapy. Cambridge, MA, Harvard University Press, 1975

Smith M, Glass G, Miller T: The Benefits of Psychotherapy. Baltimore, MD, Johns Hopkins University Press, 1980

Stiles W, Shapiro D, Elliott R: Are all psychotherapies equivalent? Am Psychol 41:165–180, 1986

Strupp H, Hadley S: Specific vs. non-specific factors in psychotherapy. Arch Gen Psychiatry 36:1125–1136, 1979

Svartberg M, Stiles T: Comparative effects of short-term psychodynamic psychotherapy: a meta-analysis. J Consult Clin Psychol 59:704–714, 1991

Weissman MM, Bothwell S: Assessment of social adjustment by patient self-report. Arch Gen Psychiatry 33:1111–1115, 1976

Woody G, Luborsky L, McLellan AT, et al: Psychotherapy for opiate addicts: does it help? Arch Gen Psychiatry 40:639–645, 1983

CHAPTER 2

Personality Factors in Brief Treatment of Depression

Further Analyses of the NIMH-Sponsored Treatment for Depression Collaborative Research Program

Sidney J. Blatt, Ph.D.

Research in psychotherapy generally indicates that most forms of therapy are more effective than nontreatment control conditions, that a few forms of therapy are particularly effective in reducing some specific symptoms, but that a general equivalence exists among most forms of therapy. Extensive meta-analyses of comparative outcome studies indicate that few differences in therapeutic efficacy exist among various forms of treatment (American Psychiatric Association 1982; Shapiro and Shapiro 1982; Smith et al. 1980). Still applicable today is Frank's 1979 observation that "no one therapy has been shown to be overall significantly superior to any other . . ." (p. 311). Luborsky (1995) and colleagues (1975) have labeled this functional equivalence of various forms of therapy the dodo bird phenomena — "all therapies have won and therefore all should have prizes." This functional equivalence (Stiles et al. 1986) suggests that either our research methods are insen-

The author is indebted to his colleagues who participated in our further analysis of data from the NIMH TDCRP: Colin M. Bondi, Paul A. Pilkonis, Donald M. Quinlan, Charles A. Sanislow III, and David C. Zuroff.

sitive to differences among treatments or various forms of a treatment share some common processes that make them functionally equivalent (Frank 1982; Strupp and Binder 1984). These assumed shared processes are often referred to as *nonspecific effects*.

Although much effort has been devoted to comparing various types of therapies, relatively little attention has been paid to differences among patients and their contribution to therapeutic outcome. Most studies assume a uniformity of patients, expecting all patients to respond to treatment in essentially the same way. Over 40 years ago, Cronbach (Cronbach 1953, 1957; Cronbach and Gleser 1953; Edwards and Cronbach 1952), however, suggested that it might be productive to differentiate among patients and to examine the interaction between patients and types of treatment, with the assumption that various types of patients might respond differently to different forms of treatment. Cronbach originally had noted in educational research that different individuals respond differently to various types of instruction and sometimes respond to the same instruction in different, but equally desirable, ways (Shoham-Salomon and Hannah 1991). Cronbach was quite clear that he regarded these issues equally applicable to psychotherapy research (Blatt and Felsen 1993). Only a few studies, however, have explored whether patient variables play a role in treatment outcome. Horowitz et al. (1984) found a significant interaction between the developmental level of patients' self-concept and their response to insight-oriented as compared to supportive, brief treatment for bereavement. Sotsky et al. (1991), in an analysis of the data of the Treatment of Depression Collaborative Research Program (TDCRP) sponsored by the National Institute of Mental Health (NIMH), found evidence of a congruence of some patient pretreatment characteristics and responses to particular forms of treatment. Sotsky et al. (1991) concluded that "each therapy relies on specific and different learning techniques to alleviate depression, and thus each may depend on an adequate capacity in the corresponding sphere of patient functioning to produce recovery with the use of that approach" (p. 1006).

Cronbach (1975) cautioned, however, that the study of the interactions between patient and treatment and between patient and outcome would not be easy because of difficulty identifying the appropriate individual qualities of patients out of the potentially infinite array of personal characteristics that might be relevant to the treatment process. A special issue of the *Journal of Consulting and Clinical Psychology* (Beutler 1991; Smith and Sechrest 1991; Snow 1991) devoted to these patient-treatment interactions stressed that if patient variables are to be included in psychotherapy research, they must be theoretically derived and/or empirically justified. Without these moorings, investigators could be drawn into what Cronbach (1975) described as a "hall of mirrors."

This chapter presents a theoretical model of personality development and psychopathology that potentially provides some guidelines for introducing patient variables into psychotherapy research. Various forms of psychopathology are conceptualized in this theoretical model, not as diseases assumed to derive from malfunctioning biological processes, but as disruptions of psychological development. Psychological development is assumed, in this theoretical model, to derive from a complex dialectic transaction between two fundamental developmental processes: 1) a relatedness (or anaclitic) developmental process that involves the development of the capacity to establish increasingly mature, mutually satisfying, reciprocal, interpersonal relationships, and 2) a self-definitional (or introjective) developmental process that involves the development of a consolidated, realistic, essentially positive, differentiated, and integrated self-identity. These two developmental processes (relatedness and self-definition) normally evolve throughout life in a reciprocal, mutually facilitating transaction. An increasingly differentiated, integrated, and mature sense of self is contingent upon establishing satisfying interpersonal relationships, and, conversely, the continued development of increasingly mature and satisfying interpersonal relationships is contingent on the development of a more mature self concept or identity. In normal psychological development, these two processes evolve in an interactive, reciprocally balanced dialectic from birth through senescence (Blatt 1974, 1990, 1991, 1995; Blatt and Blass 1990; Blatt and Shichman 1983).

These formulations about personality development are consistent with a wide range of personality theories ranging from fundamental psychoanalytic conceptualizations to basic empirical investigations of personality development that consider these two dimensions of relatedness and self-definition as central to psychological development (e.g., Angyal 1951; Bakan 1966; Balint 1952; Bowlby 1988; Freud 1930/1957; McAdams 1985; McClelland 1986; Shor and Sanville 1978; Wiggins 1991). A variety of procedures have been developed that reliably assess these two dimensions and a wide range of research demonstrates that these two dimensions have good construct validity. Extensive research has also demonstrated important differences between individuals who, within the normal range, place somewhat greater emphasis on either of these two personality dimensions (Blatt and Zuroff 1992). Thus, this theoretical model of personality development potentially offers a well-established conceptual framework for introducing personality variables into psychotherapy research.

In this theoretical model, various forms of psychopathology can be viewed as evolving from disruptions of these normal developmental processes. Many forms of psychopathology express an exaggerated overemphasis on one of these developmental processes and the defensive avoidance of the other. Two distinctly different configurations of psychopathology come from these exaggerated preoccupations, each of which contain several types of disordered behavior that range from relatively severe to relatively mild forms of psychopathology (Figure 2–1; Blatt 1974, 1990, 1991, 1995; Blatt and Shichman 1983).

Based on developmental and clinical considerations, one configuration of disorders, labeled *anaclitic psychopathology*, involves a primary preoccupation with interpersonal relations such as issues of trust, caring, intimacy, and sexuality. Patients with anaclitic disorders are intensely preoccupied with issues of relatedness at different developmental levels, ranging from a lack of differentiation between self and others, to dependent attachments, to difficulties in more mature types of relationships. Anaclitic disorders, ranging developmentally from more to less disturbed, include non-paranoid schizophrenia, borderline personality disorder, infantile (or dependent) personality disorder, anaclitic depression, and hysterical disorders. These disorders not only share a basic preoccupation with libidinal issues of relatedness, but they also all use primarily avoidant defenses to cope with psychological conflict and stress (e.g., withdrawal, denial, repression).

In contrast, a series of disorders can be identified as *introjective psychopathology* in which patients are primarily preoccupied with establishing and maintaining a viable sense of self at different developmental levels, ranging from a basic sense of separateness, through con-

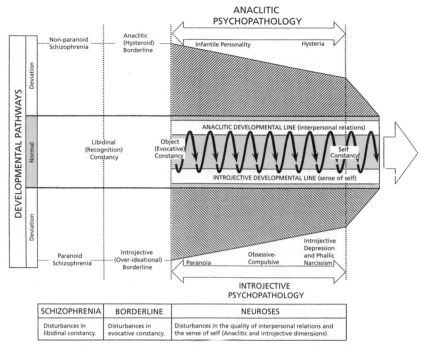

FIGURE 2–1. A model of personality development and psychopathology. Source. *Reprinted from Blatt SJ, Schichman S: Two primary configurations of psychopathology. Psychoanalysis and Contemporary Thought 6:187–254, 1983. Used with permission.*

cerns about autonomy and control, to more complex internalized issues of self-worth. Introjective patients are more ideational and concerned with establishing, protecting, and maintaining a viable self-concept than they are about the quality of their interpersonal relations and achieving feelings of trust, warmth, and affection. Issues of anger and aggression, directed toward the self or others, are usually central to their difficulties. Introjective disorders, ranging developmentally from more to less severely disturbed, include paranoid schizophrenia, the schizotypic or over-ideational borderline, paranoia, obsessive-compulsive personality disorder, introjective (guilt-ridden) depression, and phallic narcissism. Patients with these disorders not only share a preoccupation with issues of self-definition and an instinctual focus on aggression, they also use primarily counteractive defenses that transform conflicts rather than avoid them (e.g., projection, rationalization, intellectualization, doing and undoing, reaction formation, and overcompensation) (Blatt 1974, 1990, 1991, 1995; Blatt and Shichman 1983).

These two broad configurations of psychopathology can be distinguished reliably from clinical case records. In contrast to the atheoretical diagnostic scheme established in DSM-III, DSM-III-R, and DSM-IV (American Psychiatric Association 1980, 1987, 1994), which is based primarily on differences in manifest symptoms, the diagnostic differentiation between anaclitic and introjective psychopathologies derives from dynamic considerations including differences in primary instinctual focus (libidinal vs. aggressive), types of defensive organization (avoidant vs. counteractive), and predominant character style (e.g., emphasis on object vs. self-orientation and on affects vs. cognition.

Two studies have reliably differentiated between these two types of patients based on clinical case records prepared at intake and have studied the therapeutic response of these two groups of patients in long-term intensive treatment (Blatt 1992; Blatt and Ford 1994; Blatt et al. 1988). The results indicate that anaclitic and introjective patients come to treatment with different needs, respond differentially to different types of therapeutic intervention, and demonstrate different treatment outcomes.

In the first investigation, therapeutic change was studied in a sample of seriously disturbed, treatment-resistant patients in long-term, intensive, psychodynamically oriented, inpatient treatment in an open therapeutic facility (including four times weekly psychoanalytically oriented psychotherapy) (Blatt and Ford 1994; Blatt et al. 1988). Systematic differences were found in the therapeutic response of these two types of patients based on a number of independent measures of change derived from clinical case records and psychological test protocols assessed at the outset of treatment and after 15 months of intensive inpatient treatment. Generally, patients demonstrated significant improvement across multiple assessment procedures derived from the clinical case records and from the psychological test protocols. Introjective patients, those patients preoccupied primarily with issues of self-definition, autonomy, self-control, and self-worth, generally had greater overall improvement than did anaclitic patients. Independent of the degree of therapeutic gain, anaclitic and introjective patients expressed therapeutic change in different ways. Introjective patients express therapeutic change primarily in changes in the intensity of clinical symptoms (as reliably rated from clinical case reports) and in the level of cognitive functioning as independently assessed on psychological tests administered at the beginning and toward the end of treatment, including significant changes in thought disorder on the Rorschach and in intelligence. In contrast, therapeutic change in anaclitic patients, those patients preoccupied primarily with concerns about disruptions of interpersonal relatedness, was expressed primarily in the quality of their interpersonal relationships (as reliably rated from clinical case reports) and in their representation of the human form on the Rorschach. Thus, anaclitic and introjective patients appear to change primarily in the modalities that express their basic concerns and preoccupations. Anaclitic patients changed primarily in dimensions assessing interpersonal relationships; change in introjective patients was expressed primarily in cognitive functioning and in clinical symptoms.

The distinction between anaclitic and introjective patients was also applied to a further analysis of data from the Menninger Psychotherapy Research Project (MPRP). The Menninger study was designed to compare the effects of psychoanalysis and long-term, psychodynamically oriented psychotherapy with outpatients. Despite many prior analyses of data from the clinical evaluations and psychological test assessments conducted both before and after treatment, the results from the MPRP have repeatedly failed to find any systematic differences between these two types of therapeutic intervention (Wallerstein 1986). Using the distinction of two configurations of psychopathology, further analysis of data from the MPRP, however, indicate that anaclitic and introjective patients are differentially responsive to psychotherapy and psychoanalysis. Independent evaluation of psychological test data gathered at the beginning and the end of treatment indicates that anaclitic patients had significantly greater improvement in psychotherapy than they did in psychoanalysis. Introjective patients, in contrast, had significantly greater improvement in psychoanalysis than they did in psychotherapy. Not only were the differences between these two groups of patients significant within each type of treatment, but the patient-by-treatment interaction was a significant ($P < .001$) cross-over interaction (Blatt 1992). Thus, the relative therapeutic efficacy of psychoanalysis versus psychotherapy seems contingent, to a significant degree, on the nature of the patient's pathology and character structure. It seems consistent that the more dependent, interpersonally oriented anaclitic patients should respond more effectively in a therapeutic context that provided more direct personal interaction with the therapist, and that the more ideational introjective patients, preoccupied with separation, autonomy, and independence, would respond more effectively in psychoanalysis (Blatt 1992).

The findings of both these studies — of outpatients in two different forms of treatment and the long-term, intensive treatment of seriously disturbed, treatment-resistant patients — indicate the importance of including patient variables in psychotherapy research. Aspects of patients' personality appear to interact with dimensions of the therapeutic process to determine the nature of therapeutic change and the efficacy of different types of treatment. As stated earlier, patients come to treatment with different types of problems, different character styles, and different needs, and they respond in different ways to different types of therapeutic intervention. The differential response of anaclitic and introjective patients in these studies of long-term treatment of inpatients and outpatients suggests that this distinction might be useful in evaluating the differential effectiveness of various forms of brief psychotherapy.

It should be noted that the differentiation between interpersonally oriented, dependent, anaclitic patients and ideational, perfectionistic, self-critical introjective patients has been particularly useful in identifying two major subtypes of depression (Blatt 1974; Blatt et al. 1976, 1982, 1990). Investigators from both dynamic (e.g., Arieti and Bemporad 1978, 1980; Blatt 1974; Bowlby 1988) and cognitive-behavioral (Beck 1983) perspectives have discussed two major types of experiences that result in two types of depression: 1) disruptions of gratifying interpersonal relationships (e.g., loss of a significant figure) and 2) disruptions of an effective and essentially positive sense of self (e.g., feelings of failure, guilt, and worthlessness). The distinction between anaclitic (dependent) and introjective (self-critical) depressed patients has been made in a wide range of studies using three well-established scales: the Depressive Experiences Questionnaire (DEQ; Blatt et al. 1976, 1979), the Sociotropy-Autonomy Scale (S-AS; Beck 1983), and the Dysfunctional Attitudes Scale (DAS; Weissman and Beck 1978).[1] Studies using these three scales have demonstrated important differences between anaclitic (dependent or sociotropic) and introjective (self-critical or autonomous) depression (Blatt and Zuroff 1992).

The availability of empirical data from the NIMH-sponsored TDCRP provided the opportunity to explore the role of these patient dimensions in the brief treatment of depression. This exploration seemed especially appropriate given the considerable evidence indicating the reliability and validity of the distinction between relatedness and self-definition as personality dimensions and between anaclitic and introjective forms of psychopathology, especially in the study of depression.

The TDCRP was a comprehensive, well-designed, and carefully conducted, multisite collaborative clinical trial to evaluate several forms of brief (16–20 sessions) outpatient treatment of depression. The

---

1. Several factor-analytic studies of the DAS have consistently identified two major and stable factors in the DAS; one focused on issues of relatedness and the other on issues of self-definition. These factors have been labeled, respectively, "need for approval by others" and "performance evaluation" ("self worth" or "perfectionism") (Cane et al. 1986; Imber et al. 1990; Oliver and Baumgart 1985).

Pilon (1987), conducting a discriminant analysis based on these three measures of two types of depression (DEQ, S-AS, and DAS), the Beck Depression Inventory (BDI; Beck 1978) identified two fundamental dimensions that he labeled: 1) *relatedness-to-others* that included appealing to others for support, help, and advice; seeking to be loved and valued by others; and craving affection and being overly dependent and fearful of abandonment and 2) *self-definition* that included feeling unsatisfied and critical of oneself, feeling a failure for not meeting expectations, needing to be outstanding and avoid feeling inferior, and feeling ambivalent about interpersonal relationships. Pilon noted the congruence of these two dimensions with the dependency and self-criticism scales of the DEQ and with the need for approval and perfectionism scales of the DAS. Blaney and Kutcher (1991) also evaluated the relationships among these measures of two dimensions of depression (DEQ, S-AS, and DAS) and found high congruence among the three scales that assessed interpersonal relatedness (DEQ dependency, S-AS sociotropy, and DAS need for approval). The relationships among the three scales that assess individuality (DEQ self-criticism, S-AS autonomy, and DAS perfectionism) were more complex, primarily because the autonomy scale of the S-AS appears to measure primarily counterdependency rather than individuality. The relationship between the DEQ self-criticism and DAS perfectionism scales, however, was substantial and both have robust correlations with independent measures of depression (Nietzel and Harris 1990; Zuroff et al.1990).

program protocol randomly assigned 239 patients to four treatment conditions: cognitive-behavioral therapy (CBT), interpersonal therapy (IPT), imipramine plus clinical management (IMI-CM) as a standard reference, and pill-placebo plus clinical management (PLA-CM) as a double-blind control condition.[2]

The therapists in the four treatment conditions at each of the three research sites were experienced clinicians (10 each providing IPT and pharmacotherapy, and 8 providing CBT) with high levels of professional training (M.D. or Ph.D.), who had, on average, over 11 years of clinical experience. All therapists received specific training in the treatment they provided in this research protocol and only therapists who met competency criteria participated in the final study. Tapes of the treatment sessions were reviewed systematically to assure adherence to treatment protocols and therapists received monthly consultation during the study (Elkin 1994).

Patients were nonbipolar, nonpsychotic, seriously depressed outpatients who met research diagnostic criteria for major depressive disorder (Spitzer et al. 1978) and had a score of 14 or greater on a modified, 20-item, Hamilton Rating Scale for Depression (HRSD; Hamilton 1960, 1967).

Therapeutic change was assessed with an interview and a self-report measure of depression (HRSD and BDI, respectively), an interview and a self-report measure of general clinical functioning (Global Assessment Scale [GAS; Spitzer et al. 1973] and Hopkins Symptom Checklist [HSCL-90; Derogatis et al. 1974], respectively), and an interview measure of social adjustment (Social Adjustment Scale [SAS]; Weissman and Paykel 1974). Factor analysis of the residualized gain scores of these five primary outcome measures at termination (HRSD, BDI, GAS, HSCL-90, and SAS) indicated that they load substantially ($P > .79$) on a single factor with an eigenvalue of 3.78, accounting for 75.6% of the variance (Blatt et al. 1996). No other eigenvalue ap-

2. Clinical management was included in the imipramine and placebo conditions to monitor possible side effects of the medication and to provide general support and encouragement as a minimal therapeutic condition to deal with ethical concerns about treating severely depressed patients with placebo (Elkin 1994). Clinical management (CM) included "clinically indicated and appropriate supportive psychotherapeutic measures and interventions . . . interventions related to specific organized systems of psychotherapy [however, were] . . . not permitted" (Fawcett et al. 1987, p. 320).

proached 1.0, indicating that this factor is a consistent measure of therapeutic change. Thus, a composite of these five residualized gain scores can be used as the measure of therapeutic outcome for each patient (Blatt et al. 1996).

Prior analyses of the TDCRP data (Elkin et al. 1989) indicated some differences in therapeutic outcome among the three brief treatments for depression; IPT and IMI-CM were more effective than CBT, but only with more severely depressed patients. In our analyses of data from the TDCRP, we sought to differentiate anaclitic from introjective patients within the TDCRP, based on our findings that patient dimensions play a central role in determining treatment effects in the study of therapeutic change in the long-term intensive treatment of seriously disturbed, treatment-resistant patients at the Austen Riggs Center, in our comparison of the effects of psychoanalysis and psychotherapy in the data of the MPRP, and in the findings of Sotsky et al. (1991). Review of the intake evaluations of the TDCRP by an experienced judge indicated, however, that these case reports contained primarily descriptions of the patients' symptoms of depression and lacked sufficient detail about aspects of the patients' lives to allow the anaclitic-introjective distinction to be made reliably from these clinical case records. Fortunately, the DAS had been administered as part of the TDCRP protocol primarily to assess the effects of treatment on dysfunctional cognitions. The fact that the DAS is composed of two primary factors — concerns about issues of relatedness (i. e., need for approval [NFA]) and issues of self-definition (i.e., perfectionism [PFT]) — enabled us to assess the contribution of pretreatment levels of these two types of concerns to differential outcome in the four treatment conditions (CBT, IPT, IMI-CM, PLA-CM) of the TDCRP.

Whereas NFA and PFT did not interact significantly with the different forms of treatment in predicting outcome, PFT was negatively related to outcome ($P = .032$ to $.004$) as assessed by all five primary measures of clinical change (HRSD, BDI, GAS, HSCL-90, and SAS), across all four treatment groups (Blatt et al. 1995a). Combining all five outcome measures into a single factor, PFT predicted the combined residualized gain score at a highly significant level ($t = 3.90$, $P < .0001$). NFA, in contrast, had a consistent but only a marginally positive relationship to treatment outcome on all five outcome measures. Combining all five residualized gain scores into a single measure, NFA was only marginally related to outcome ($t = 1.59$, $P = .114$). Thus, pre-occupation with issues of self-definition and self-worth, as measured by the DAS PFT scale, is a significant disruptive factor that interferes with the capacity to benefit from short-term treatment whether the treatment is pharmacotherapy (IMI-CM), psychotherapy (CBT and IPT), or placebo (Blatt et al. 1995b; Table 2–1).

Additionally, pretreatment PFT had consistent and significant negative relationships with ratings made by the therapists, independent clinical evaluators, and by the patients themselves at termination and at follow-up assessments at 18 months. Pretreatment PFT had significant correlations with estimates at follow-up of the patients' clinical condition, need for further treatment, and their satisfaction with their treatment (S. J. Blatt, C. A. Sanislow, D. C. Zuroff, C. A. Bondi, P. A. Pilkonis, unpublished data, June 1996) indicating that the disruptive effects of pretreatment PFT persisted even at the follow-up evaluation conducted 18 months after the termination of treatment (Tables 2–2 and 2–3).

The extensive data gathered as part of the NIMH TDCRP also provided an opportunity to evaluate if some circumstances within the various treatments in the TDCRP served to reduce the negative effects of pretreatment PFT. We were particularly interested in whether the quality of the therapeutic relationship as experienced by the patient might mitigate the negative effects of PFT on treatment outcome (Blatt et al. 1996). The Barrett-Lennard Relationship Inventory (B-L RI; Barrett-Lennard 1962) had been administered as part of the research protocol to assess the quality of the therapeutic relationship at the beginning of treatment (after two sessions) and at termination. The B-L RI is based on Carl Rogers' (1951, 1957, 1959) concepts that the therapist's empathic understanding, positive regard, and congruence are the "necessary and sufficient conditions" for therapeutic change. Based on these formulations, Barrett-Lennard (1962) developed several scales (empathic understanding, level of positive regard, and congruence) to assess the patient's perception of the therapeutic relationship. Several reviews (Barrett-Lennard 1985; Gurman 1977) indicate acceptable levels of reliability and validity for these scales of the B-L RI. Prior research, for example, indicates that these scales predict thera-

TABLE 2–1

Analysis of covariance: regression of DAS PFT and NFA on residualized change scores (effects of treatments and marital status partialled out)

Measure	Standard regression weight	SE	t	P
Depression measures				
BDI (N = 153)				
PFT	.222	.006	2.18	.031
NFA	−.033	.008	−0.32	NS
HRSD (N = 153)				
PFT	.296	.006	2.93	.004
NFA	−.075	.008	−0.74	NS
General clinical functioning				
HSCL-90 Total (N = 153)				
PFT	.274	.006	2.74	.007
NFA	−.025	.008	−0.24	NS
GAS (N = 153)				
PFT	−.328	.006	−3.28	.001
NFA	.122	.008	1.22	NS
Social adjustment				
SAS (N = 153)				
PFT	.250	.006	2.50	.014
NFA	−.085	.008	−0.85	NS

Note. *Based on an analysis of covariance for treatment groups with marriage dummy variables also as covariates, residual change scores as dependent variables, using SPSS/PC + V.401. All coefficients for marriage variables were nonsignificant (P > .10).*

Source. *The results presented in this table differ in several ways from the original presentation of these findings in Table 1 of Blatt et al. (1995a). The original presentation of this table had several errors that were subsequently corrected (see Blatt et al. 1995b).*

peutic change and are related significantly to independent estimates of the therapist's competence (Barrett-Lennard 1962; Table 2–4).

The degree to which patients perceived their therapist at the end of the second treatment hour as empathic, caring, open, and sincere, as assessed by the B-L RI, had a significant (P < .05) overall relationship to therapeutic outcome on 4 of the 5 outcome measures (HSCL-90, GAS, and SAS) in the TDCRP (Blatt et al.

TABLE 2–2

t-test of pretreatment DAS pure NFA and PFT and degree of satisfaction with treatment as rated by therapists and clinical evaluators at termination

	Means	
	NFA	PFT
Therapist		
Patient satisfied with treatment		
Yes	0.12	−0.53
No	−0.32	3.31
t	0.18	−1.52
Therapist satisfied with treatment		
Yes	0.40	−1.36
No	−0.76	3.49
t	0.79	−1.89*
Needs further treatment		
Yes	0.42	1.34
No	−0.39	−1.45
t	0.45	1.18
Clinical evaluator		
Patient satisfied with treatment		
Yes	0.49	−1.00
No	−3.08	6.30
t	1.71	−2.51**
Needs further treatment		
Yes	−0.52	2.87
No	0.57	−3.15
t	−0.70	2.74***

* P = .06.　　** P < .05.　　*** P < .01.

1996).[3] The perceived level of the therapeutic relationship at the end of the second treatment hour was independent of the patients' pretreatment level of DAS PFT ($r = -.09$). Though highly perfectionistic patients appear to be capable of perceiving their therapist positively, nevertheless they are relatively less able to benefit from treatment. Because

---

3. This finding is consistent with the report by Krupnick et al. (1996) who, using the Vanderbilt Therapeutic Alliance Scale (Hartley and Strupp 1983), found that mean therapeutic alliance, assessed in the 3rd, 9th, and 15th sessions, was significantly related to outcome across treatment groups. This relationship was determined, however, primarily by the contributions of the patient rather than by the therapist to the therapeutic alliance.

TABLE 2–3

Correlation of pretreatment pure DAS NFA and PFT and therapeutic effects at termination and 18-month follow-up as rated by therapist, clinical evaluator, and patient

	Termination		Follow-up[a]	
	NFA	PFT	NFA	PFT
Composite gain score	−.07	.29****	−.04	.11
Therapist				
I (Clinical change) (+)[b]	−.04	−.16**	—	—
II (Current functioning) (+)	.01	.04	—	—
Clinical evaluator				
Current condition	−.04	.21***	−.10	.17**
Degree of change (+)	.05	−.24***	.15*	−.14
Liking of patient (+)	.06	−.09	.03	−.07
Patient				
Treatment satisfaction	−.07	.15*	−.11	.23***
Current condition	.00	.11	.00	.16*
Degree of therapeutic change[c]	−.03	.26****	.19*	−.21***
Change related to treatment (+)	.09	−.11	—	—

[a] *Therapists did not participate in the follow-up assessments.*

[b] *7-point Likert scales were usually reversed scales, a higher number indicate poorer functioning. Scales with a positive direction are indicated by a plus sign (+) at the end of the question.*

[c] *Therapeutic change at 18-month follow-up assessed by extensive questionnaire about a number of specific types of changes (i.e., symptoms of depression, interpersonal relations, negative self attitudes).*

* P < .10.   ** P < .05.   *** P < .01.   **** P < .001.

DAS PFT and B-L RI scores are not significantly correlated, they each appear to contribute independent variance to the prediction of therapeutic outcome. Surprisingly, however, the interaction of DAS PFT and B-L RI does not add significantly to the prediction of therapeutic outcome. Exploratory analyses, however, indicated a significant curvilinear (quadratic) component to the interaction between DAS PFT and B-L RI in predicting therapeutic outcome. As indicated in Figure 2–2, the level of B-L RI at the end of the second hour had only marginal effects on the relation of DAS PFT to therapeutic outcome at low and high levels of PFT (P < .10 and .15, respectively), but the level of the B-L RI significantly (P < .001) reduced the negative effects of PFT on treatment outcome at the midlevel of PFT (Blatt et al. 1996).

TABLE 2–4

Correlation of B-L RI with residualized therapeutic gain scores at termination

Measures of depression	
HRSD	−.11
BDI	−.15[t]*
Measures of general clinical functioning	
GAS[a]	.24**
HSCL-90	−.22**
Social adjustment	
SAS	−.26**

*[t] < .10.   ** P < .01.

[a] *The GAS is a positive scale, higher scores indicate better functioning.*

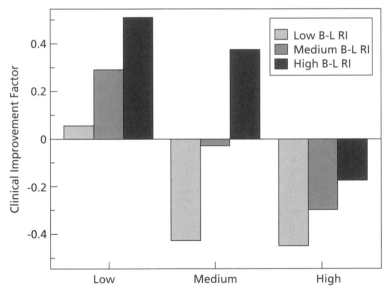

FIGURE 2–2. *Clinical improvement as a function of the level of pretreatment perfectionism and the quality of the therapeutic alliance at the second treatment session.* Source. *Reprinted from Blatt SJ, Zuroff DC, Quinlan DM et al: Interpersonal factors in brief treatment of depression: further analyses of the NIMH Treatment of Depression Collaborative Research Program.* J Consult Clin Psychol *64:162–171, 1996. Used with permission.*

In summary, these analyses indicated that the effects of brief treatment for depression, as assessed in the NIMH-sponsored TDCRP, are significantly determined by patient dimensions, especially by pretreatment levels of perfectionism or self-criticism, independent of the type of treatment the patient received. This negative effect of PFT in brief treatment stands in contrast with the findings that perfectionistic, self-critical, introjective outpatients did relatively well in long-term, intensive, outpatient treatment (Blatt 1992) as well as in long-term, intensive, inpatient treatment of seriously disturbed, treatment-resistant patients (Blatt and Ford 1994). The findings of the three investigations presented here indicate that patient characteristics significantly influence the relative efficacy of therapeutic interventions. The distinction between two primary dimensions of personality development, relatedness and self-definition, and between two parallel types of psychopathology, anaclitic and introjective, have enabled us to introduce central dimensions of the patient into studies of the treatment process and to evaluate their interaction with the mutative forces that potentially exist in both short- and long-term treatment. These findings, consistent with prior research (e.g., Crits-Christoph 1992; Crits-Christoph and Mintz 1991; Luborsky et al. 1986; Miller and Berman 1983; Smith et al. 1980; Stiles et al. 1986), indicate that therapeutic outcome is significantly influenced by interpersonal dimensions of the treatment process—by patient characteristics and by the capacity of the patient and therapist to establish an effective therapeutic relationship (e.g., Blatt et al. 1996; Burns and Nolen-Hoeksema 1992; Horvath and Symonds 1991; Krupnick et al. 1996). Research should be devoted to studying more fully these interpersonal dimensions of the treatment process.

References

American Psychiatric Association Commission on Psychotherapies: Psychotherapy Research: Methodological and Efficacy Issues. Washington, DC, American Psychiatric Association, 1982

American Psychiatric Association: Diagnostic and Statistical Manual of Mental Disorders, 3rd Edition. Washington, DC, American Psychiatric Association, 1980

American Psychiatric Association: Diagnostic and Statistical Manual of Mental Disorders, 3rd Edition, Revised. Washington, DC, American Psychiatric Association, 1987

American Psychiatric Association: Diagnostic and Statistical Manual of Mental Disorders, 4th Edition. Washington, DC, American Psychiatric Association, 1994

Angyal A: Neurosis and Treatment: A Holistic Theory. Edited by Hanfmann E, Jones RM. New York, Wiley, 1951

Arieti S, Bemporad JR: Severe and Mild Depression: The Therapeutic Approach. New York, Basic Books, 1978

Arieti S, Bemporad JR: The psychological organization of depression. Am J Psychiatry 137:1360–1365, 1980

Bakan D: The Duality of Human Existence: An Essay on Psychology and Religion. Chicago, IL, Rand McNally, 1966

Balint M: Primary Love and Psychoanalytic Technique. London, Hogarth Press, 1952

Barrett-Lennard GT: Dimensions of therapist responses as causal factors in therapeutic change. Psychol Monogr 76 (Whole No. 562), 1962

Barrett-Lennard GT: The Relationship Inventory now: issues and advances in theory, method, and use, in The Psychoanalytic Process: A Research Handbook. Edited by Greenberg LS, Pinsof WM. New York, Guilford 1985, pp 439–476

Beck AT: Depression Inventory. Philadelphia, PA, Philadelphia Center for Cognitive Therapy, 1978

Beck AT: Cognitive therapy of depression: new perspectives, in Treatment of Depression: Old Controversies and New Approaches. Edited by Barrett JE, Clayton PJ. New York, Raven, 1983, pp 265–290

Beutler LE: Have all won and must all have prizes? Revisiting Luborsky et al.'s verdict. J Consult Clin Psychol 59:226–232, 1991

Blaney PH, Kutcher GS: Measures of depressive dimensions: are they interchangeable? J Pers Assess 56:502–512, 1991

Blatt SJ: Levels of object representation in anaclitic and introjective depression. Psychoanal Study Child 29:107–157, 1974

Blatt SJ: Interpersonal relatedness and self-definition: two personality configurations and their implications for psychopathology and psychotherapy, in Repression and Dissociation: Implications for Personality Theory, Psychopathology & Health. Edited by Singer JL. Chicago, IL, University of Chicago Press, 1990, pp 299–335

Blatt SJ: A cognitive morphology of psychopathology. J Nerv Ment Dis 179:449–458, 1991

Blatt SJ: The differential effect of psychotherapy and psychoanalysis on anaclitic and introjective patients: the Menninger Psychotherapy Research Project revisited. J Am Psychoanal Assoc 40:691–724, 1992

Blatt SJ: Representational structures in psychopathology, in Rochester Symposium on Developmental Psychopathology, Vol VI: Emotion, Cognition, and Representation. Edited by Cicchetti D, Toth S. Rochester, NY, University of Rochester Press, 1995, pp 1–33

Blatt SJ, Blass RB: Attachment and separateness: a dialectic model of the products and processes of psychological development. Psychoanal Study Child 45:107–127, 1990

Blatt SJ, Felsen I: "Different kinds of folks may need different kinds of strokes": the effect of patients' characteristics on therapeutic process and outcome. Psychother Res 3:245–259, 1993

Blatt SJ, Ford R: Therapeutic Change: An Object Relations Perspective. New York, Plenum, 1994

Blatt SJ, Shichman S: Two primary configurations of psychopathology. Psychoanalysis and Contemporary Thought 6:187–254, 1983

Blatt SJ, Zuroff DC: Interpersonal relatedness and self-definition: two prototypes for depression. Clin Psychol Rev 12:527–562, 1992

Blatt SJ, D'Afflitti JP, Quinlan DM: Experiences of depression in normal young adults. J Abnorm Psychol 85:383–389, 1976

Blatt SJ, D'Afflitti JP, Quinlan DM: Depressive Experiences Questionnaire. New Haven, CT, Yale University, 1979

Blatt SJ, Ford RQ, Berman W, et al: The assessment of therapeutic change in schizophrenic and borderline young adults. Psychoanalytic Psychology 5:127–158, 1988

Blatt SJ, Quinlan DM, Chevron ES, et al: Dependency and self-criticism: psychological dimensions of depression. J Consult Clin Psychol 50:113–124, 1982

Blatt SJ, Quinlan DM, Chevron E: Empirical investigations of a psychoanalytic theory of depression, in Empirical Studies of Psychoanalytic Theories, Vol 3. Edited by Masling J. Hillsdale, NJ, Analytic Press, 1990, pp 89–147

Blatt SJ, Quinlan DM, Pilkonis PA, et al: Impact of perfectionism and need for approval on the brief treatment of depression. J Consult Clin Psychol 63:125–132, 1995a

Blatt SJ, Zuroff DC, Quinlan DM, et al: Patient and therapist characteristics in the brief treatment of depression: further analyses of the NIMH TDCRP. Paper presented at the annual meeting of the Society for Psychotherapy Research, Vancouver, British Columbia, July 1995b

Blatt SJ, Zuroff DC, Quinlan DM, et al: Interpersonal factors in brief treatment of depression: further analyses of the NIMH Treatment of Depression Collaborative Research Program. J Consult Clin Psychol 64:162–171, 1996

Bowlby J: A Secure Base: Clinical Applications of Attachment Theory. London, Routledge & Kegan Paul, 1988

Burns DD, Nolen-Hoeksema S: Therapeutic empathy and recovery from depression in cognitive-behavioral therapy: a structural equation model. J Consult Clin Psychol 60:441–449, 1992

Cane DB, Olinger LJ, Gotlib IH, et al: Factor structure of the Dysfunctional Attitude Scale in a student population. J Clin Psychol 42:307–309, 1986

Crits-Christoph P: The efficacy of brief dynamic psychotherapy: a meta-analysis. Am J Psychiatry 149:151–158, 1992

Crits-Christoph P, Mintz J: Implications of therapists effects for the design and analysis of comparative studies of psychotherapies. J Consult Clin Psychol 45:1001–1004, 1991

Cronbach LJ: Correlation between persons as a research tool, in Psychotherapy: Theory and Research. Edited by Mowrer OH. New York, Roland, 1953, pp 376–389

Cronbach LJ: The two disciplines of scientific psychology. Am Psychol 12:671–684, 1957

Cronbach LJ: Beyond the two disciplines of scientific psychology. Am Psychol 30:116–127, 1975

Cronbach LJ, Gleser GG: Assessing similarity between profiles. Psychol Bull 50:456–474, 1953

Derogatis LR, Lipman RS, Rickels K, et al: The Hopkins Symptom Checklist (HSCL): a self-report symptom inventory. Behav Sci 19:1–15, 1974

Edwards AL, Cronbach LJ: Experimental design for research in psychotherapy. J Clin Psychol 8:51–59, 1952

Elkin I: The NIMH Treatment of Depression Collaborative Research Program: where we began and where we are now, in Handbook of Psychotherapy and Behavior Change, 4th Edition. Edited by Bergin AE, Garfield SL. New York, Wiley, 1994, pp 114–135

Elkin I, Shea MT, Watkins JT, et al: NIMH Treatment of Depression Collaborative Research Program: general effectiveness of treatments. Arch Gen Psychiatry 46:971–983, 1989

Fawcett J, Epstein P, Fiester SJ, et al: Clinical management-Imipramine/Placebo Administration Manual: NIMH Treatment of Depression Collaborative Research Program. Psychopharmacol Bull 23:309–324, 1987

Frank JD: The present status of outcome studies. J Consult Clin Psychol 47:310–316, 1979

Frank JD: Therapeutic components shared by all psychotherapies, in Psychotherapy Research and Behavior Change, Vol 1. Edited by Harvey JH,

Parks MM. Washington, DC, American Psychological Association, 1982, pp 5–37

Freud S: Civilization and its discontents (1930), in The Standard Edition of the Complete Psychological Works of Sigmund Freud, Vol 21. Translated and edited by Strachey J. London, Hogarth Press, 1957, pp 64–145

Gurman AS: The patient's perception of the therapeutic relationship, in Effective Psychotherapy: A Handbook of Research. Edited by Furman AS, Razin AM. New York, Pergamon, 1977

Hamilton M: A rating scale for depression. J Neurol Neurosurg Psychiatry 23:56–62, 1960

Hamilton MA: Development of a rating scale for primary depressive illness. British Journal of Social and Clinical Psychology 6:278–296, 1967

Hartley D, Strupp H: The therapeutic alliance: its relationship to outcome in brief psychotherapy, in Empirical Studies of Psychoanalytic Theories. Edited by Masling J. Hillsdale, NJ, Lawrence Erlbaum Associates, 1993, pp 1–27

Horowitz MJ, Marmar C, Weiss DS, et al: Brief psychotherapy of bereavement reactions: the relationship of process to outcome. Arch Gen Psychiatry 41:438–448, 1984

Horvath AO, Symonds BD: Relation between working alliance and outcome in psychotherapy: a meta-analysis. Journal of Counseling Psychology 38:139–149, 1991

Imber SD, Pilkonis PA, Sotsky SM, et al: Mode-specific effects among three treatments for depression. J Consult Clin Psychol 58:352–359, 1990

Krupnick JL, Sotsky SM, Simmens S, et al: The role of the therapeutic alliance in psychotherapy and pharmacotherapy outcome: findings in the NIMH Treatment of Depression Collaborative Research Program. J Consult Clin Psychol 64:532–539, 1996

Luborsky L, Singer B, Luborsky L: Comparative studies of psychotherapies: is it true that "Everyone has won and all must have prizes"? Arch Gen Psychiatry 32:995–1008, 1975

Luborsky L: Are common factors across different psychotherapies the main explanation for the Dodo Bird verdict that "Everyone has won so all shall have prizes." Clinical Psychology: Science and Practice 2:106–109, 1995

Luborsky L, Crits-Christoph P, McLellan AT, et al: Do therapists vary much in their success? Findings from four outcome studies. Am J Orthopsychiatry 56:501–512, 1986

McAdams DP: Power, Intimacy, and the Life Story: Personological Inquiries into Identity. Homewood, IL, Dorsey, 1985

McClelland DC: Some reflections on the two psychologies of love. J Pers 54:334–353, 1986

Miller RC, Berman JS: The efficacy of cognitive behavior therapies: a quantitative review of the research evidence. Psychol Bull 94:39–53, 1983

Nietzel MT, Harris MJ: Relationship of dependency and achievement/autonomy to depression. Clin Psychol Rev 10:279–297, 1990

Oliver JM, Baumgart BP: The Dysfunctional Attitude Scale: Psychometric properties in an unselected adult population. Cognitive Theory and Research 9:161–169, 1985

Pilon D: Validation of Beck's sociotropic and autonomous modes of depression. Paper presented at the meeting of the American Psychological Association, New York City, August 1987

Rogers CR: Client-Centered Therapy. Boston, MA, Houghton Mifflin, 1951

Rogers CR: The necessary and sufficient conditions of therapeutic personality change. Journal of Consulting Psychology 21:95–103, 1957

Rogers CR: A theory of therapy, personality, and interpersonal relationships as developed in the client-centered framework in psychology: a study of science, in Formulations of the Person and the Social Context. Edited by Koch S. New York, McGraw-Hill, 1959, pp 184–256

Shapiro DA, Shapiro D: Meta-analysis of comparative therapy outcome studies: A replication and refinement. Psychol Bull 92:581–604, 1982

Shoham-Salomon V, Hannah MT: Client-treatment interactions in the study of differential change processes. J Consult Clin Psychol 59:217–225, 1991

Shor J, Sanville J: Illusions in Loving: A Psychoanalytic Approach to Intimacy and Autonomy. Los Angeles, CA, Double Helix, 1978

Smith B, Sechrest L: The treatment of aptitude x treatment interactions. J Consult Clin Psychol 59:233–244, 1991

Smith ML, Glass GV, Miller TI: The Benefits of Psychotherapy. Baltimore, MD, John Hopkins University Press, 1980

Snow RE: Aptitude-treatment interactions as a framework for research on individual differences in psychotherapy. J Consult Clin Psychol 59:205–216, 1991

Sotsky SM, Glass DR, Shea MT, et al: Patient predictors of response to psychotherapy and pharmacotherapy: findings in the NIMH Treatment of Depression Collaborative Research Program. Am J Psychiatry 148:997–1008, 1991

Spitzer RL, Gibson M, Endicott J: Global Assessment Scale, New York, New York State Department of Mental Hygiene, 1973

Spitzer RL, Endicott J, Robins E: Research diagnostic criteria: rationale and reliability. Arch Gen Psychiatry 35:773–782, 1978

Stiles WB, Shapiro DA, Elliot R: Are all psychotherapies equivalent? Am Psychol 41:161–180, 1986

Strupp HH, Binder JL: Psychotherapy in a New Key: A Guide to Time Limited Dynamic Psychotherapy. New York, Basic Books, 1984

Wallerstein RS: Forty-two Lives in Treatment: A Study of Psychoanalysis and Psychotherapy. New York, Guilford, 1986

Weissman AN, Beck AT: Development and validation of the Dysfunctional Attitude Scale: a preliminary investigation. Paper presented at the meeting of the American Psychological Association, Toronto, Canada, August–September 1978

Weissman MM, Paykel ES: The Depressed Women: Study of Social Relationships. Chicago, IL, University of Chicago Press, 1974

Wiggins JS: Agency and communion as conceptual coordinates for the understanding and measurement of interpersonal behavior, in Thinking Clearly about Psychology, Vol 2: Personality and Psychotherapy. Edited by Grove WW, Cicchetti D. Minneapolis, MN, University of Minnesota Press, 1991, pp 89–113

Zuroff DC, Quinlan DM, Blatt SJ: Psychometric properties of the Depressive Experiences Questionnaire. J Pers Assess 55:65–72, 1990

Therapist and Patient Personality Characteristics and the Nature, Quality, and Outcome of Psychotherapy

Focus on the Myers Briggs Type Indicator

David S. Janowsky, M.D.

In recent years the academic study of psychotherapy has become progressively more focused on evaluating the efficacy and cost effectiveness of specific psychotherapies or psychotherapy-pharmacotherapy combinations for formally diagnosable psychiatric disorders. In part, this evolution has occurred because we now have tools, such as DSM-IV (American Psychiatric Association 1994), which allow for effective, reliable, categorical diagnoses of emotional disorders. Probably supportive of categorical diagnostic descriptions is an emerging psychobiology of emotional disorders that demonstrates central and peripheral serotonergic, noradrenergic, cholinergic, peptide, genetic, and other neuromodulator and associated biological changes as representative of a given psychiatric diagnosis. In parallel, codification of treatment techniques has produced focused manuals that describe specific psychotherapeutic maneuvers and strategies for specific disorders.

In contrast to this neat and scientific approach, when the psycho-

Supported by a grant from the Richard King Mellon Family Foundation and NIMH MHCRC Grant MH 33127.

therapeutic and pharmacotherapeutic treatment literature is carefully evaluated, it is increasingly clear that a given psychotherapy, applied carefully, even with the use of a manual, can be efficacious for a variety of disorders. For example, both cognitive-behavioral therapy and interpersonal therapy are useful for the treatment of depression, panic disorder, social phobia, bulimia, obsessive-compulsive disorder, and generalized anxiety disorder. Similarly, selective serotonin reuptake inhibitors, monoamine oxidase inhibitors, and some tricyclic antidepressants are generally, and probably nonspecifically, helpful in these psychiatric disorders. Conversely, a significant number of patients with a specific and carefully diagnosed disorder fail to respond to a so-called proven treatment.

Also against the tide toward categorization and diagnostic and psychopharmacological specificity is a growing body of information suggesting that core or underlying personality variables, not formally linked to specific emotional disorders, such as introversion, neuroticism, and interpersonal dependency, correlate with diagnosis (Akiskal et al. 1983) and may determine the effectiveness of pharmacological and psychosocial therapies (Clayton et al. 1994; Hirschfeld et al. 1983, 1986). For example, Joyce et al. (1994a) have used the Tridimensional Personality Questionnaire (TPQ; Cloninger 1987) to show that depressed individuals who score low in a combination of novelty seeking, harm avoidance, and reward dependence, or who are reward dependent and harm avoidant do best on a variety of antidepressants, whereas other TPQ combinations do not respond as well. Joyce et al. (1994a) also noted that harm avoidant depressed women selectively did best on the noradrenergic antidepressant, desipramine, while reward dependent depressed women did best on the serotonergic antidepressant, clomipramine. Similarly, Peselow et al. (1992a, 1992b) have shown that depressed, sociotropic patients who scored low in autonomy did poorly on antidepressant drugs compared with placebo, while more highly autonomous individuals who were low in sociotropy did best on antidepressants and poorly on placebo. Ansseau et al. (1991) found that compulsive personality traits predicted a selective positive response to serotonergic antidepressants. In addition, Blatt et al. (1995, and Chapter 2, this volume) have shown that highly autonomous, perfectionistic depressed patients did poorly in short-term tricyclic pharmacotherapy and psychotherapy.

Even the biology of emotional disorders appears to be strongly linked to personality (Dabbs and Hopper 1990). For example, Joyce et al. (1994b) noted that subjects with depression, not differing in the severity of their symptoms on other variables, were more prone to have elevated morning cortisol levels if they scored high on the extravagance subscale of TPQ novelty seeking, high on the fatigue subscale of harm avoidance, and high on reward dependence. In addition, patients with bipolar disorder were shown to have increased physiologic reactivity to stress if they were introverted and obsessional (Swendsen et al. 1995), and to have higher cortisol activity as part of this reactivity. Introverted individuals, even as small children (Kagan et al. 1988), have relatively higher resting cortisol levels than those who are less introverted, and such introverts tend to be more anxious and possibly more depressed in childhood and as they grow older.

The possibility exists that some psychiatric illnesses, such as the affective and anxiety disorders, are less treatment specific than has been generally thought true, and that for psychotherapy and pharmacotherapy, diagnosis as such may matter less than other underlying features, including personality, which itself may be linked to biology. The focus of this chapter is to review and present information suggesting that personality factors in the psychotherapist and in the patient, alone and interacting, may be exerting important influences that effect the formation of therapeutic relationships and determine therapeutic outcome.

In our current socioeconomic climate, third-party-supported psychotherapy is becoming ever more constricted in time and scope. Furthermore, the growing use of paraprofessionals has deprofessionalized and changed the practice of psychotherapy, as case managers and other less rigorously trained mental health workers become major contacts for emotionally disturbed individuals. The lack of extensive formal training of such paraprofessionals may make reliance on their basic personality a major variable in determining patient compliance, the quality of the therapeutic relationship, bonding, and therapeutic outcome. At the least, if the personality match between the patient and the therapist or case manager is poor, it seems logical that the patient may be less likely to keep appointments and the therapist may be less inclined to be committed to working with the patient. Thus, the significance of the personality fit between the patient and the therapist in today's world of psychiatric treatment may be especially significant, since there is often less time to form relationships, for therapists to learn to tolerate their patients, and for patients to accept the idiosyncrasies of their therapists.

Personality Surveys

A plethora of psychological tests and surveys are used to define the personalities of normal people and psychiatric patients, but in this chapter, we limit ourselves to considering two well-intercorrelated surveys that have been more recently used to evaluate basic personality and temperament, especially in normal subjects, believed to have relevance to the psychotherapeutic process. Our major focus is on the Myers Briggs Type Indicator (MBTI; Myers and McCaulley 1985), with a secondary focus on the five-factor NEO Personality Inventory (NEO-PI; Costa and McCrae [1990, 1992]) scale. The MBTI is widely used by the lay public in business, management, counseling, and educational circles. It has been given to hundreds of thousands of people, and the acquired normative and occupational data is extensive (Myers and McCaulley 1985). In addition, insights gained over the past several decades from MBTI-focused research are extensive, and these findings have been operationalized into several popular lay books (Myers and Myers 1980). Such books discuss in a very readable and understandable way how different MBTI types prefer to respond and interact with at work, in school, in marriage, and in social settings. Therefore, since the possibility that insights gained from application of the MBTI to psychiatric populations could be easily understood, and since the test is widely used, a certain practicality and usefulness not so easily found with the plethora of other personality tests generally used by professional personnel in research exists. In addition, MBTI profiles appear relatively stable over time in a given individual, and they correlate with the variables of other psychometric tests of personality, as shown in Table 3–1.

The MBTI is a Jungian-based scale that divides individuals categorically by their preferences for extroversion or introversion (E vs. I), sensing or intuitive (S vs. N), thinking or feeling (T vs. F), and judging or perceiving (J vs. P). Operationally, extroverts are most at home in the outer world of people and things than in the inner world of ideas; sensing types generally would rather work with known facts than look into possibilities and relationships; thinking types generally base their judgments more on impersonal analysis than on personal values; judging types generally like a planned, decided, orderly way of life better than a flexible and spontaneous way. The preferences of introverted, intuitive, feeling, and perceiving types each oppose their companion typez (Myers and McCaulley 1985). Although each of the eight types is considered a distinct entity, continuum scores along a given dichot-

TABLE 3–1

MBTI types significantly correlated with other personality variables

MBTI type	Positive correlations	Negative correlations
Extroversion Introversion	Extroversion, Sociability, Outgoing, Venturesome, Social Adjustment, Self-Confidence, Gregarious	Depression, Guilt Process, Social Introversion, Neuroticism
Sensing-Intuitive	Orderliness, Conscientiousness	Openness, Tenderness, Lability, Dyscontrol, Flexibility, Tolerance for Complexity, Blame Avoidance
Thinking-Feeling	Autonomy, Orderliness, Aggression	Nurturance, Empathy, Blame Avoidance, Succorance, Tenderness, Agreeableness, Abasement, Deference, Affiliation
Judging-Perceiving	Conscientiousness, Self-Control, Autonomy, Achievement, Depression, Aggression	Lability, Deference, Flexibility

omy (i.e., extroversion to introversion) can be derived (Myers and McCaulley 1985).

The MBTI has been found to correlate highly with several more scientifically popular personality rating scales, including the NEO-PI scale, which divides individuals along five dimensions: neuroticism, extroversion, openness to experience, agreeableness, and conscientiousness. Each of the NEO-PI factors is described by a single descriptor, and a low score implies the opposite set of characteristics. Significantly, the extroversion, openness to experience, agreeableness, and conscientiousness scales of the NEO-PI correlate quite well ($r = 0.43-0.73$) with extroversion-introversion, intuitive-sensing, feeling-thinking, and judging-perceiving continuum on the MBTI, respectively (McCrae and Costa 1989; MacDonald et al. 1994). The TPQ measures individuals as to degree of novelty seeking, harm avoidance, and reward dependence. These factors correlate highly with several aspects of the NEO-PI, and thereby would be quite likely to correlate with MBTI types.

Therapist Personality Type and Choice of Preferred Therapy

As reviewed by Myers and McCaulley (1985), therapists such as counseling clergymen, clinical psychologists, and psychiatrists have been found predominantly to be intuitive (as opposed to sensing) types on the MBTI. Thus, they are probably high in openness to experience on the NEO-PI. They have also been found to more often be MBTI feeling types, and thus probably are high in NEO-PI agreeableness. In some studies they are more frequently perceptive types and are probably low on NEO-PI conscientiousness . However, Carskadon (1979) has reviewed information suggesting that there are, in spite of these generalities, different MBTI personality characteristics among therapists interested in different forms of psychotherapy. Levin (L. S. Levin, "Jungian personality variables in psychotherapists of five different theoretical orientations," unpublished doctoral dissertation, Georgia State University, 1978), studying 90 psychologists and psychiatrists (as reviewed by Carskadon 1979), noted that therapists preferring rational-emotive therapy and/or behavioral therapies were most often MBTI thinking types and that there was an underrepresentation of feeling or perceiving types in these therapists. Also, behavioral therapists were the least intuitive of MBTI types. Perceiving types and intuitive plus perceiving types preferred Gestalt therapy, and judging types were underrepresented among Gestalt therapists. Intuitive plus feeling types and feeling plus perceiving types were overrepresented among those who preferred experiential therapies, with thinking types being underrepresented. For those using psychoanalytic approaches, a combination of introverted plus judging types and intuitive plus judging types were overrepresented, and perceiving types were underrepresented. These results are summarized in Table 3–2.

Similarly, Hirschfeld et al. (1977) noted that the Sotoria House treatment staff, intensively treating schizophrenic patients without the use of pharmacotherapy in a group living situation, tended to be INFP MBTI types. This group differed somewhat from the treatment staff of a university psychiatric teaching ward, who were statistically more extroverted, and numerically relatively less often intuitive, feeling, and perceiving types, although these latter types continued to be predominant in both groups. Thus, there is considerable core personality variability among therapists and among those who select different therapies as their preferred mode of practice.

Therapist Personality Style and Therapeutic Outcome

The relationship of psychotherapeutic outcome and the quality of psychotherapeutic relationships have been linked to the nature of the psychotherapist's personality. The evidence from the literature of the 1950s and early 1960s suggests that schizophrenic inpatients and depressed neurotic outpatients respectively show different treatment responses according to the personalities of their therapists (Betz 1963; McNair et al. 1962; Whitehorn and Betz 1954, 1957, 1960). In this early work, therapists were divided into two types, designated Type A

TABLE 3–2

The relationship of MBTI scales to preferred psychotherapy orientation

Type of therapist	Overrepresented scales	Underrepresented scales
Rational-emotive therapists[a] (least intuitive and most thinking)	T, SP, NT	F, NF, NP, EP
Gestalt therapists	P, NP	J, NJ
Experiential therapists (most feeling)	F, NF, FP	T, NT
Psychoanalytic therapists (most judging)	J, IJ, NJ	P

[a] *Includes behavioral therapists (Levin 1978; as reviewed by Carskadon 1979).*

and Type B. Type A therapists were found to do best with *process* schizophrenics, who were generally psychotic, suspicious, and distrustful (Betz and Whitehorn 1956; Whitehorn and Betz 1954, 1957, 1960). Type B therapists were found by McNair et al. (1962) to do best with more introjective, intrapunitive, depressed, neurotic patients. It was found that the personality of Type A therapists was one that showed a dislike for activities of a mechanical, technical, or manual nature, and these individuals had interests more like those of lawyers, accountants, and journalists. Type B therapists, in contrast, were found to prefer mechanical activities and had interests similar to math or physical science teachers, carpenters, plumbers, and other manual workers.

The differences in outcome due to having a Type A versus Type B profile as a therapist were most significant when psychiatrists were studied early in their training, and the differences tended to diffuse as training progressed. Furthermore, as the use of neuroleptics and antidepressants became more widespread, the differences in response to Type A and Type B therapists in schizophrenics tended to disappear. Nevertheless, the Type A-Type B dichotomy was a well-documented phenomena in the years preceding and leading into the era of psychiatric drug treatment, and it probably has significance for the present time, given current conditions.

Kuder and Strong Vocational Interest Inventory occupational interest profiles relevant to Type A and Type B therapists have been correlated with MBTI profiles (Myers and McCaulley 1985). Kuder

Interest Inventory (Kuder, 1968) profiles of auto mechanics, brick-layers, engineers, farmers, machinists, printers, television repairmen, and truck drivers tend to correlate significantly with sensing, thinking, and judging preferences on the MBTI. Therefore, therapists who score as relatively more sensing (i.e., presumably scoring low on openness to experience on the NEO-PI), thinking (presumably scoring low on agreeableness on the NEO-PI), and judging (presumably scoring high on conscientiousness on the NEO-PI) would be expected to have been Type B therapists in the earlier studies. Conversely, Kuder and Strong Vocational Interest Inventory profiles demonstrating greater interest in more abstract, nonmechanical, nontechnical pursuits are more intuitive, feeling, and perceiving MBTI types. Jobs that correlate with these Type A MBTI characteristics include artists, musicians, art and music educators, English students, psychologists, sociologists, ministers, psychoanalysts, and clinical psychologists. These relationships are outlined in Table 3–3.

Truax (1963), Truax et al. (1966), Blatt and Zuroff (1992), Nelson and Stake (1994) and a variety of other authors exploring therapist personality have noted that patient satisfaction and positive evaluation of the quality of therapy by patients and therapists tends to be related to a number of interpersonal variables in the therapists, as does outcome. These so-called positive therapeutic qualities include perceived therapist empathy, genuineness, openness, and acceptance of the patient (Barrett-Lennard 1972). Significantly, Jenkins et al. (1992) has noted that empathy in graduate students studying to be therapists correlated with being a feeling type on the MBTI.

The importance of these interpersonal qualities has been reemphasized in the Collaborative Depression Study. Blatt et al. (1995) noted that subjects who were depressed, especially those who have a medium amount of perfectionism, showed greater improvement in their depression in the 3-month treatment trial if their therapist was rated as having the already described positive therapeutic qualities early in the therapeutic process, and this phenomenon occurred regardless of whether the type of treatment assigned to the patient was pharmacological or psychotherapeutic. Similarly, Nelson and Stake (1994) found that for patients seen in medium- to long-term therapy, those

TABLE 3–3

MBTI *preferences correlating with Type A and Type B therapists and with occupations*

Occupations	MBTI scales
Type A	
Journalist	N, F, P
Personnel manager	E, P
Lawyer	N, T
Artist	N, P
Minister	E, N, F
Advertising executive	N
Type B	
Auto mechanic	S, J
Bricklayer	S, J
Math teacher	S, T, J
Mechanical engineer	T
Plumber	S, J
TV repairman	E, S, T, J
Craftsman	S, T, J
Printer	S
Forester	I, T
Personnel director	E
Carpenter	S, J
Firemen	S, J
Electrician	S, J

therapists who were rated on the MBTI as extroverted and feeling types were the ones whose patients rated themselves as experiencing the most positive therapeutic experience.

Fit Between Patient Personality and Therapeutic Modalities

In addition to therapist personality relating to patient outcome, a growing literature suggests that the fit between patient personality and specific treatments may influence psychotherapeutic outcome. For example, Fairbanks (1987) showed that imagery rehearsal plus relaxation therapy was most effective in treating anxiety disorder patients who were MBTI intuitive types. In contrast, cognitive restructuring therapy techniques plus relaxation therapy were most effective in treating patients who were sensing types. Also, it has been noted by Cline (1985) that cardiac patients did best in a rehabilitation program if they scored on the MBTI as a combination of extroverted, thinking, and judging types, rather than other types.

In addition to these findings, several other observations corroborate a relationship between MBTI patient personality and outcome. Graff (W. S. Graff, "The effectiveness of systematic desensitization in the reduction of test anxiety in Jungian thinking versus feeling personality types," unpublished doctoral dissertation, Auburn University, 1975) found that MBTI thinking males and feeling females experienced significant test anxiety reduction with systematic desensitization, with the converse relationship not occurring. Giroux (J. T. Giroux, "Selection of a therapeutic technique according to Myers-Briggs type: an investigative study," unpublished master's thesis, Mississippi State University, 1979) noted that rational-emotive group therapy worked best for MBTI feeling types, but did not work well for thinking types. Also, patients with anxiety disorder who scored high on novelty seeking (high on the disorderliness and impulsivity subscales) on the TPQ were found to be those who were most likely to drop out of an antidepressant drug treatment trial (Wingerson et al. 1993).

In addition to these studies, Blatt et al. (1995) noted that patients with high levels of perfectionism (i.e., probably those who would be judging types on the MBTI and those who would have scored high on conscientiousness on the NEO-PI) have tended to have relatively poor psychotherapeutic and psychopharmacologic outcomes in the 12-week experimental phase of the Collaborative Depression Study. In a contrasting study, Blatt (1990) found that those subjects who were depressed and also had high levels of perfectionism did very well in intensive, 5-day per week psychoanalytic therapy.

Finally, with respect to the type of therapy individuals with different personalities prefer, Carskadon (1977), studying students completing a questionnaire describing different therapies, found that MBTI thinking types (presumably those who are low on agreeableness on the

NEO-PI scale), rated themselves as preferring descriptions of behavioral approaches, whereas feeling types (i.e., individuals probably high on agreeableness on the NEO-PI) overwhelmingly preferred humanistic approaches. Carskadon (1977, 1979) found feeling types, listening to a tape of therapy involving high levels of unconditional regard, preferred the high unconditional positive regard therapy, whereas thinking types did not value this quality. Finally, Arain (1968) noted that MBTI thinking-type high school students preferred cognitive characteristics in prospective counselors, whereas feeling types preferred counselors with affective and more emotional characteristics.

Patient-Therapist Personality Fit and Therapeutic Outcome

Over the years a number of studies have attempted to link patient-therapist personality fit or concordance to the outcome and/or the appreciation of the quality of psychotherapy by patients. Generally, these studies have not been shown to have overly dramatic results. However, there are several studies that have suggested that a match between the patient's and the therapist's personality is indeed important. As described earlier, it has been noted that most therapists are intuitive types on the MBTI. Mendelsohn (1966) noted that students electing counseling were most often also intuitive types. Furthermore, MBTI intuitiveness in trainees was found to correlate highly with the positive rating that psychotherapy supervisors gave to them. Therefore there may be a quiet conspiracy for like intuitive types to elect each other in the therapist-client relationship, and for intuitive psychotherapy supervisors to most appreciate their more intuitive students. This bias may explain the tendency of many therapists to most appreciate insight oriented, "psychologically minded" (i.e., MBTI intuitive) patients.

As described earlier, Nelson and Stake (1994) noted that patients tend to rate the quality of their therapy highest if the therapists tend toward being MBTI extroverted and feeling types. However, another important factor determining ratings of the quality of therapy is a positive correlation between therapists and their patients on the MBTI thinking-feeling continuum, as well as on the judging-perceiving continuum. Concordance of these variables between patient and therapist was shown by Nelson and Stake (1994) to predict positive patient ratings as to the quality of therapy. Thus, there appears to be room for variability with respect to the patient-therapist fit in determining the evaluation of the quality of therapy by the patient, and possibly, because positive therapeutic qualities have been shown to predict outcome in many studies, in determining the continuation and outcome of therapy.

Related to patient-therapist fit is the observation by Blatt et al. (1995) that there are two major types of individuals with depression: the anaclitic type (i.e., individuals who are seeking to be cared for by others, who find relating through interpersonal interactions very important, and who become depressed due to a withdrawal of caring, probable sociotropic types) and the introjective type (i.e., those who are perfectionistic, autonomous, high achieving individuals who work hard and are hard on themselves and who become depressed because they do not live up to their ideals, probable autonomous types). One may speculate that anaclitic types represent feeling types on the MBTI and people high in agreeableness on the NEO-PI. Conversely, introjective, intrapunitive people are probably thinking and/or judging types on the MBTI and are probably high on conscientiousness on the NEO-PI.

As mentioned earlier (Blatt 1990), patients who are depressed and perfectionistic seem to do poorly in short-term therapies of a number of types. However, these patients appear to do very well in intensive, long-term psychoanalytic therapy. As described already, psychoanalysts, in contrast to more supportively and experientially (i.e., humanistically) oriented therapists, tend to more often be judging types on the MBTI. Therefore, it would not be surprising if those perfectionistic individuals who do well in psychoanalytic psychotherapy have relatively similar personalities to those of their psychoanalytic therapists, and those perfectionistic types who tend to do poorly in short-term therapies are interacting with the majority of psychotherapist types, who are dissimilar to themselves (i.e., the usual feeling, perceiving, nonjudgmental MBTI types).

Supportive of the relationship between patient and therapist fit and outcome is a study not involving patients or therapists at all. Andrews et al. (1979) have studied the rates of recidivism of probationers whose probation officers were either professional or voluntary officers. In one part of their study, these authors divided the probationers and the probation officers into those who were high and low on empathy, respectively. Low empathy probation officers did better with low empathy probationers. This relationship was especially strong among probationers who were poorly socialized. Likewise, the match of a probation officer and a probationer who both scored high in empathy yielded low rates of recidivism. A highly empathetic officer and a probationer low in empathy led to dramatically high rates of recidivism.

Psychotherapeutic Implications of MBTI Profiles in Suicidal Patients

The author and his colleagues have begun a program to determine whether suicidality is related to specific MBTI personality types. Ultimately, the hope is to relate these types to psychotherapeutic treatment strategies and outcomes. We have studied a total of 94 suicidal psychiatric inpatients. All subjects were given the MBTI and were diagnosed using DSM III-R (American Psychiatric Association 1987) criteria. Diagnoses included major depression, bipolar disorder, substance abuse without depression, major depression plus substance abuse, dysthymia, schizophrenia, and schizoaffective schizophrenia, several personality disorder diagnoses, and other diagnoses. The majority of the patients had some form of affective disorder. We classified patients as having had suicidal ideation and/or having made a current or past suicide attempt. Of the 94 subjects who had experienced serious suicidal ideation and/or made an attempt, as noted in a chart review, 47 had actually made a suicidal attempt just before the current hospitalization or during previous years.

Table 3–4 shows the percentage and numbers of the population of 94 suicidal patients studied who fit into the 16 possible MBTI categories. A significantly higher number of suicidal individuals than

TABLE 3–4

Distribution of MBTI types among 94 suicidal psychiatric inpatients

MBTI type	n	%	I[a]
ISTJ*	3	3.19	0.31
ISFJ**	16	17.02	1.88
INFJ	3	3.19	0.67
INTJ	3	3.19	0.67
ISTP	4	4.26	1.29
ISFP***	21	22.34	4.98
INFP***	14	14.89	2.42
INTP	3	3.19	0.80
ESTP	2	2.13	0.65
ESFP	3	3.19	0.60
ENFP	4	4.26	0.45
ENTP	2	2.13	0.46
ESTJ	4	4.26	0.41
ESFJ	11	11.70	1.24
ENFJ	1	1.06	0.19
ENTJ*	1	1.06	0.18

[a] *Ratio of patient distribution to normative distribution.*
*P < .05.   **P < .01.   ***P < .001.

would be expected from population norms (expressed as *I* in Table 3–4) were clustered in three of the MBTI categories. Individuals who were most often suicidal were INFP, ISFP, and ISFJ. Overall, dramatically more introverted patients were found in the suicidal group. In addition, ESFJ types were slightly more represented in the suicidal patient population than in the general population (Granade et al. 1987). In addition, when patients who actually had a history of making a suicide attempt were evaluated separately, an even higher frequently was found for those who were in the ISFJ category. In contrast, generally, being an extroverted and/or intuitive and/or especially a thinking type protected against suicidality.

Our data concerning suicidality is generally consistent with the results of a similar study (Street and Kromrey 1994) of suicidality in college students, comparing students who noted on a questionnaire survey that they had previously had suicidal ideation, or made suicide attempts with students who had not done so, using the MBTI. Results from that study reflected gender as well as main effects. As with our study, Street and Kromrey (1994) present data and review evidence that INFP students in general, IP women, ISF males, and INP males predominated in the more suicidal students. Differing from our data, ENJ males also predominated. In contrast, individuals who were thinking types were very unlikely to be suicidal, a finding also noted by our study of inpatients. The relationship of our observations to those of Street and Kromrey (1994) is illustrated in Table 3–5.

The use of core or underlying personality testing and its application to the practice of psychotherapy and/or pharmacotherapy has not been a major component of the treatment of seriously disturbed and/ or suicidal patients. Such testing, using the MBTI, has generally been applied in management, education, and counseling circles. However, it is likely that understanding a patient's core personality may be helpful in working with that patient with respect to intrapsychic dynamics and interpersonal interactions with family, friends, and colleagues. In

TABLE 3–5

Comparison of Street and Kromrey's (1994) high and low suicide risk students with University of North Carolina (UNC) inpatients

Street and Kromrey (1994)		Concordance with UNC inpatient data
Sex	MBTI type	
High-risk groups		
Male	ISF	Yes
	INP	Yes
	ENJ	No
Females	IP	Yes
Low-risk groups		
Males	ISTJ	Yes
Females	INTP ($\pm$)	$\pm$
	ISTP ($\pm$)	$\pm$
Both	INTJ	Yes
	ESTJ	Yes
	ESTP	Yes
	ENTJ	Yes
	ENTP	Yes

a very insightful article primarily based on his clinical experience, Miller (1991) linked the five-factor NEO-PI model to the most effective therapeutic stance to be taken by a therapist for a given patient. For example, he noted that patients who were low scorers on the NEO-PI openness to experience scale (i.e., probably MBTI sensing types) generally preferred and did best with more behaviorally oriented and cognitively oriented therapies in which concrete direction and guidance were given. He also noted that these individuals did not do as well with more abstract therapies, such as psychodynamically and psychoanalytically oriented treatments. The converse occurred in patients who were high on openness to experience on the NEO-PI scale (i.e., probably MBTI intuitive types). These patients seemed to appreciate the creative flux and explorative nature of dynamically oriented psychotherapy. Miller (1991) similarly noted that individuals who are high on the NEO-PI extroversion scale seem to prefer group and emotive therapies, whereas introverts do not. Highly conscientious individuals (probably MBTI judging types), generally work hard in therapy and do well. Low conscientiousness types (probably perceiving types on the MBTI) did less well and tend to drop out of therapy earlier and more often.

Seriously suicidal patients who are INFP types would be expected to do well with therapists who are also NFP types, at least in the short run, and who are therapists who practice more supportively oriented therapies. Significantly, many, even most, therapists fit this profile. Treatment of such patients might thus best be accomplished using a rather supportive, experiential, and humanistic approach. However, not all suicidal and/or depressed patients are INFP types. Indeed, the greatest number of our patients attempting suicide were ISFJ types. Such individuals might feel more comfortable with therapists who are also more sensing and/or judging and/or possibly feeling types themselves, and might do best in therapies which tend to attract more sensing and judging oriented therapists, such as the behaviorally oriented therapies. Quite possibly, suicidal patients who are intuitive rather than sensing types, but who are also thinking and judging types as well, might ultimately do best in more intensive, long-term, psychoanalytically oriented therapies, having been paired with practitioners who also tend to be N, T, and J types. Obviously, the converse possibility may be true. The efficacy of pairing opposite patients and therapist MBTI types in psychotherapy ultimately may prove most effective in causing change and improvement, assuming that initial bonding in the relationship allows continuation.

Considering an individual's MBTI profile may allow a theoretical framework from which to be able to interact with suicidal and other patients concerning their various problems. For example, knowing that a given patient is both sensing and judging would suggest working in a rather concrete way to address the patient's need to control and need for order. A patient who is a thinking type may have difficulty easily relating to questions as to how they feel. They may do better initially to consider issues from a cognitive or thinking point of view. Helping a patient who is a perceiving type to understand how he or she may be thought of by a spouse or superior at work of the opposite type may be helpful. Put in that context, differences may be considered from a nonjudgmental point of view. Such a perspective may allow patients to consider their interactions in a different light, thinking of significant others as having varying personality perspectives and acting on these rather than thinking about good or bad, right or wrong, success or failure. For feeling types, issues related to loss of significant others and withdrawal of caring may predominate as a major cause of emotional problems. Attending to the need for interpersonal support, warmth, and caring could thus at least be the initial focus of therapy in these patients.

The Interface of Psychobiology, Personality, and Psychotherapy

Finally, it is worth elaborating upon the interface between psychotherapy and the biology of emotional disorders. There is considerable evidence that the NEO-PI scales, especially neuroticism, openness to experience, conscientiousness, and extroversion are significantly determined by genetics (Bergeman et al. 1993). Indeed, the relationship of the dopamine-receptor gene to higher levels of extroversion (i.e., warmth, excitement seeking, positive emotions) and lower conscientiousness (i.e., deliberation) on the NEO-PI scale has been identified

(Ebstein et al. 1996). It may be that genetic or neurochemical predispositions to a significant extent determine the styles of and/or preferences for psychotherapy in the psychotherapist and in the patient. Such genetic predispositions may indeed determine who goes into such fields as counseling, psychology, and psychiatry and who finds a given therapeutic modality most appealing, both as a therapist and as a patient.

Furthermore, in addition to the actual therapeutic qualities and personality characteristics of the therapist, there is evidence that patient neurochemical state may determine his or her perception of the interpersonal skills (therapeutic qualities) of a therapist. Patients high in depression and/or other negative affects were found (Janowsky et al. 1981) to experience low interpersonal skills such as empathy, genuineness, and acceptance in their therapists. This phenomena could be immediately reversed by infusion of intravenous methylphenidate, a dopamine releasing agent. Thus, biological state in part seemed to determine the *quality* of the therapeutic relationship.

It is therefore quite possible that certain characteristics of personality in the psychotherapist, partially genetically determined and biochemically expressed, resonate with similar and/or opposing genetically determined characteristics in the patient to determine the perception of quality of therapy by the patient and/or the positivity of therapeutic outcome. Ultimately, it may be that such resonance between patient and therapist may determine the ability of a psychotherapeutic intervention and/or a given therapist to effectively alleviate symptoms and cause therapeutic change. Conversely, a patient's genetics, neurotransmitters, and neuromodulators may obviously be altered by psychotropic drugs, leading, in a similar way, to symptom alleviation. Although these possibilities remain quite speculative and do not account for obvious environmental and technical considerations, they are certainly worthy of consideration in developing a coherent hypothesis as to the mechanisms of pharmacotherapy and psychotherapy.

Conclusion

In this chapter I reviewed many aspects of patient and therapist personality: how their interactions relate to therapeutic outcome and how they affect the perception of the quality of therapy. This focus has been relatively neglected in the psychotherapeutic literature, especially in recent years. Enough information has now accumulated to make personality considerations a more central focus of the study of the science of psychotherapy. More specifically, since the MBTI is widely used in our society, has high face validity, and is easily accessible to patients and practitioners alike, the MBTI may be an excellent instrument to include in such investigations and consider using as a tool to develop therapeutic strategies. Similar comments are relevant to the use of the NEO-PI and the TPQ.

References

Akiskal HS, Hirschfeld RMA, Yerevanian BI: The relationship of personality to affective disorders. Arch Gen Psychiatry 40:801–810, 1983

American Psychiatric Association: Diagnostic and Statistical Manual of Mental Disorders, 3rd Edition, Revised. Washington, DC, American Psychiatric Association, 1987

American Psychiatric Association: Diagnostic and Statistical Manual of Mental Disorders, 4th Edition. Washington, DC, American Psychiatric Association, 1994

Andrews DA, Kiessling JJ, Russell RJ, et al: Volunteers and the one-to-one supervision of adult probationers. Toronto, Ontario Ministry of Correctional Services, 1979

Ansseau M, Troistantaines B, Papart B, et al: Compulsive personality as a predictor of response to serotonergic antidepressants. BMJ 303:760–761, 1991

Arain AA: Relationships among counseling clients' personalities, expectations, and problems (doctoral dissertation, Rutgers University, 1967). Dissertation Abstracts 29:4903A–4904A, 1968

Barrett-Lennard GT: Dimensions of therapist change as causal factors in therapeutic change. Psychological Monographs 76, 1972

Bergeman CS, Chipuar HM, Plomin R, et al: Genetic and environmental effects on openness to experience, agreeableness and conscientiousness: an adoption/twin study. J Pers 61:159–179, 1993

Betz BJ: Differential success rates of psychotherapists with "process" and "nonprocess" schizophrenic patients. Am J Psychiatry 11:2090–1091, 1963

Betz BJ, Whitehorn JC: The relationship of the therapist to the outcome of therapy in schizophrenia. Psychiatry Research Reports 5:89–105, 1956

Blatt SJ: Interpersonal relatedness and self-definition: two personality configurations and their implications for psychopathology and psychotherapy, in Repression and Dissociation: Implications for Personality Theory, Psychopathology, and Health. Edited by Singer JL. Chicago, IL, University of Chicago Press, 1990, pp 229–336

Blatt SJ, Zuroff DC: Interpersonal relatedness and self-definition: Two prototypes for depression. Clin Psychol Rev 12:527–562, 1992

Blatt SJ, Quinlan DM, Pilkonis PA, et al: Impact of perfectionism and need for approval on the brief treatment of depression: The National Institute of Mental Health Treatment of Depression Collaborative Research Program revisited. J Consult Clin Psychol 63:125–132, 1995

Carskadon TG: Relationship of psychological type to therapy preferences and willingness to seek help. Paper presented at the Second National Conference on the Uses of the Myers-Briggs Type Indicator, East Lansing, MI, November 1977

Carskadon TG: Clinical and counseling aspects of the Myers-Briggs Type Indicator: a research review. Research in Psychological Type 2:2–31, 1979

Clayton PJ, Ernst C, Angst J: Premorbid personality traits of men who develop unipolar or bipolar disorders. Eur Arch Psychiatry Clin Neurosci 243:340–346, 1994

Cline JA: Cardiac rehabilitation program compliance and personality type (Myers Briggs Type Indicators, socioeconomic status). Dissertation Abstracts International 46(10A):2930, 1985

Cloninger CR: A systematic method for clinical description and classification of personality variants. Arch Gen Psychiatry 44:573–588, 1987

Costa PT, McCrae RR: Personality disorders and the five-factor model of personality. J Personal Disord 4:362–371, 1990

Costa PT, McCrae RR: The five-factor model of personality and its relevance to personality disorders. J Personal Disord 6(4):343–359, 1992

Dabbs JM, Hopper CII: Cortisol, arousal, and personality in two groups of normal men. Personality and Individual Differences 11(9):931–935, 1990

Ebstein RP, Novick O, Umansky R, et al: Dopamine D4 receptor (D_4DR) exon III polymorphism associated with the human personality trait of novelty seeking. Nat Genet 12:78–80, 1996

Fairbanks WD: A comparison study of two cognitive treatment modalities crossed with selected Myers-Briggs Personality typologies in the reduction of anxiety (Ph.D. Thesis, Univ of Wyoming, Publication #AAC8813301), in CAPT Abstracts, Gainesville, Fl, 1987

Granade JG, Hatfield HH, Smith SS, et al: The selection ratio type table pc program. Gainesville, FL, Center for Applications of Psychological Type, 1987

Hirschfeld RM, Matthews SM, Mosher LR, et al: Being with madness: personality characteristics of three treatment staffs. Hosp Community Psychiatry 28(4):267–273, 1977

Hirschfeld RM, Klerman G, Clayton P, et al: Assessing personality: effects of the depressive state on trait assessment. Am J Psychiatry 140:695–699, 1983

Hirschfeld RM, Klerman GL, Keller MB, et al: Personality of recovered patients with bipolar affective disorder. J Affect Disord 11:81–89, 1986

Janowsky DS, Clopton PL, Huey L, et al: Effects of methylphenidate on interpersonal perceptions. Psychopharmacol Bull 17(3):183–185, 1981

Jenkins SI, Stephens, JC, Chew AL, et al: Examination of the relationship between the Myers-Briggs Type Indicator and empathetic response. Percept Mot Skills 74(3 Pt 1):1003–1009, 1992

Joyce PR, Mulder R, Cloninger CR: Temperament predicts clomipramine and desipramine response in major depression. J Affect Disord 30:35–46, 1994a

Joyce PR, Mulder R, Cloninger R: Temperament and hypercortisolemia in depression. Am J Psychiatry 151:195–198, 1994b

Kagan JP, Reznick JS, Snidman N: Biologic basis of childhood shyness. Science 240:167–171, 1988

Kuder GF: Kuder occupational interest survey: manual. Chicago, IL, Scientific Research Associates, 1968

McCrae RR, Costa PT: Reinterpreting the Myers-Briggs Type Indicator from the perspective of the five-factor model of personality. J Pers 57:17–40, 1989

MacDonald DA, Anderson PE, Tsagarakis CI, et al: Examination of the relationship between the Myers-Briggs Type Indicator and the NEO Personality Inventory. Psychological Reports 74:339–344, 1994

McNair DM, Callahan DM, Lorr M: Therapist "type" and the patient response to psychotherapy. J Consult Clin Psychol 26(5):425–429, 1962

Mendelsohn GA: Effects of client/counselor similarity on the duration of counseling: a replication and extension. Journal of Consulting Psychology 13:228–234, 1966

Miller T: The psychotherapeutic utility of the five-factor model of personality. J Pers Assess 57:415–433, 1991

Myers IB, McCaulley MH: Manual: A Guide to the Development and Use of the Myers-Briggs Type Indicator. Palo Alto, CA: Consulting Psychologists Press, 1985

Myers IB, Myers PB: Gifts Differing. Palo Alto, CA: Consulting Psychologists Press, 1980, pp 1–9

Nelson BA, Stake JE: The Myers-Briggs Type Indicator personality dimensions and perceptions of quality of therapy relationships. Psychotherapy 31(3):449–455, 1994

Peselow ED, Robins CJ, Sanfilipo MP, et al: Sociotropy and autonomy: relationship to antidepressant drug treatment response and endogenous-non-endogenous dichotomy. J Abnorm Psychol 101:479–486, 1992a

Peselow ED, Fieve RR, DiFiglia C: Personality traits and response to desipramine. J Affective Disord 24:209–216, 1992b

Street S, Kromrey JD: Relationships between suicidal behavior and personality types. Suicide Life Threat Behav 24(3):282–292, 1994

Swendsen J, Hammen C, Heller T, et al: Correlates of stress reactivity in patients with bipolar disorder. Am J Psychiatry 152:795–797, 1995

Truax CB: Effective ingredients in psychotherapy: an approach to unraveling the patient-therapist interaction. Journal of Counseling Psychology 3:256–263, 1963

Truax CB, Wargo DG, Frank JD, et al: Therapist empathy, genuineness, and warmth and patient therapeutic outcome. J Consult Clin Psychol 30(5):395–401, 1966

Whitehorn JC, Betz BJ: A study of psychotherapeutic relationships between physicians and schizophrenic patients. Am J Psychiatry 111:321–331, 1954

Whitehorn JC, Betz BJ: A comparison of psychotherapeutic relationships between physicians and schizophrenic patients when insulin is combined with psychotherapy and when psychotherapy is used alone. Am J Psychiatry 113:901–910, 1957

Whitehorn JC, Betz BJ: Further studies of the doctor as a crucial variable in the outcome of treatment with schizophrenic patients. Am J Psychiatry 117:215–223, 1960

Wingerson D, Sullivan M, Dager S, et al: Personality traits and early discontinuation from clinical trials in anxious patients. J Clin Psychopharmacol 13(3):194–197, 1993

CHAPTER 4

Patient Characteristics Associated With Successful Treatment

Outcome Findings From the NIMH Treatment of Depression Collaborative Research Program

M. Tracie Shea, Ph.D.

Irene Elkin, Ph.D.

Stuart M. Sotsky, M.D., M.P.H.

The search for patient characteristics associated with a positive treatment outcome has a long history. Clinical observations have emphasized the importance of patient qualities in determining treatment outcome, but the empirical search for consistent predictors has proven to be elusive (Garfield 1994). A notable impediment has been the substantial differences across studies in terms of types of patient samples, patient variables assessed, methods of assessment, types and duration of treatments, and definition of positive outcome. The increasing use of standardized treatments, including assessments of adherence to prescribed and proscribed interventions, as well as clearer definitions and assessments of patient samples, should be helpful in producing clearer and more consistent findings.

This chapter examines the question of patient features associated with successful treatment outcome in outpatients with major depressive disorder (MDD), studied in the NIMH Treatment of Depression Collaborative Research Program (TDCRP; Elkin et al. 1985, 1989). The design of the TDCRP included a carefully defined patient sample, standardization of the treatments, assessments of adherence and competence of therapists in delivering the treatments, inclusion of multiple treatment approaches (including two different forms of psychotherapy), and a relatively large patient sample.

There are, of course, many ways to define success in terms of treatment outcome. Often, the degree of change from pretreatment to posttreatment is used as an outcome measure, with more change obviously reflecting more successful outcome. When outcome is examined in this way, partial, as well as complete, response is included. Another approach is to define outcome categorically, such as the occurrence of complete recovery or full remission of symptoms. A definition of outcome that involves full recovery may more closely represent the notion of success than does improvement measured continuously. In this chapter, we summarize earlier findings from the TDCRP examining patient features and outcome defined continuously and categorically at the termination of treatment (Blatt et al. 1995; Elkin et al. 1989, 1995; Shea et al. 1990; Sotsky et al. 1991). Then we focus on patient features associated with successful treatment outcome (defined categorically as full recovery and remission), when longer-term outcome over an 18-month, posttreatment follow-up period is considered. Two questions are of interest for both the shorter- and longer-term outcome: 1) What patient features are general predictors of more favorable outcome (i.e., are associated with a more positive outcome regardless of treatment condition)? 2) What patient features are differentially predictive of favorable outcome, depending upon treatment condition?

Methods

The TDCRP has been described in detail elsewhere (Elkin et al. 1985, 1989). Briefly, it was a multisite clinical trial of the efficacy of two forms of brief psychotherapy: cognitive-behavioral therapy (CBT; Beck et al. 1979) and interpersonal psychotherapy (IPT; Klerman et al.

1984). Also included were a standard reference condition consisting of imipramine plus clinical management (IMI-CM) and a pill-placebo plus clinical management control condition (PLA-CM). All treatments were 16 weeks in length. Experienced therapists received further training in their respective study treatments, and therapist competency and adherence to the treatment approaches were assessed throughout the study. Different therapists conducted treatment in the different treatment conditions, except for the pharmacotherapy condition, which was double-blind. To be included, patients had to meet research diagnostic criteria for MDD and have a minimum score of 14 on a modified version of the 17-item Hamilton Rating Scale for Depression (HRSD; Hamilton 1960), in addition to passing several exclusion criteria (Elkin et al. 1989). At the outset of the study, 250 patients were randomly assigned to one of the four treatment conditions, 239 actually entered treatment, and 162 completed treatment.

Patients were assessed at 4-week intervals during the 16-week treatment phase. Termination evaluations were generally completed at 16 weeks; patients not completing treatment were given early termination evaluations when possible. Following completion of treatment, patients entered an 18-month, naturalistic follow-up phase, with comprehensive assessments at 6-month intervals. The course of MDD and other Axis I disorders over the interval since the previous interview were assessed using the Longitudinal Interval Follow-up Evaluation (LIFE; Keller et al. 1987). Treatment was not controlled during the follow-up phase.

Patient Predictors of Outcome at Termination of Treatment

General Predictors

With the exception of severity, described later in this chapter, the primary analyses examining patient characteristics as predictors of outcome at termination of treatment were reported by Sotsky et al. (1991).

An initial set of 26 variables, selected on the basis of previous findings in the literature, were examined (Table 4–1) in two samples: 1) patients completing treatment and 2) the total sample of all patient entering treatment. Two indices of outcome were used: a continuous measure (total score on the 23-item HRSD), and a categorical measure

TABLE 4–1

Patient variables examined in primary predictor analyses of outcome at termination of treatment

---

Sociodemographic variables
    Age*
    Sex*
    Marital status*
    Social class*

Diagnostic and course variables
    Endogenous depression*
    Recurrent depression
    Primary depression
    Situational depression
    Double depression*
    Melancholia
    Family history of affective disorder*
    Age at onset of first episode
    Duration of current episode*
    Acuteness of onset of current episode*
    Number of previous episodes

Functioning, personality, and symptom variables
    Social functioning*
    Work functioning*
    Social satisfaction
    Patient expectation of improvement*
    Dramatic personality disorder
    Odd personality disorder
    Number of personality disorders
    Anxiety*
    Somatization/hypochondriasis
    Interpersonal sensitivity

Note. Variables included in main predictor analyses are indicated here with an asterisk and are described in greater detail in the text.

of "complete response" (17-item HRSD of 6 or less and a BDI score of 9 or less). Whereas the continuous measure reflects degree of positive change, the categorical measure of complete response more closely captures the notion of successful treatment outcome (i.e., absence of symptoms).

To reduce the number of independent variables from the initial set of 26 for the main predictor analyses across treatments, preliminary multiple regression analyses, with variables grouped by domain (sociodemographic, diagnostic and course, and personality and functioning), were first conducted within each individual treatment condition. The most consistent predictors of outcome from these analyses were selected for the main analyses, which examined predictors of outcome across all treatments, as well as predictors of differential outcome among treatments (described later in this chapter). The 13 variables included in these latter analyses are indicated with an asterisk in Table 4–1.

For the continuous measure of outcome, ANCOVAs with two factors (treatment and predictor variable) were used. For continuous predictor variables, patients were divided into two groups using a median split. Significant main effects for predictor variables identified those variables associated with outcome across treatment conditions; predictor by treatment condition interactions identified differential treatment effects. For the categorical (complete response) measure of outcome, log linear analyses (treatment by predictor by response level) were used, with best-fit models examined to determine main effects and predictor by treatment interactions.

Table 4–2 summarizes the findings reported by Sotsky et al. (1991) for predictors across treatments in the sample of patients completing treatment. Predictors of complete response included age (younger age was associated with complete response, but in the completer sample only), dysfunctional attitudes (lower levels of dysfunction were associated with complete response), social functioning (better functioning was associated with complete response), and duration of the intake episode of MDD (longer duration was associated with poorer outcome in the total sample of patients). Dysfunctional attitudes were also associated with outcome on the continuous measure, whereas age and

TABLE 4–2

Patient variables predicting outcome at termination across treatments

	Continuous outcome	Categorical outcome
Age[a]		**
Dysfunctional attitudes	*	***
Social functioning		*
Endogenous depression	**	
Duration of episode[b]	**	*
Double depression	**	
Patient expectation of improvement	**	

[a] *Sample of patients completing treatment only*
[b] *Total sample of patients only*
*P < .10. **P < .05. ***P < .01.

social functioning were not. Other variables associated with outcome on the continuous measures, but not with complete response, included endogenous depression and more positive expectations of improvement (both associated with better outcome), and the presence of an underlying chronic intermittent or minor (double) depression (associated with poorer outcome).

In a separate paper, the association between personality disorders and outcome was examined in more detail (Shea et al. 1990). The presence of personality disorder features, present "to a considerable extent," "to a marked degree," or "to an extreme degree" (assessed by the Personality Assessment Form [Shea et al. 1987]), was associated with a lower rate of recovery, defined as a score of 6 or less on the 17-item HRSD at termination. Personality disorder features were also associated with less improvement in social functioning. Each of the three Axis II clusters (odd/eccentric, dramatic/erratic, and anxious/fearful) were similarly predictive of a poorer outcome on these measures.

In later analyses by Blatt et al. (1995) (see also Chapter 2), two factors from the Dysfunctional Attitude Scale (DAS; Weissman and Beck 1978) (perfectionism and need for social approval) as predictors of outcome in patients completing treatment were examined. Higher scores on the perfectionism but not on the social approval factor were found to be associated with poorer outcome on several measures.

Interactions With Treatment

Patient variables that were found to interact with treatment condition (i.e., predict differential treatment response) included two measures of severity of depression, social functioning, work functioning, and dysfunctional attitudes.

Severity of depression was examined in the initial paper reporting TDCRP outcome findings, as it was seen from the outset as a potentially important factor in differential treatment outcome (Elkin et al. 1989). Preliminary analyses were reported in the first outcome article (Elkin et al. 1989), and subsequent analyses using the recent and more sophisticated data analytic approach (random regression models) were published later (Elkin et al. 1995). In both reports, the role of pretreatment severity in terms of symptoms of depression (17-item HRSD), as well as symptom severity and impairment in functioning (Global Assessment Scale [GAS; Spitzer et al. 1973]), was shown to be important to treatment response, with significant interactions with treatment condition.

It was in the more severely impaired subsamples that treatment differences emerged. For the more severe subsample on the GAS (GAS < 50), the later (Elkin et al. 1995) analyses showed the IMI-CM condition to be significantly superior to CBT and IPT, in addition to PLA-CM. Among the less severely impaired, there were no significant differences among the treatments, although the ordering of treatments was different, with CBT and IPT doing somewhat better (but not significantly so) than the IMI-CM and PAL-CM conditions.

A similar interaction was present for symptom severity based on the HRSD, although for the more severely depressed group as defined by the HRSD (HRSD ≥ 20), the outcome for IPT was quite similar to that for IMI-CM. In addition, for this group of more severely depressed patients, IPT was sometimes found to be superior to PLA-CM (Elkin et al. 1989, 1995). In the later analyses (Elkin et al. 1995), IMI-CM was superior to CBT for the HRSD-defined more severely depressed patients.

Findings of treatment interactions on the DAS, social functioning, and work functioning (functioning measures assessed by the Social

Adjustment Scale [SAS; Weissman and Paykel 1974]) were reported by Sotsky et al. (1991). On the DAS and on measures of social functioning, significant interactions with treatment were present on both the continuous and complete response measures of outcome. For work functioning, the interaction was significant only on the categorical (complete response) measure of outcome. Pretreatment scores on the DAS predicted differential treatment outcome as follows: both CBT and IMI-CM (but particularly IMI-CM) tended to do better for patients with lower (less dysfunctional) DAS scores and relatively worse for patients with higher (more dysfunctional) scores. The opposite was true for IPT and PLA-CM (i.e., the direction was for better outcome to occur for those with higher DAS scores).

The interaction of pretreatment social functioning with treatment condition was due to a better outcome occurring for IPT and CBT (but particularly IPT) for patients with less social dysfunction, in contrast to IMI-CM, which did better for those patients with higher levels of social dysfunction at pretreatment. Thus, for both of these two patient features, patients with relatively less dysfunction in the area targeted by the treatment condition (i.e., cognitive dysfunction and CBT, social functioning and IPT) did relatively better than those with higher levels of dysfunction in that treatment. As suggested by Sotsky et al. (1991), one interpretation of these findings is that depressed patients need to have a minimal capacity in the area of functioning targeted by the treatment approach to benefit from a short-term treatment. The better outcome for IMI-CM for patients with lower DAS scores, however, requires a different explanation. It is interesting to note that the pattern for IMI-CM on the DAS differs from that on measures of other types of functioning, where the direction for IMI-CM is to do better for patients with more severe dysfunction (i.e., GAS, social functioning).

The pattern of differential outcome for the other variable with a significant interaction with treatment, work functioning, was consistent with the GAS and social functioning for IMI-CM. For patients with higher levels of work dysfunction at pretreatment, over 70% reached a score of 6 or less on the HRSD at termination, compared with just over 30% of those with relatively less severe work dysfunction. For

PLA-CM, outcome relative to level of work dysfunction was in the opposite direction.

Patient Predictors of Longer-Term Outcome

Incorporating the posttreatment period in the measure of outcome addresses a somewhat different question. By extending the definition of *successful* treatment outcome to include maintenance of recovery following treatment, such outcome is more stringently defined. Examining predictors of outcome so defined can be viewed as a search to identify patients having the best chance of being adequately treated with a short-term treatment. Given the increasing recognition of major depression being an often chronic and recurrent disorder, it is important to identify patient features that are associated with an increased likelihood of a complete response that is maintained following completion of treatment.

To address this question, we defined the following three longer-term outcome groups. The first is the successful longer-term outcome group, defined as completion of treatment, achievement of a stable recovery extending a minimum of eight weeks following treatment termination, and maintenance of the recovery (i.e., absence of symptoms at full MDD criteria) during the 18-month follow-up period. Of all patients entering treatment, 49 patients (21%) met these criteria. The second group is defined similarly to the first group in the short-term (i.e., complete treatment and recovery), but these patients ($n = 30$) relapsed (had an episode of MDD) during the follow-up. The third group includes all others (i.e., those who failed to complete treatment, or completed treatment but failed to meet the recovery criteria). Seven patients who had completed treatment, but did not complete the follow-up assessments were excluded. It should be noted that by requiring completion of treatment as a requirement for the successful longer-term outcome group, we are focusing on patient features associated with successful *treatment* outcome extended over the longer term, which may be distinct from general prognostic predictors. For example, included in the "all other" group are 8 patients who did not complete treatment, but were in remission from MDD throughout the follow-up. Because these patients dropped out of treatment and/or received too few sessions to presume lasting effects of the study treatments, it would be inappropriate to consider them as treatment successes.

General Predictors

Demographic and clinical features as potential predictors of longer-term outcome across treatment conditions were examined, first by univariate analyses and then using a discriminant function analysis including all of the predictors. We examined a similar set of variables as those investigated in the outcome at termination analyses, although we excluded some that were not predictive of outcome in those analyses. Table 4–3 shows the patient variables that differed significantly or at a trend level $(P < .10)$ among the three longer-term outcome groups. There were no significant differences among the outcome groups on demographic variables (age, sex, race, marital status, occupation). In terms of severity of depression, both of the groups that recovered are characterized by lower scores at pretreatment on the HRSD, compared with the group of subjects failing to complete treatment or to recover. The groups did not differ on the pretreatment GAS scores. They did differ on the proportion with definite endogenous depression, with the recover/no relapse group having a higher proportion of patients with endogenous depression (43%) than the subjects who recovered but relapsed (17%). There was a trend toward differences on double depression, with the recover/no relapse group having a lower proportion of patients with double depression (16%), less than half the rate of the other two groups (37% in the recover/relapse group and 33% in the "all other" group).

Patients in the recover/relapse group are also characterized by a younger age at first episode of depression, compared with the other two groups. With regard to prior episodes of depression, the groups differed at a trend level. The relapse group had a history of more prior

TABLE 4-3

Patient variables distinguishing longer-term outcome groups

| | Recover | | | | |
	No Relapse ($n = 49$)	Relapse ($n = 30$)	All Other ($n = 153$)	F	P
HRSD-17 score					
Mean	17.9	18.6	20.2	6.17	<.003
(SD)	(3.5)	(3.4)	(4.8)		
Age at first episode					
Mean	30.1	22.8	25.8	5.34	<.006
(SD)	(10.9)	(9.7)	(10.0)		
Endogenous depression					
n	21	5	47	6.04	.049
(%)	(43)	(17)	(31)		
Double depression					
n	8	11	50	5.54	.063
(%)	(16)	(37)	(33)		
Prior episodes					
None					
n	22	7	53		
(%)	(45)	(23)	(35)		
1–2					
n	15	8	58		
(%)	(31)	(27)	(38)		
3 or more					
n	12	15	42	8.61	.072
(%)	(24)	(50)	(27)		

episodes compared with the group that recovered and did not relapse, with the relapse group having double the rate of three or more prior episodes (50%) compared with the subjects who recovered and remained well (24%).

There was a tendency for scores on the Personality Assessment Form (PAF; Shea et al. 1987) to distinguish the groups, but only at a trend level and only when groups 2 and 3 (recover and relapse, "all other") were combined. Trends appeared for the total score ($\chi^2 = 2.74$, df = 2, $P = .099$), for the odd cluster ($\chi^2 = 3.78$, df = 2, $P = .053$), and for the dramatic cluster ($\chi^2 = 3.85$, df = 2, $P = .051$).

In addition to the demographic variables and the GAS, other variables investigated that did not show an association with longer-term outcome as defined here include pretreatment social functioning, work functioning, dysfunctional attitudes (total score or either of the two factors), duration of the index episode of major depression at intake, and expectations about improvement.

The patient variables that were predictive of longer-term outcome in the univariate analyses were next examined using a stepwise discriminant analysis to explore the strength and independence of relationship to outcome. Age at first episode and the pretreatment HRSD scores showed the strongest relationship and were independently significant predictors (Table 4–4).

Differential Predictors

Following up on the findings at termination of treatment, we examined the interaction between patient features assessed at pretreatment and treatment condition in predicting longer-term outcome for four measures: cognitive functioning (DAS total), social functioning (SAS social leisure scale), severity of symptoms (17-item HRSD) and severity/impairment (GAS). Groups 2 and 3 were combined for these analyses, because of the reduced sample sizes when broken down by treatment condition. None of the variables investigated showed a significant interaction with treatment condition in the prediction of our categorically defined longer-term outcome.

The direction of the longer-term pattern on the DAS is similar to the pattern at termination. In the best outcome (recover/no relapse)

TABLE 4–4

Prediction of longer-term outcome stepwise discriminant function analyses

Variable	Partial R²	F	P
HRSD-17 score	.044	4.99	.008
Age at first episode	.052	5.96	.003

group, patients in the CBT and IMI-CM conditions were characterized by lower (healthier) pretreatment DAS scores; unlike those in IPT
or PLA-CM. However, for pretreatment social functioning, the direction of findings is not the same as the termination findings. The relative
advantage for IPT for the less socially impaired patients found at termination is not evident in the longer-term outcome groups.

With regard to the pretreatment severity measures, it should be
noted that the short-term advantage of IMI-CM should not necessarily
be expected to hold when the longer-term outcome is considered, because patients were tapered and discontinued from the medication at
the end of the treatment phase. Discontinuing medication after 16
weeks resembles current clinical practice far less now than it did when
the TDCRP was designed. Pretreatment symptom severity measured
by the HRSD is lower for all treatment conditions for the recover/no
relapse patients. This is consistent with the univariate and discriminant
function analyses that showed a main effect for pretreatment HRSD.

On the GAS, those patients receiving IPT and CBT who recovered
and remained well (Group 1) tended to have higher (less impaired)
GAS scores at pretreatment; this was not characteristic of patients in
IMI-CM or PLA-CM. Figure 4–1 shows the percentage of subjects in
each treatment who recovered and remained well by the pretreatment
GAS groups of more and less severe symptoms or impairment (GAS
score of <50 and ≥50, respectively). Although not statistically significant, the direction is for CBT and IPT to show the best outcome for
the less severely impaired, similar to the short-term (termination) findings.

Summary and Discussion

Our findings suggest that patients starting treatment with less severe
depression, less chronicity, and less personality disturbance do better
in both the shorter and longer term, regardless of treatment condition.
Endogenous depression was also associated with a more favorable
short- and long-term outcome. Older age at first episode of depression
and fewer prior episodes of depression, features not predictive of short-

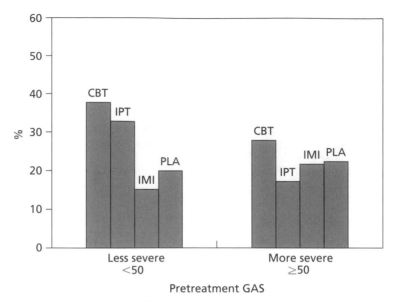

FIGURE 4–1. *Percentage of patients who recover and remain well (no relapse) by GAS and treatment.*

term outcome, were associated with better outcome when the longer term is included. Other variables associated with a better outcome at the end of treatment, including younger current age, less impairment in social functioning, and lower (less impaired) scores on the GAS, were not predictive of longer-term recovery.

The extent to which these general (across treatments) predictors may reflect an increased ability to enter and benefit from treatment, versus a tendency towards a more favorable course regardless of interventions of any type, is unclear. Considering features that were predictive of a better outcome in the PLA-CM condition, considered to be a less active treatment, suggests that younger current age and more positive expectations of improvement may be general prognostic variables, at least in the short term. It is likely that many of the other variables also reflect general prognostic features as well. It is also likely that features that predict a favorable prognosis more generally overlap with features that predispose to completing and benefiting from treatment, so to some extent this distinction may be arbitrary. Many of the current findings are consistent with other studies in the literature, including studies of naturalistic course as well as controlled treatment studies. Personality disorders have frequently been demonstrated to predict a poorer outcome in both types of studies (Shea et al. 1992b). More chronic or double depression has been found to be associated with a longer time to full recovery (Keller et al. 1982a), and to a shorter time to relapse (Keller et al. 1982b) in the NIMH Collaborative Program on the Psychobiology of Depression. This large naturalistic longitudinal study of affective disorders has also shown that having three or more prior episodes of depression is a strong predictor of relapse (Keller et al. 1982b), consistent with our finding that patients who recovered and relapsed were twice as likely to have had three or more prior episodes than those who recovered and remained well. Older age at first episode was among the strongest predictors of recovery 12 months after discharge in a sample of depressed inpatients (Keitner et al. 1992). Age at first episode of depression is often correlated with chronicity and with personality disorders, including in the current (TDCRP) sample (Shea et al. 1987); thus, it is likely that there is shared variance among these three variables in predicting outcome. In the TDCRP sample, the discriminant function analyses showed age at first episode as the more powerful predictor of the three variables.

Endogenous depression has been less consistent as a predictor of outcome in depression. A review of studies examining endogenous or melancholic depression and treatment outcome (Peselow 1992), showed that findings are mixed, but the majority of studies have found no differences in endogenous versus nonendogenous patients in response to somatic or nonsomatic treatments. In his own study, Peselow (1992) found that patients with DSM-III (American Psychiatric Association 1980) melancholia and moderate (vs. severe) depression had the best response rates to active medication and to placebo.

Patient features that may be associated with differential treatment response are of particular interest, for theoretical reasons because of the possible clues to mechanisms of change, and for clinical reasons because of the practical implications for choosing different treatment paths for patients. The majority of studies addressing this question in the area of depression have focused on psychotherapy versus drug treatments. The early belief of the existence of a preferential response to antidepressants for endogenous depression has not held up empirically, as noted earlier in this chapter. In the TDCRP, the most consistent finding for differential treatment response was on the GAS, a global index of severity of symptoms together with impairment in functioning, with IMI-CM showing a differentially superior response for the more severely depressed or impaired patients (Elkin et al. 1989, 1995). Although this finding was most consistent on the GAS, it also appeared on other measures assessing aspects of functioning, including social and work functioning (Sotsky et al. 1991). Not only does IMI-CM tend to be better than the other treatments for patients with more impairment in functioning, but IMI-CM does better for those with more impaired functioning than it does for those with less impaired functioning. This finding did not hold up in the long-term analyses, but that would not be expected because IMI-CM was discontinued following the treatment phase. It would be of interest to examine whether this differential response to antidepressants replicates in other studies (including different types of antidepressants), as well as whether impairment would remain differentially predictive in longer-term studies including maintenance treatments.

A question raised by the current investigation of longer-term outcome is whether the psychotherapies studied here may be more effective for those patients with less severe symptoms and impairment, when the posttreatment course is considered. For those patients starting treatment with a GAS of greater than 50, the proportion recovering and remaining well is twice as high for CBT and IPT than for IMI-CM, and close to twice as high than for PLA-CM. These differences were not statistically significant, but the pattern may be suggestive enough to be pursued in future studies.

The other finding that may be worth pursuing in future studies concerns the interactions relating to the DAS and SAS. At least three other studies have similarly reported a poorer outcome for patients with higher DAS scores in CBT (Keller et al. 1987; Jarrett et al. 1988; Simons et al. 1995). However, this finding does not appear to be specific to CBT. In the current study, the association of lower DAS scores and better outcome was also characteristic, and more strikingly so, for IMI-CM. Peselow and colleagues (1992) similarly reported an association between lower DAS scores and better response to antidepressants. The findings of the opposite direction for IPT and for PLA-CM argue against this variable as a general prognostic factor, but the lack of specificity of the finding for CBT makes the hypothesis that such patients (with less impairment in thinking patterns) are better able to benefit from CBT interventions less compelling. It would be interesting to explore this question using process analyses of in-session behavior for patients with high and low DAS scores in CBT and in IPT, using indicators of "absorption" of the treatment as developed by Moras (1993).

Several limiting factors in interpreting the findings presented here must be noted. First, in the longer-term outcome analyses, we did not address the issue of receiving further treatment during the follow-up phase. This probably has the strongest implications for our exploratory analyses examining differential prediction of longer-term outcome by treatment condition. A significant number of those patients who recovered and remained well received some treatment during the follow-up, so the longer-term outcome may have been influenced by treatment received over the follow-up. However, treatment rates and amounts over follow-up tended to be lower in CBT and IPT (Shea et al. 1992a), so this factor would not account for the pattern suggestive of better outcome of CBT and IPT for the GAS less impaired patients.

It is notable that, similar to other studies examining prediction of outcome, the amount of variance associated with the predictor variables is quite modest; less than 10% in our discriminant function analyses of longer-term outcome. The small amount of variance typically found in predictor analyses such as the current one, as well as the difficulty in establishing consistent predictors across studies, may be due to the strategy of examining several variables assessed in various ways in post hoc analyses. This is an argument made by Beutler (1991), who advocates using a stronger theoretical base for hypothesizing interactions among patient features and treatment approaches, and designing treatment studies to test the specific hypotheses. Beutler also advocates examining treatment procedures rather than treatment packages. At the time that the TDCRP was designed and initiated, it was concluded that there were no patient variables with sufficient theoretical or empirical basis to warrant a design incorporating stratification. Thus, although there was a strong interest in examining possible interactions of treatments with patient features, and measures were included to allow such examinations, these analyses are exploratory. Although useful for hypothesis generation, findings from such analyses require replication. The findings from the TDCRP that may be most fruitful to pursue in future studies include the interactions with measures that assess impairment in functioning (differential response for drug vs. psychotherapy), and measures that assess the area of functioning targeted by the treatment (differential response for one form of psychotherapy vs. another).

Another issue concerns the definition of successful treatment outcome. A categorical index of successful outcome is always arbitrary to some extent. In addition, we focused here only on symptomatic outcome and did not examine other important aspects of outcome, such as functioning or satisfaction with treatment (patient as well as therapist). Even though our definition of outcome excludes such other aspects, it is notable that the rates of success so defined are as low as they are. The proportion of patients entering treatment that achieve a full recovery and do not relapse over 18 months following treatment is disappointingly small (Shea et al. 1992a). Of course, this definition of success excludes the substantial improvement in symptoms for many patients who nonetheless do not meet the criteria for this definition of success, and in that sense is a pessimistic view of treatment outcome. On the other hand, even our stringent definition of treatment success does not exclude receiving further treatment, or having symptoms of depression that do not meet full criteria for major depression over the follow-up. It has become increasingly clear that although the short-term psychotherapies developed to treat depression are associated with significant improvement for many patients, treatment of depression for the majority of individuals needs to be longer-term to be fully successful.

References

American Psychiatric Association: Diagnostic and Statistical Manual of Mental Disorders, 3rd Edition. Washington, DC, American Psychiatric Association, 1980

Beck AT, Rush AJ, Shaw BF, et al: Cognitive Therapy of Depression. New York, Guilford, 1979

Beutler LE: Have all won and must all have prizes? Revisiting Luborsky et al's verdict. J Consult Clin Psychol 59:226–232, 1991

Blatt SJ, Quinlan DM, Pilkonis PA, et al: Impact of perfectionism and need for approval on the brief treatment of depression: the National Institute of Mental Health Treatment of Depression Collaborative Research Program revisited. J Consult Clin Psychol 63:841–847, 1995

Elkin I, Parloff MB, Hadley SW, et al: NIMH Treatment of Depression Research Program: background and research plan. Arch Gen Psychiatry 42:305–316, 1985

Elkin I, Shea MT, Watkins JT, et al: National Institute of Mental Health Treatment of Depression Collaborative Research Program. Arch Gen Psychiatry 46:971–983, 1989

Elkin I, Shea MT, Watkins JT, et al: Initial severity and differential treatment outcome in the National Institute of Mental Health Treatment of Depression Collaborative Research Program. J Consult Clin Psychol 63:841–847, 1995

Garfield SL: Research on client variables in psychotherapy, in Handbook of Psychotherapy and Behavior Change, 4th Edition. Edited by Bergin AE, Garfield SL. New York, Wiley, 1994

Halbreich U, Endicott J, Schachet S, et al: The diversity of premenstrual changes as reflected in the Premenstrual Assessment Form. Acta Psychiatr Scand 65:46–65, 1982

Hamilton M: A rating scale for depression. J Neurol Neurosurg Psychiatry 231:56–62, 1960

Jarrett RB, Rush AJ, Giles DE, et al: Predictors of response to cognitive therapy or tricyclic antidepressants in depressed outpatients. Paper presented at the annual meeting of the Society for Psychotherapy Research, Santa Fe, NM, June 1988

Keitner GI, Ryan CE, Miller IW, et al: Recovery and major depression: factors associated with twelve-month outcome. Am J Psychiatry 149:93–99, 1992

Keller MB, Shapiro RW, Lavori PW, et al: Recovery in major depressive disorder. Arch Gen Psychiatry 39:905–910, 1982a

Keller MB, Shapiro RW, Lavori PW, et al: Relapse in major depressive disorder. Arch Gen Psychiatry 39:911–915, 1982b

Keller MB, Lavori PW, Friedman B, et al: The longitudinal interval follow-up evaluation. Arch Gen Psychiatry 44:540–548, 1987

Klerman GL, Weissman MM, Rounsaville BJ, et al: Interpersonal Psychotherapy of Depression. New York, Basic Books, 1984

Moras K, Telfer LA, Barlow DH: Efficacy and specific effects data on new treatments: a case study strategy with mixed anxiety-depression. J Consult Clin Psychol 61:412–420, 1993

Peselow ED, Sanfilipo MP, Difiglia C, et al: Melancholic/endogenous depression and response to somatic treatment and placebo. Am J Psychiatry 149:1324–1334, 1992

Shea MT, Glass DR, Pilkonis PA, et al: Frequency and implications of personality disorders in a sample of depressed outpatients. J Personal Disord 1:27–42, 1987

Shea MT, Pilkonis PA, Beckham E, et al: Personality disorders and treatment outcome in the NIMH Treatment of Depression Collaborative Research Program. Am J Psychiatry 147:711–718, 1990

Shea MT, Elkin I, Imber SD, et al: Course of depressive symptoms over follow-up: findings from the NIMH Treatment of Depression Collaborative Research Program. Arch Gen Psychiatry 49:782–787, 1992a

Shea MT, Widiger TA, Klein MH: Comorbidity of personality disorders and depression: implications for treatment. J Consult Clin Psychol 60:857–868, 1992b

Simons AD, Gordon JS, Monroe SM, et al: Toward an integration of psychologic, social, and biologic factors in depression: effects on outcome and course of cognitive therapy. J Consult Clin Psychol 63:369–377, 1995

Sotsky SM, Glass DR, Shea MT, et al: Patient predictors of response to psychotherapy and pharmacotherapy: findings in the NIMH Treatment of Depression Collaborative Research Program. Am J Psychiatry 148:997–1008, 1991

Spitzer RL, Gibson M, Endicott J: Global Assessment Scale, New York, New York State Department of Mental Hygiene, 1973

Weissman AN, Beck AT: Development and validation of the Dysfunctional Attitude Scale: a preliminary investigation. Paper presented at the meeting of the American Psychological Association, Toronto, Canada, August-September 1978

Weissman MM, Paykel ES: The Depressed Women: Study of Social Relationships. Chicago, IL, University of Chicago Press, 1974

PART II

Dialectical Behavioral Therapy

CHAPTER 5

Dialectical Behavior Therapy for Borderline Personality Disorder

Efficacy, Specificity, and Cost Effectiveness

Marsha M. Linehan, Ph.D.

Jonathan W. Kanter, M.A.

Katherine Anne Comtois, Ph.D.

Introduction

Borderline personality disorder (BPD) is a major public health problem. It is prevalent, chronic, painful, and expensive. Although many psychosocial treatments for BPD exist, almost none have been empirically validated. This is true for the disorder as a whole as well as for the specific behavioral patterns that make up the criteria for the disorder (e.g., suicidal behavior and drug abuse). Even when there are effective treatments for criterion problems (for example, depression), standard treatment methods for these problems may be less effective when the disorder as a whole is present. In this chapter, we review the problem of BPD, its prevalence, chronicity, comorbidity, and costs to the health care system. We review the theory and strategies of the most effective treatment for BPD, dialectical behavior therapy (DBT). Finally, we review and discuss the clinical outcomes, cost effectiveness, and specificity of DBT.

The Problem

BPD is a psychiatric disorder characterized by intense negative emotions including depression, anger, self-hatred, and despair. In dealing with these emotions, individuals with BPD often engage in impulsive behaviors including drug or alcohol abuse, eating binges, and parasuicide, which is defined as any intentional, acute, self-injurious behavior with or without suicidal intent, including both suicide attempts and self-mutilating behaviors. BPD is the only psychiatric diagnosis for which parasuicide is a criterion, and parasuicide is thus considered a hallmark of BPD. Rates of parasuicide in patients diagnosed with BPD range from 69% to 80% (Clarkin et al. 1983; Cowdry et al. 1985; Gunderson 1984). The suicide rate among all individuals meeting criteria for BPD (including those with no parasuicide) is 5% to 10% (Frances et al. 1986), and that rate doubles when only those with a history of parasuicide are included (Stone 1987). Finally, patients with BPD are notoriously difficult to treat. In fact, one study has estimated that almost all (97%) of patients with BPD have received outpatient psychiatric treatment (Perry et al. 1990), and another found they average 6.1 therapists in their lifetime (Skodol et al. 1983). The emotional and behavioral dysregulation experienced by these patients results in chaotic and unstable interpersonal relationships, including psychotherapeutic relationships. Problems in treating these patients have been included in the *Diagnostic Interview for Borderlines* (Gunderson et al. 1981), and evidence of these problems is another hallmark of BPD.

Prevalence and Chronicity

BPD has been found to exist in 0.2%–1.8% of the general population. Higher prevalence of the disorder is found among psychiatric patients: 8%–11% of outpatients (Widiger and Frances 1989; Widiger and Weissman 1991) and 14%–20% of inpatients (Kroll et al. 1981; Modestin et al. 1997; Widiger and Weissman 1999) are estimated to be diagnosed with BPD. However, these estimates may be low. Because

BPD is a DSM-IV (American Psychiatric Association 1994) Axis II disorder, it is rarely the primary diagnosis. Often a clinician does not assess for BPD or make an Axis II diagnosis at all. Alternatively, BPD may not be diagnosed because the clinician is conscious of the stigma associated with the BPD label, and the diagnosis is not required. Most medical claims and many mental health databases have no record of BPD. Skodol and Oldham (1991) found that only 1.9% of public mental health patients in New York State were diagnosed with BPD. They concluded that BPD, like other personality disorders, is greatly underdiagnosed in the public system.

Follow-up studies consistently indicate that the diagnosis of BPD is chronic, although the number of individuals who continue to meet diagnostic criteria slowly decreases over the life span. Two to 3 years after index assessment, 60%–70% of patients continued to meet criteria (Barasch et al. 1985; Stevenson and Meares 1992). Other short-term follow-up studies found little change in functional level and consistently high rates of psychiatric hospitalization over 2 to 5 years (Barasch et al. 1985; Dahl, 1986; Richman and Charles 1976). Four to 7 years after index assessment, 57%–67% of patients continued to meet criteria (Kullgren, 1992; Pope et al. 1983). An average of 15 years after index assessment, 25%–44% of patients continued to meet criteria (McGlashan 1986; Paris et al. 1987).

BPD disproportionately affects women who present for services. In their review of the literature, Widiger and Weissman (1991) found that 76% of individuals diagnosed with BPD were women. BPD is seen more frequently among Caucasians although the reasons why are not clear (Akhtar et al. 1986; Castaneda and Franco 1985). In their review of seven studies of BPD, Akhtar and colleagues (1986) found that the percentage of black patients ranged from 3% to18% with a mean of 10%. Castaneda and Franco (1985), studying an inpatient sample in the Bronx, found that 25% of patients with BPD were African-American, 35% were Hispanic, and 41% were Caucasian. In our own pilot study (M. M. Linehan, K. A. Comtois, and L. A. Dimeff, unpublished data, July, 1996), we collected ethnicity data on 50.2% of referral calls (other callers either refused to report ethnicity or called for information only and therefore were not asked). One-quarter (26.7%) of these calls were from ethnic subjects (3.8% Native American or Alaska

Native, 11.4% African-American, 1.0% Asian or Pacific Islander, 4.8% Latino, and 5.7% other or mixed). Among the 27 subjects accepted into the pilot study, 70.4% were Caucasian, 7.4% Native American or Alaska Native, 11.1% African-American, 7.4% Latino, and 3.7% other or mixed.

BPD is particularly prevalent among substance abusers. In a study of 64 female, psychiatric outpatients meeting criteria for substance abuse, Vaglum and Vaglum (1985) found that 66% also met criteria for BPD. In a more restricted sample, Nace and colleagues (1983) found that 13% of 94 people consecutively admitted to an alcohol treatment program also met criteria for BPD. Kosten and colleagues (1989) report a similar percentage (12%) of BPD patients among a sample of 150 individuals treated for opiate addiction. Tousignant and Kovess (1989) found that one-third of substance abusers showed a high number of BPD traits. Substance abusers with BPD are uniformly more disturbed than are those abusers who do not meet criteria for BPD. They are more likely to be polydrug abusers (usually combining drug and alcohol abuse), are more likely to be comorbid for depressive disorders, have more frequent suicide attempts and accidents, and score higher on measures of impulse dyscontrol and antisocial tendencies and lower on reality testing (Inman et al. 1985; Nace et al. 1983; Tousignant and Kovess 1989).

Individuals with BPD are more likely to meet criteria for current substance abuse than are all other psychiatric patients except those with antisocial disorder (Koenigsberg et al. 1985; Loranger and Tulis 1985; McCann et al. 1992; Pitts et al. 1985; Zanarini et al. 1989), and patients with BPD more commonly report a history of substance abuse than do other patients (Akiskal et al. 1985). Koenigsberg and colleagues (1985), reporting on a sample of 2,462 inpatients and outpatients, found that 21% of patients diagnosed with BPD had a primary Axis I diagnosis of substance abuse. This overlap is not surprising because impulsiveness that leads to self-damage, including substance abuse, is one of the criteria for BPD. The comorbidity is not due entirely to this overlap in criteria, however. For example, Dulit and colleagues (1990) found that 67% of patients with BPD currently met criteria for substance abuse disorder. When substance abuse was not used as a criterion of BPD, the incidence dropped to 57%, still a substantial portion of the population.

In addition to substance abuse, comorbidity of BPD with other disorders further complicates and exacerbates the clinical picture. Comorbidity estimates vary widely as samples are drawn from different clinical sites. Estimates for depression are high, ranging from 81% to 100% comorbidity with BPD (Zanarini et al. 1989; Prasad et al. 1997). Estimates for comorbid psychotic diagnoses are lower but more variable, ranging from 0% to 44% (Fyer et al. 1997; Prasad et al. 1997; Zanarini et al. 1989). Estimates for comorbid anxiety disorders were quite different across two sites, 24% (Zanarini et al. 1989) and 81% (Prasad et al. 1997). One study assessed comorbidity with eating disorders at 14% (Zanarini et al. 1989). In a preliminary analysis of our data of parasuicidal women with BPD, we found 89% comorbid with major depression, 48% with alcohol dependence, 26% with stimulant dependence, 29% with cocaine dependence, 38% with panic, 36% with posttraumatic stress disorder, 17% with bulimia, and 12% with anorexia nervosa (Comtois et al. 1996).

Costs to the System

Research over the last 20 years has shown that among the mentally ill who are served by public mental health agencies, there is a subpopulation that uses a disproportionate amount of inpatient psychiatric treatment. Studies have indicated that 6%–18% of all patients admitted to inpatient psychiatric treatment account for 20%–42% of admissions (Carpenter et al. 1985; Geller 1986; Green 1988; Hadley et al. 1990; Surber et al. 1987; Woogh 1986). Hadley and colleagues (1992) have shown that, across sites, a stable 30%–35% of patients receiving inpatient psychiatric treatment use 75%–80% of the inpatient treatment dollars; 5% use 26% of inpatient resources (Hadley et al. 1990).

Studies have reported from 9% to 40% of those who highly use inpatient psychiatric treatment have been diagnosed with BPD (Geller 1986; Surber et al. 1987; Widiger and Weissman 1991; Woogh 1986), and thus much of the health care costs of patients with BPD are due to their lengthy and repeated hospitalizations. Exact cost estimates are limited because follow-up studies have varied widely in methodology, ascertainment, tracking, method of obtaining follow-up information, length of time between index and follow-up, and treatment of subject morbidity. McGlashan (1986) reported an average of 6 months of pre-index psychiatric hospitalization, but Skodol and colleagues (1983) reported only 10.8 weeks. Linehan and colleagues (1991), by assigning control subjects to treatment as usual in the community, created a natural follow-along condition. Of these subjects, 55% had at least one psychiatric hospitalization during the first year of follow-up, and the average subject spent 11% of the year in a psychiatric unit. Stevenson and Meares (1992) reported that their average subject spent 14% of the year in a psychiatric unit.

Two factors that result in increased hospitalization for patients with BPD are discussed in the literature. First, several authors noted that the outpatient services available for these patients do not match well with their needs. Historically, individuals with BPD have not benefited from outpatient services—both medication (Brinkley 1993; Soloff 1990) and psychotherapy (Perry et al. 1990; Skodol et al. 1983). Swigar and colleagues (1991) and Rascati (1990) noted that public mental health outpatient services were focused on the needs of patients with schizophrenia and bipolar disorder and did not meet the needs of patients with BPD (and, therefore, were unlikely to prevent rehospitalization). Kofoed and colleagues (1986) noted that patients with BPD quickly dropped out of their program (day treatment and dual diagnosis programming, respectively). Although 97% of patients with BPD have received outpatient psychiatric contact, with an average of 6.1 therapists per lifetime, lack of improvement or decompensation in psychotherapy and long-term hospitalization have been hallmarks of BPD throughout its history (Perry et al. 1990; Skodol et al. 1983).

Second, individuals with BPD frequently engage in parasuicidal behaviors, and these behaviors frequently result in inpatient hospitalizations. Comparing parasuicide rates across studies is difficult, not only because of methodological differences, but also due to different definitions—or lack of definitions—of *parasuicide*. Kreitman (1977) defines parasuicidal behavior as overt, acute, intentional, self-injurious acts, including suicide attempts as well as acts with no suicide intent, but other researchers have variously used the terms *parasuicide, self-harm, suicide attempt, suicide gesture,* and *self-mutilation* as synonymous, overlapping, or mutually exclusive. With this in mind, Mc-Glashan (1986) reported 21% of subjects parasuicided at least once during follow-up; Tucker and colleagues (1987) reported 30% of subjects parasuicided in the first year of follow-up; and Stevenson and Meares (1992) reported an average of 0.83 parasuicides per subject in the first year of follow-up.

Because of legal and ethical concerns about patient suicide, it is difficult to limit the hospitalization of parasuicidal patients with BPD (Fine and Sansone 1990; Rissmiller et al. 1994). In addition, the legal system for involuntary commitment focuses little attention on outpatient treatment, leading to revolving-door use of involuntary inpatient facilities. In part, this represents an inability to discriminate between acute and chronic suicidality, but as Rissmiller and colleagues (1994) point out, public inpatient and outpatient psychiatric benefits are already so limited that further cost-reduction strategies at this point may lead to an increase in completed suicides. In addition, many clinicians and service providers also believe that patients with BPD incur a host of costly secondary problems, such as involvement with social service agencies, employment problems, problems with housing, and involvement with the legal system; however, there is little data on the prevalence or costliness of these problems.

In sum, patients with BPD can present special difficulties due to their high suicidality, frequent parasuicidal acts, high drug abuse and other comorbidity, as well as their high dropout and failure rates in outpatient treatments, which they frequently seek. These difficulties often lead them into inpatient treatment services, which are costly and, it seems, also largely ineffective at preventing subsequent rehospitalizations or at reducing dysfunctional behaviors. Unfortunately, BPD is a relatively chronic condition, and patients with this disorder continue to seek outpatient treatments, continue to parasuicide in the face of unremitting emotional dysfunction, and continue to be placed in costly, inpatient treatment programs, and possibly to use a host of other public services.

Dialectical Behavior Therapy

DBT is a comprehensive outpatient treatment program developed specifically to treat chronic and severely dysfunctional individuals with BPD. The foundation of DBT is a biosocial model of BPD that emphasizes a causal interaction between biological and environmental factors in the etiology of BPD, similar to Millon's (1987) social learning thesis. The fundamental biological factor in BPD etiology is a deficit in emotion regulation, possibly caused by genetics, prenatal factors, early traumatic events, or a combination of these factors. The fundamental environmental factor is an *invalidating* environment. BPD results from a reciprocal transaction between the individual and the environment over time (i.e., the individual becomes progressively more emotionally dysregulated over time in response to the invalidating environment, and the environment becomes progressively more invalidating over time in response to the individual's dysregulation). Over time, individuals with BPD develop emotional difficulties whose etiologies can be characterized by two factors: 1) these individuals lack important interpersonal, self-regulation (including behavioral and emotional regulation) and distress tolerance skills, and 2) personal and environmental factors inhibit the use of behavioral skills the individual does have and often reinforce inappropriate dysfunctional behaviors.

DBT is defined by its philosophical base, *dialectics*, a term which is meant to convey two meanings. It implies that multiple tensions coexist and are dealt with in therapy with patients who are severely suicidal and who are diagnosed with BPD. It also conveys the emphasis in DBT on enhancing dialectical thinking patterns and on replacing rigid, dichotomous thinking characteristic of patients who are suicidal and who are diagnosed with BPD with dialectical thinking. The overriding dialectic is the necessity of acceptance of patients as they are within the context of trying to help them to change the way they act and think. Treatment strategies are divided into those most related to acceptance and those most related to change, and DBT requires that the therapist balance use of these two types of strategies within each treatment interaction. The emphasis on acceptance, even of dysfunctional behaviors, is similar to a relapse prevention model that assumes and even plans for dysfunctional behavior. It incorporates a nonjudg-mental, nonevaluative stance toward both the patient and his or her behavior. Thus, accepting a parasuicidal subject and assuming that the behavior might reoccur is an example of acceptance of parasuicidal behavior. The emphasis on change, more typical of traditional behav-ior therapy, suggests that the behavior must improve. Requiring a com-mitment to work on improving the behavior during the first session is an example of using a change procedure.

Stages of Disorder: Targets of Treatment

Although a considerable literature exists regarding the appropriate treatment for many DSM-IV disorders, factors other than diagnosis often affect treatment outcome. For example, the complexity and se-verity of an individual's disorder and the individual's concomitant an-cillary issues and other life problems can complicate the picture and obstruct potentially successful treatments. In DBT, a staging frame-work is useful for summarizing an individual's dysfunction and match-ing treatment to the whole individual, not just the disorder. An indi-vidual with BPD (or other disorders) can be at different stages of disorder, conceptualized by the severity, pervasiveness, and complexity of the individual's level of dysfunction and comorbidity of disorder. Four major stages of disorder have been suggested, each with a cor-responding set of treatment targets and problems to be solved (Linehan 1993, 1997, in press).

Stage One is the most severe stage of disorder. Patients at this stage present with complex, multiple problems and meet criteria for severe BPD and/or multiple Axis I and/or Axis IV disorders under the DSM classification system. Behavioral dyscontrol is the immediate problem at this stage, and treatment necessarily targets helping the patient re-gain basic control of behavior, reducing life-threatening behaviors, keeping the patient in treatment, and helping the patient acquire at least the basic capabilities needed to meet other goals. Stage One treat-ment targets are arranged in the following hierarchy :

1. Reduced high-risk suicidal and life-threatening behaviors, including parasuicide.
2. Reduced therapy-interfering behaviors, including attendance at treatment and compliance with treatment requirements.
3. Reduced quality-of-life interfering behaviors, such as drug abuse, excessive hospitalizations, homelessness, unemployment, economic difficulties, health problems, depression, and anxiety.
4. Replacement of maladaptive responses with skillful interpersonal behaviors, emotion regulation, and distress tolerance.
5. Individual patient goals not related to other targeted behavior patterns.

If maladaptive behaviors in the first three target areas have occurred since the previous sessions, then those behaviors are the focus of the session until they are dealt with. Woven throughout all work is a therapeutic emphasis on a dialectical stance and replacing maladaptive behaviors with the DBT behavioral skills, which are explicitly taught in DBT group skills training. Stage One treatment targets have been developed most fully and have been focused on in treatment outcome research, as discussed later in this chapter.

At Stage Two, patients have actions under reasonable control but are still in a great deal of pervasive emotional pain for individuals diagnosed with BPD, often because of posttraumatic stress. This stage can be thought of as *quiet desperation*. At this stage, the experience of emotions and associated cues is traumatic, and avoidance of emotional cues and emotional experiencing is a key problem. In general, Stage Two treatment targets reducing posttraumatic stress through exposure to trauma-related cues and enhancing the patient's ability to experience and process emotions nontraumatically. If Stage Two treatment is not successful, a life of quiet desperation may be intolerable for some individuals, who are at risk for eventually deteriorating back to Stage One.

Stage Three is conceptualized as problems in living and/or general unhappiness, which may be serious but are not disabling and do not seriously interfere with life functioning. Patients at this stage either have done the work necessary to progress out of earlier stages or were never severely disordered enough to need this work; and treatment targets achieving *ordinary* happiness and unhappiness as well as a stable sense of self-respect. If problems in higher stages have not recurred or developed, then treatment targets are determined by the problems or issues that the patient wants to emphasize. Stage Four, the final stage, involves the residual sense of incompleteness that many, if not most, individuals feel from time to time. Individuals at Stage Four seek a sense of completeness and the capacity for sustained joy through expanded awareness, spiritual fulfillment, deep psychological insight, or other life pursuits.

Functions of Treatment: Modes of Service Delivery

DBT is organized around five functions of successful treatment: capability enhancement, motivational enhancement, enhancement of generalization of gains, enhancement of capabilities and motivation of therapists, and structuring of the environment to support clinical progress.

The need for *capability enhancement* is based on the premise that the emotional difficulties of an individual diagnosed with BPD stem in part from behavioral skills deficits; this idea is similar to Kohut's (1984) deficit model of BPD. Capability enhancement is addressed in standard DBT with skills training, which focuses primarily on the acquisition and strengthening of specific behavioral skills theoretically related to BPD behaviors. Emphasis is on modeling, instructions, behavioral rehearsal, feedback and coaching, and homework assignments. DBT systematically teaches four sets of skills: mindfulness, interpersonal effectiveness, emotional regulation, and distress tolerance. A fifth skill, self-regulation, is woven into all areas of skills training. Mindfulness skills include focusing attention on observing one's self or one's immediate context, describing observations, spontaneously participating, being nonjudgmental, focusing awareness, and being effective (focusing on what works). Interpersonal effectiveness training is a mixed regimen of skills for maximizing effectiveness in interpersonal conflict situations. Emotion regulation training teaches a range of behavioral and cognitive strategies for reducing unwanted emotional responses as well as urges to engage in emotion-dependent actions. It focuses primarily on teaching how to identify and describe emotions, how to avoid situations and cues associated with previous dysfunctional behavior, how to stop avoiding negative emotions and reduce their intensity, and how to increase positive emotions. Distress tolerance training teaches a number of delay of gratification and self-soothing techniques aimed at surviving crises without attempting suicide, using drugs, or engaging in other dysfunctional behaviors. In other clinical applications, and in a modified form of DBT for substance abusers, capability enhancement also is addressed with medications, which, when successful, increase the capability of an individual's biological systems to regulate or self-regulate.

Teaching of new skills often is not enough for patients with BPD. The need for *motivational enhancement* is based on the premise that individuals with BPD often do not engage in functional behaviors, such as those learned in skills training, because these behaviors are blocked by automatic or overlearned emotional responses (which trigger avoidance) or by dysfunctional cognitions, or are not sufficiently reinforced by natural contingencies. The overall goal of motivational enhancement is to make sure that clinical progress is reinforced and not punished, that maladaptive behavior is not reinforced, and that emotions, cognitions, and other factors that inhibit or interfere with clinical progress are reduced. Exposure, cognitive restructuring, and contingency management techniques are used by DBT therapists to address problematic or excessive emotional responses, dysfunctional cognitions, and/or contingencies of reinforcement. Although the techniques used differ, this focus on motivational enhancement in DBT is similar in spirit to the motivational model of BPD of Kernberg and colleagues (1989).

The need for *enhancing generalization* is based on the premise that active efforts by the therapist and the patient are required to ensure generalization of new behaviors to everyday life settings; that sometimes a patient needs his or her therapist to stop interpreting and start coaching. Enhancing generalization is addressed by homework assignments, in vivo interventions, and phone consultations. For example, DBT therapists use explicit phone consultation strategies designed to help patients generalize skills learned in therapy to everyday problem situations. Patients are encouraged to call during crises when they may be unable to generalize skills without help. In settings such as day treatment, inpatient units, and residential programs, on-site consultations during office hours may supplement (or sometimes replace) phone consultations.

Structuring the environment addresses the need for the patient's natural and therapeutic environments to be maximally supportive of treatment progress. The therapist's goal here is to assist the patient in developing environments that reinforce clinical progress and not dysfunctional behavior. DBT therapists create a treatment environment that encourages progress and does not encourage relapse. Family sessions may be prescribed if the therapist thinks communication with the family might be helpful.

Enhancing therapist's capability and motivation is seen as an important, and often overlooked, function of successful treatment in that the extreme emotionality, unremitting crises, and other behaviors characteristic of BPD often results in therapist burnout and feelings of hopelessness. In DBT, treating the therapist is an integral part of the therapy. Weekly team meetings of all DBT therapists address this function by providing consultation and support for therapists in their efforts. By addressing each other's capabilities and motivation, DBT therapists keep each other doing good therapy.

Strategies of Treatment

DBT comprises five sets of strategies: three sets of technical strategies concern the organization and application of therapeutic techniques, one set of stylistic strategies describes communication styles for how DBT therapists implement techniques and interact with patients, and one set of case management strategies outlines effective communication with the patient's networks outside of therapy and with the therapist's support network. There are, as well, a number of specific, behavioral treatment protocols covering suicidal behavior, crisis management, therapy-interfering behavior and compliance issues, relationship problem solving, and ancillary treatment issues, including medication management.

The three technical strategies are dialectical strategies, validation strategies, and problem-solving strategies. Dialectical strategies involve balancing acceptance (validation strategies) and change (problem-solving strategies) in all interactions, always searching for a synthesis, and looking to shift the frame of problems that resist solution. Validation consists of a set of strategies that emphasize acceptance and validation of the patient: listening empathetically, reflecting accurately, articulating that which is experienced but not necessarily said, clarifying those disordered behaviors that are due to disordered biology or past learning history, and finding and highlighting those behaviors that are valid because they fit current facts or are effective for the patient's long-term goals. The essence of validation is *radical genuineness*, which involves seeing and responding to the patient as a person of equal status and value and recognizing the patient as he or she is, always keeping firmly in mind an empathic understanding of the patient's deficits and difficulties. Problem-solving strategies are designed to assess the specific problems of the individual, determine what factors are controlling or maintaining the problem behaviors, and then systematically apply therapeutic interventions. These interventions include behavioral analysis, insight and pattern recognition, didactic strategies, solution analysis, orienting and commitment strategies.

Efficacy

Outcomes With Suicidal Patients

DBT was first evaluated with a 1-year clinical trial involving 47 chronically parasuicidal women meeting criteria for BPD (Linehan et al. 1991). Specific inclusion criteria for this study were meeting BPD criteria on DSM-III (American Psychiatric Association 1980), having at least 2 incidents of parasuicide in the last 5 years (with one during the last 8 weeks), and being between the ages of 18 and 45 years. Exclusion criteria were meeting the DSM-III criteria for schizophrenia, bipolar disorder, substance dependence, or mental retardation. Subjects were matched on age, number of lifetime parasuicides and psychiatric hospitalizations, and on an indicator of good versus poor prognosis. Statistical tests did not find significant differences at pretreatment between conditions on BPD severity scores, number of previous parasuicides, number of psychiatric hospitalizations, depression, hopelessness, suicide ideation, reasons for living, employment, or marital status.

Subjects were randomly assigned to either DBT or treatment-as-usual (TAU). TAU was a naturalistic condition: Subjects were given an alternative therapy referral and allowed to participate in any type of treatment available in the community. DBT therapists included the first author (M.M.L.), who saw one patient, and other psychologists, psychiatrists, and mental health professionals. All therapists were trained and supervised by M.M.L. Treatment lasted 1 year, with blind assessments given every 4 months, followed by two posttreatment assessments given at 6-month intervals. Except for analysis of treatment dropout rates, only those DBT subjects who stayed in treatment long enough to be considered treated, defined as four or more sessions ($n = 22$), were included in the analyses.

Treatment Effectiveness

DBT was more effective at achieving each of the specific treatment targets, as already defined, than was TAU (Linehan et al. 1991). Regarding the first target, reduction of parasuicide and other life-threatening behaviors, TAU subjects engaged in significantly more parasuicides than did DBT subjects during the year of treatment. Significantly more subjects in the DBT group than the TAU group completely stopped parasuicidal behaviors during treatment. Looking only at those subjects who parasuicided, parasuicides in the TAU subject group were of significantly higher medical risk and required significantly more medical treatment than were those parasuicides by subjects in the DBT group. The second target, reduction of behaviors that interfere with the process of therapy, was operationalized as the number of subjects who dropped their first therapist during the study, as dropping therapy obviously is the most serious therapy-interfering behavior. DBT was significantly better than TAU at maintaining subjects in therapy: 58% of subjects in the TAU group dropped their first therapist, compared with 17% of those in the DBT group. Subjects undergoing DBT also stayed in therapy significantly longer than did subjects receiving TAU. The third target, reduction of behaviors that seriously interfere with quality of life, was operationalized as reductions in days spent in psychiatric inpatient units and in number of admissions to inpatient units. Subjects in the DBT group spent significantly less days in psychiatric inpatient units and had significantly less inpatient admissions than did subjects in the TAU group. Interpersonal outcomes also favored DBT. Those subjects receiving DBT scored significantly lower than did subjects undergoing TAU on a measure of state anger, and scored significantly higher on measures of global adjustment and interviewer-rated and self-reported social adjustment (Linehan et al. 1994). Regression and other analyses indicated that the superiority of DBT over TAU on these outcomes was not due to lower fees in the DBT condition, more hours of therapy received by the DBT group, telephone availability of DBT therapists, or the sense of being part of a team developing a new treatment (Linehan and Heard 1993). However, no significant differences between conditions were found on measures of depression, hopelessness, reasons for living, or suicide ideation.

As a general outcome measure, psychiatric hospitalizations and parasuicide episodes were combined into a single variable with values of good, moderate, and poor based on the following criteria. Subjects with neither a psychiatric hospitalization nor a parasuicide episode during the last 4 months were labeled good. Subjects with either one or more hospitalizations or one or more parasuicide episodes were labeled moderate. Subjects with both one or more hospitalizations and one or more parasuicide episodes were labeled poor. Significant results favoring DBT were found using this general outcome measure (Figure 5–1). Of those subjects receiving DBT, 55% had good outcomes and 9% had poor outcomes, compared with 32% good outcomes and 23% poor outcomes in the TAU group.

Thirty-seven (37) subjects were located for 6-month follow-up interviews, and 35 were located for 12-month follow-up interviews. Many

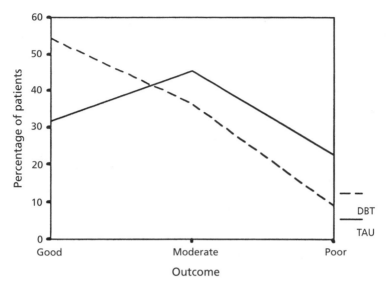

FIGURE 5-1. *General outcomes by condition.*

were unwilling to complete the entire assessment battery but agreed to an abbreviated interview covering essential outcome data. Overall, the superiority of DBT over TAU achieved during the treatment year was maintained during the year following treatment (Linehan et al. 1993). Subjects in the DBT group maintained gains over subjects in the TAU group on global adjustment, social adjustment, and work performance. In every area where DBT was superior to TAU at post-treatment, DBT gains were maintained for at least 6 months. DBT superiority was stronger during the first 6 months of follow-up for measures of parasuicidal behavior and anger and was stronger during the latter 6 months in reducing psychiatric inpatient days.

Cost Effectiveness

When compared with TAU, DBT significantly improved outcomes of a number of variables implicated in the costliness of BPD, including psychiatric inpatient admissions, length of inpatient stays, and number of parasuicides. A preliminary analysis of cost effectiveness, with outcomes converted into average yearly health care costs, suggests that

DBT is cost effective, saving $9000 per patient during the first year of treatment compared with TAU (Linehan and Heard, in press). Although outpatient therapy cost subjects in the DBT group over $1,000 per subject more than it did subjects in the TAU group, DBT saved over $9,000 per subject in costs of psychiatric and medical hospitalization days.

A replication and extension study of this clinical trial currently is underway. Eighty (80) chronically parasuicidal women will be followed for 1 year of treatment and 1 year of follow-up. A more rigorous control condition is being used, community individual psychotherapy, rather than TAU. DBT therapists have received more training than have previous DBT therapists, and adherence to therapy is now being measured.

Outcomes With Drug Abusers

DBT also has been evaluated with a 1-year treatment development study involving 29 substance-dependent women meeting criteria for BPD. To treat substance abusers (Linehan and Dimeff 1995), the DBT treatment target hierarchy was modified to focus on substance abuse behaviors and urges. High-risk suicidal and parasuicidal behaviors, and behaviors that interfered with or threatened the continuation of therapy were still targeted first and second, as no treatment works with a client who is dead or not in the treatment. However, if no high-risk suicidal behaviors or therapy-interfering behaviors occurred, drug-abusing behaviors and urges were at the top of the session agenda. The problem-solving strategies developed for parasuicidal behavior were modified for substance abuse. If substance abuse or an urge to abuse was reported, the therapist conducted an extremely detailed behavioral chain analysis of the episode followed by a solution analysis that focused on alternate behaviors that could have been used to avert the problem behavior. This was followed by use of a number of detailed commitment strategies designed to elicit and strengthen the client's recommitment to stop the problem behaviors and replace them with skillful behaviors.

Patients were randomly assigned to either DBT for substance abusers (DBT-S; $n = 8$) or TAU ($n = 10$). Subjects were matched on age, motivation to stop using drugs, severity of highest drug dependence, and global assessment of functioning scores. Inclusion and exclusion criteria were the same as in the previous study, with the additional inclusion criteria of meeting criteria for DSM-IV polysubstance use disorder or substance use disorder in one or more of the following areas: cocaine, amphetamines, opiates, sedative-hypnotics, hallucinogens, or anxiolytics.

Although the sample size was small, restricting statistical power to detect real differences, preliminary results are encouraging (Linehan et al. 1997). Regarding the first target, reduction of parasuicide and other life-threatening behaviors, DBT-S and TAU conditions both showed significant reductions in parasuicidal behavior over the treatment year, but no significant between-group differences were found. However, significantly more subjects in the TAU than DBT group were on selective serotonin reuptake inhibitors; this was not the case in the first study. A more detailed analysis of parasuicidal behavior taking into account this potential confound has not yet been undertaken. Regarding the second target, reduction of behaviors that interfere with the process of therapy, 39% of patients in the DBT-S group dropped their first therapist, and 69% of patients in the TAU group dropped their first therapist. This suggests that DBT-S remains effective at maintaining patients in treatment. Regarding the third target, reduction of behaviors that seriously interfere with quality of life, patients receiving DBT-S engaged in significantly less substance abuse over the treatment year, measured with scheduled and random urinalyses and with self-report, than did patients receiving TAU. A trend in favor of DBT-S over TAU was also found at the 4- and 8-month assessments in global adjustment. No differences were found in inpatient psychiatric hospitalization days or admissions. Analyses of cost effectiveness have not been completed as of this writing.

A replication and extension study of the efficacy of DBT-S currently is underway. Thirty-two (32) subjects will be randomly assigned to a 1-year treatment of DBT-S or a new comparison condition, comprehensive 12-step validation (CTSV), which will control for threats to internal validity, including the readiness to seek out treatment, the provision of psychotherapy and of emotional empathy and validation, and clinical assessment. All clients receiving CTSV will be required to attend either additional weekly 12-step groups or meet with a 12-step sponsor weekly.

Other Outcomes

Two studies suggest that DBT group skills training alone is not enough for positive outcomes; individual therapy is a necessary component of the treatment. Barley and colleagues (1993), using a controlled non-randomized design, compared components of DBT with standard treatment (TAU) on a psychiatric inpatient unit. First, they compared DBT group skills training only to TAU and found no differences in rates of parasuicidal behavior. Next, they added coaching techniques and other aspects of individual therapy to DBT group skills training and found that this combination resulted in significantly lower rates of parasuicidal behavior for patients receiving DBT. In a different study, in which DBT group skills training only was compared with a no-skills-training control condition, no significant differences were found between groups (Linehan et al. 1993).

Specificity

In the studies already described, only Stage One targets of DBT treatment were studied, given the severity of the inclusion criteria and the 1-year, time-limited treatment. For individuals with BPD, Stage One is characterized by parasuicidal behavior, repeated hospitalizations, drug abuse, unemployment, and disrupted relationships, all extremely costly and troubling problems. DBT appears to be effective at treating what it targets. In the study of chronically parasuicidal women with BPD, DBT, compared with TAU, was superior at reducing parasuicidal behavior, keeping patients out of the hospital, maintaining patients in treatment, reducing anger and improving social adjustment. In the study of drug-dependent women with BPD, treatment targets were modified to focus more on substance abuse and urges to abuse. In this study, DBT, compared with TAU, was superior at reducing drug abuse but not parasuicidal behavior. In this research, DBT was not as successful with the Stage Two target of reducing emotional distress. For example, DBT compared with TAU did not reduce depression, hopelessness, or suicide ideation and neither did it increase reasons for living in either study. Further research is needed to determine DBT's effectiveness with stages Two and Three, as well as to determine the components of DBT that lead to the outcomes for each target.

Conclusion

DBT was developed to treat the chronic and severe problems of patients with BPD. As a behavioral treatment, it was designed to target specific problem behaviors, most particularly parasuicide and drug abuse. A hierarchy of targets was developed to address dysfunction in each of four stages of disorder; from Stage One, severe behavioral dyscontrol, to Stage Four, a sense of incompleteness. Strategies of DBT reflecting the dialectic between acceptance and change are used to assist patients toward more functional behaviors to move up through the stages. Clinical trials of DBT versus TAU show that DBT is more effective at decreasing targeted behaviors, including parasuicide, hospitalization, therapy dropout, and drug abuse. DBT also has been shown to be cost effective. DBT has not been shown to be more effective with dysfunctional behaviors not explicitly targeted. Further research is being conducted to replicate outcomes with more rigorous control groups and clarify the components of DBT related to specific outcomes.

References

Akhtar S, Byrne JP, Doghramji K: The demographic profile of borderline personality disorder. J Clin Psychiatry 47(4):196–198, 1986

Akiskal HS, Yerevanian BI, Davis GC, et al: The nosologic status of borderline personality: clinical and polysomnograph study. Am J Psychiatry 142:192–198, 1985

American Psychiatric Association: Diagnostic and Statistical Manual of Mental Disorders, 3rd Edition. Washington, DC, American Psychiatric Association, 1980

American Psychiatric Association: Diagnostic and Statistical Manual of Mental Disorders, 4th Edition. Washington, DC, American Psychiatric Association, 1994

Barasch A, Frances A, Hurt S, et al: Stability and distinctness of borderline personality disorder. Am J Psychiatry 142:1484–1486, 1985

Barley WD, Buie SE, Peterson EW, et al: The development of an inpatient cognitive-behavioral treatment program for borderline personality disorder. J Personal Disord 7(3):232–240, 1993

Brinkley JR: Pharmacotherapy of borderline states. Psychiatr Clin North Am 16(4):853–854, 1993

Carpenter MD, Mulligan JC, Brader IA, et al: Multiple admissions to an urban psychiatric center: a comparative study. Hosp Community Psychiatry 36(12):1305–1308, 1985

Castaneda R, Franco H: Sex and ethnic distribution of borderline personality disorder in an inpatient sample. Am J Psychiatry 42:1202–1203, 1985

Clarkin JF, Widiger TA, Frances A, et al: Prototypic typology and the borderline personality disorder. J Abnorm Psychol 92(3):263–275, 1983

Comtois KA, Linehan MM, Schmidt HS: Diagnostic comparison of drug-dependent and parasuicidal patients with borderline personality disorder. Paper presented at the Association for the Advancement of Behavior Therapy Meeting, New York, 1996

Cowdry RW, Pickar D, Davies R: Symptoms and EEG findings in the borderline syndrome. Int J Psychiatry Med 15:201–211, 1985

Dahl AA: Prognosis of the borderline disorders. Psychopathology 19:68–79, 1986

Dulit RA, Fyer MR, Haas GL, et al: Substance use in borderline personality disorder. Am J Psychiatry 147:1002–1007, 1990

Fine MA, Sansone RA: Dilemmas in the management of suicidal behavior in individuals with borderline personality disorder. Am J Psychother 44(2):160–171, 1990

Frances A, Fyer M, Clarkin JF: Personality and suicide. Ann N Y Acad Sci 487:281–293, 1986

Fyer MR, Frances AJ, Sullivan T, et al: Comorbidity of borderline personality disorder. Arch Gen Psychiatry 45:348–352, 1997

Geller JL: In again, out again: preliminary evaluation of a state hospital's worst recidivists. Hosp Community Psychiatry 37(4):386–390, 1986

Green JH: Frequent rehospitalization and noncompliance with treatment. Hosp Community Psychiatry 39(9):963–966, 1988

Gunderson JG, Kolb JE, Austin V: The diagnostic interview for borderline patients. Am J Psychiatry 138(7):896–903, 1981

Hadley TR, McGurrin MC, Pulice RT, et al: Using fiscal data to identify heavy service users. Psychiatr Q 61(1):41–48, 1990

Hadley TR, Culhane DP, McGurrin MC: Identifying and tracking "heavy users" of acute psychiatric inpatient services. Adm Policy Ment Health 19(4):279–290, 1992

Inman DJ, Bascue LO, Skoloda T: Identification of borderline personality disorders among substance abuse inpatients. J Subst Abuse Treat 2:229–232, 1985

Kernberg OF, Selzer MA, Koenigsberg HW, et al: Psychodynamic Psychotherapy of Borderline Patients. New York, Basic Books, 1989

Koenigsberg H, Kaplan R, Gilmore M, et al: The relationship between syndrome and personality disorder in DSM-III: experience with 2,462 patients. Am J Psychiatry 142(2):207–212, 1985

Kofoed L, Kania J, Walsh T, et al: Outpatient treatment of patients with substance abuse and coexisting psychiatric disorders. Am J Psychiatry 143(7):867–872, 1986

Kohut H: How Does Analysis Cure? Chicago, IL, University of Chicago Press, 1984

Kosten RA, Kosten TR, Rounsaville BJ: Personality disorders in opiate addicts show prognostic specificity. J Subst Abuse Treat 6:163–168, 1989

Kreitman N: Parasuicide. London, England, Wiley, 1977

Kroll JL, Sines LK, Martin K: Borderline personality disorder: construct validity of the concept. Arch Gen Psychiatry 39:60–63, 1981

Kullgren G: Personality disorders among psychiatric inpatients. Nord Psykiatr Tidsskr 46(1):27–32, 1992

Linehan MM: Cognitive Behavioral Therapy of Borderline Personality Disorder. New York, Guilford, 1993

Linehan MM: Dialectical behavior therapy (DBT) for borderline personality disorder. California Alliance for the Mentally Ill's The Journal 8:44–46, 1997

Linehan MM: Development, evaluation, and dissemination of effective psychosocial treatments: stages of disorder, levels of care, and states of treatment research, in Drug Abuse: Origins and Interventions. Edited by Glantz MG, Hartel CR. Washington, DC, American Psychological Association, in press

Linehan MM, Dimeff LA: Extension of Standard Dialectical Behavior Therapy to Treatment of Substance Abusers With Borderline Personality Disorder. Seattle, WA: University of Washington.

Linehan MM, Heard HL: Impact of treatment accessibility on clinical course of parasuicidal patients: in reply to Hoffman RE [letter]. Arch Gen Psychiatry 50:157–158, 1993

Linehan MM, Heard HL: Borderline personality disorder: costs, course, and treatment outcomes, in Cost-Effectiveness of Psychotherapy: A Guide for Practitioners, Researchers and Policy-Makers. New York, Oxford University Press, in press

Linehan MM, Armstrong HE, Suarez A, et al: Cognitive-behavioral treatment of chronically parasuicidal borderline patients. Arch Gen Psychiatry 49:1060–1064, 1991

Linehan MM, Heard HL, Armstrong HE: Naturalistic follow-up of a behavioral treatment for chronically parasuicidal borderline patients. Arch Gen Psychiatry 50:971–974, 1993

Linehan MM, Tutek DA, Heard HL, et al: Interpersonal outcome of cognitive behavioral treatment for chronically suicidal borderline patients. Am J Psychiatry 151:1771–1776, 1994

Loranger AW, Tulis EH: Family history of alcoholism in borderline personality disorder. Arch Gen Psychiatry 42:153–157, 1985

McCann JT, Flynn PM, Gersh DM: MCMI-II diagnosis of borderline personality disorder: base rates versus prototypic items. J Pers Assess 58:105–114, 1992

McGlashan TH: The Chestnut Lodge follow-up study, III: long-term outcome of borderline personality disorder. Arch Gen Psychiatry 43:20–30, 1986

Millon T: On the genesis and prevalence of the borderline personality disorder: a social learning thesis. J Personal Disord 1(4):354–372, 1987

Modestin J, Abrecht I, Tschaggelar W, et al: Diagnosing borderline: a contribution to the question of its conceptual validity. Arch Psychiatr Nervenkr 233:359–370, 1997

Nace EP, Saxon JJ, Shore N: A comparison of borderline and nonborderline alcoholic patients. Arch Gen Psychiatry 40:54–56, 1983

Paris J, Brown R, Nowlis D: Long-term follow-up of borderline patients in a general hospital. Compr Psychiatry 28:530–535, 1987

Perry JC, Herman JL, van der Kolk BA, et al: Psychotherapy and psychological trauma in borderline personality disorder. Psychiatric Annals 20(1):33–43, 1990

Pitts WM, Gustin QL, Mitchell C, et al: MMPI critical item characteristics of the DSM-III borderline personality disorder. J Nerv Ment Dis 173(10):628–631, 1985

Pope HG, Jonas JM, Hudson JI, et al: The validity of DSM-III borderline personality disorder: a phenomenologic, family history, treatment response, and long-term follow-up study. Arch Gen Psychiatry 40:23–30, 1983

Prasad RB, Val ER, Lahmeyer HW, et al: Associated diagnoses (comorbidity) in patients with borderline personality disorder. J Psychiatry Neurosci 15(1):22–27, 1997

Rascati JN: "Managed care and the discharge dilemma": commentary. Psychiatry 53(2):124–126, 1990

Richman J, Charles E: Patient dissatisfaction and attempted suicide. Community Ment Health J 12:301–305, 1976

Rissmiller DJ, Steer R, Ranieri WF, et al: Factors complicating cost containment in the treatment of suicidal patients. Hosp Community Psychiatry 45(8):782–788, 1994

Skodol AE, Oldham JM: Assessment and diagnosis of borderline personality disorder. Hosp Community Psychiatry 42(10):1021–1028, 1991

Skodol et al: 1983

Skodol AE, Buckley P, Charles E: Is there a characteristic pattern in the treatment history of clinic outpatients with borderline personality? J Nerv Ment Dis 171:405–410, 1983

Soloff PH: What's new in personality disorders?: an update on pharmacologic treatment. J Personal Disord 4(3):233–243, 1990

Stevenson J, Meares R: An outcome study of psychotherapy for patients with borderline personality disorder. Am J Psychiatry 149(3):358–362, 1992

Stone MH: Constitution and temperament in borderline conditions: biological and genetic explanatory formulations, in The Borderline Patient: Emerging Concepts in Diagnosis, Psychodynamics, and Treatment. Edited by Grotstein JS, Solomon MF, Lang JA. Hillsdale, NJ, Analytic Press, 1987, pp 25–287

Surber RW, Winkler EL, Monteleone M, et al: Characteristics of high users of acute inpatient services. Hosp Community Psychiatry 38(10):1112–1116, 1987

Swigar ME, Astrachan B, Levine MA, et al: Single and repeated admissions to a mental health center: demographic, clinical and use of service characteristics. Int J Soc Psychiatry 37(4):259–266, 1991

Tousignant M, Kovess V: Borderline traits among community alcoholics and problem-drinkers: rural urban differences. Can J Psychiatry 34:796–799, 1989

Tucker L, Bauer SF, Wagner S, et al: Long-term hospital treatment of borderline patients: a descriptive outcome study. Am J Psychiatry 144(11):1443–1448, 1987

Vaglum S, Vaglum P: Borderline and other mental disorders in alcoholic female psychiatric patients: a case control study. Psychopathology 18(1):50–60, 1985

Widiger TA, Frances AJ: Epidemiology, diagnosis, and comorbidity of borderline personality disorder, in American Psychiatric Press Review of Psychiatry, Vol. 8. Edited by Tasman A, Hales RE, Frances AJ. Washington, DC, American Psychiatric Press, 1989, pp 8–24

Widiger TA, Weissman MM: Epidemiology of borderline personality disorder. Hosp Community Psychiatry 42(10):1015–1021, 1991

Woogh CM: A cohort through the revolving door. Can J Psychiatry 31:214–221, 1986

Zanarini MC, Gunderson JG, Frankenburg FR: Axis I phenomenology of borderline personality disorder. Compr Psychiatry 30(2):149–156, 1989

PART III

Cognitive-Behavioral Therapy

Cognitive and Behavioral Therapies Alone or Combined With Antidepressant Medication in the Treatment of Depression

Melanie M. Biggs, Ph.D.

A. John Rush, M.D.

Epidemiology of Depression

Major depressive disorder is characterized by affective, somatic, and cognitive difficulties that impair psychosocial functioning (e.g., occupational, marital, parental roles). The lifetime incidence of major depressive disorder is estimated to be 15% (Meyers et al. 1984), whereas as many as eight million individuals in the United States are afflicted with a major depressive illness in a given year (Regier et al. 1993).

The factors that place individuals at risk for developing a major

This research was supported in part by a grant from the National Institute of Mental Health (MH-53799) and Mental Health Connections, a partnership between Dallas County Mental Health and Mental Retardation and the Department of Psychiatry of the University of Texas Southwestern Medical Center. Funding is from the Texas State Legislature and the Dallas County Hospital District.

The authors wish to thank Steven R. Krebaum, M.S., Shannon M. Baker, M.A., and Christine A. McKenzie, M.Ed., for their technical assistance. The authors also appreciate the secretarial support of Fast Word, Inc., of Dallas and David Savage, and the administrative support of Kenneth Z. Altshuler, M.D., Chairman, Department of Psychiatry, University of Texas Southwestern Medical Center.

depressive disorder include female gender; family history of depressive illness; history of previous depressive episodes; prior suicide attempts; 40 years of age or younger; experiencing a postpartum period, stressful life event, lack of social support, or a general medical condition; and current alcohol and/or substance abuse (Depression Guideline Panel 1993). Women are more than twice as likely as men to develop depressive disorders. The lifetime risk of developing a major depressive illness is as high as 25% in women and 12% in men. The point prevalence rates for major depressive disorders in Western industrialized nations are estimated to be as high as 9% for women and 3% for men (Depression Guideline Panel 1993).

Course of Illness

Most major depressive disorders are recurrent, lifelong illnesses. Patients who have experienced one major depressive episode have more than a 30% chance of having a second within 12 months. Within 10 years following the first episode of depression at least 75% of patients will have experienced a recurrence (Lavori et al. 1994). The risk of subsequent depressive episodes increases as the number of depressive episodes increases. Thus, the risk of a third episode of depression is as high as 90% following a second depressive episode (Kupfer 1991).

Poor interepisode recovery or chronic prolonged episodes account for 25% of all patients with major depressive disorder. Depressive episodes associated with poor interepisode recovery are associated with a greater risk of a subsequent episode, increased need for long-term treatment, greater consideration of combination treatment, and a poorer prognosis (Depression Guideline Panel 1993).

A growing body of evidence suggests that the more chronic forms of depression may be more difficult to treat pharmacologically and psychotherapeutically (Harpin et al. 1982; Hoberman et al. 1988; Mason et al. 1993; Mercier et al. 1992; Rush et al. 1978; Scott 1992; Sotsky et al. 1991). Howland's (1991) comprehensive review revealed that depressive disorders with full interepisode recovery and shorter episodes had a higher response rate to pharmacotherapy than chronic depressions (i.e., chronic major depressions and double depressions [dysthymic disorders with superimposed major depression]). Similarly, Thase and colleagues (1994) reported that chronically depressed patients (i.e., patients with chronic major depression or double depression) were slower to respond and evidenced more partial responses to cognitive behavioral therapy. Mason and colleagues (1993) report similar findings with a group of patients with double depression who were treated either with interpersonal psychotherapy or desipramine.

Thus, adaptations of cognitive, behavioral, and interpersonal psychotherapies may be called for to treat patients more effectively who suffer from chronic depressions. In addition, these findings raise the as yet unanswered question of whether patients with chronic depressions benefit preferentially from the combination of psychotherapy and antidepressant medications (Blackburn et al. 1981; Miller et al. 1990) or whether sequential trials of psychotherapy and antidepressant medications are needed (see Markowitz 1994 for review; Stewart et al. 1993).

The Role of Stress

Much research has been conducted on the relationship between psychosocial stressors and the onset of depressive episodes. In a comprehensive review, Brown and Harris (1978) suggest that women with a predisposition or vulnerability toward developing a depressive episode endorsed the following factors: early loss of a mother, having three or more children, lack of employment outside the home, and lack of a confiding relationship with a husband or boyfriend. In contrast, Rodgers (1991) reported women to be vulnerable to depressive disorders because of financial hardship and childhood risk (e.g., negative attributional style, truancy, negative self-esteem), whereas men were reported to be at higher risk for depression when they experienced financial hardship and unemployment (Rodgers 1991). Brown and colleagues (1992) reported that intrapersonal factors may convert events into stresses that precipitate depressive episodes. The literature supports a significant role of psychosocial stressors in the development of depressive illnesses.

Retrospective, and some prospective, studies are consistent with the notion that psychosocial stressors play significant roles in the onset of a depressive disorder but lesser roles in precipitating subsequent depressive episodes (Paykel et al. 1996; Post 1992). It has been suggested that psychosocial stressors trigger the onset of the initial episodes of depression that, in turn, result in initiating neurobiological changes that make patients vulnerable to subsequent recurrences (Post 1992). However, acceptance of this notion is not universal.

Furthermore, positive psychosocial events have been associated with recovery or improvement in depressive episodes in patients depressed for at least 20 previous weeks (Brown et al. 1992). Specifically, anchoring or increased security (e.g., finalizing a divorce; obtaining employment) and fresh starts (e.g., events that indicate a change in a situation that gives hope) have been related to the recovery and improvement of depressive episodes (Brown et al. 1992).

Secular Trends

The literature suggests a cohort effect such that those born in more recent decades have an earlier onset of both bipolar and unipolar recurrent major depressive disorder (Giles et al. 1989; Hagnell et al. 1982; Klerman 1976; Lavori et al. 1987, 1993; Robins et al. 1984; Weissman and Myers 1978). Lavori and colleagues (1987, 1993) investigated the birth cohort effect to determine if the rising numbers of patients affected with major depressive episodes at an earlier age was due to artifacts of measurement, time period, or age effects. The results suggested a consistent pattern of increasing rates and earlier ages of onset with successive birth cohorts across all strata assessed in the United States (Lavori et al. 1993).

Morbidity and Mortality

There is increasing evidence that the presence of depressive disorder in conjunction with major general medical conditions worsens the morbidity and/or mortality associated with them. For example, Frasure-Smith and colleagues (1994) found a 5.7 times greater likelihood of death in patients within 6 months of their myocardial infarction (MI) if depression was present as opposed to absent. At 18 months, patients with major depression post-MI continued to have a higher mortality rate (3.6 times), as compared with post-MI patients who were not diagnosed with a major depression (Frasure-Smith et al. 1995). Similarly, Rovner et al. (1991), in a study of recent nursing home admissions, found a 59% greater death rate in patients diagnosed with depression as opposed to patients who were not depressed within 12 months of admission.

Recent Estimates of Cost

Cost estimates indicate the economic burden of depression to be $43.7 billion per year (in 1990 dollars) (Greenberg et al. 1993). The total cost of depression in the United States is comprised of approximately $12 billion (28%) in annual direct costs, $7.5 billion (17%) in annual mortality costs, and $23.8 billion (55%) in annual morbidity costs due to absenteeism and loss of productivity while on the job. Although these estimates are large, it has been suggested that they probably underestimate the costs of depression, because the figures do not include costs due to other factors (e.g., lack of detection and treatment of this disorder, which increases health services utilization; the decline in quality of life associated with this disorder; and the financial costs on family and friends) (Greenberg et al. 1993).

Thus, depressive conditions are common, costly, disabling, typically recurrent, and not infrequently chronic. The rationale to develop and evaluate alternative treatments for these disorders is obvious. Several psychological theories and the derivative therapies have been developed and evaluated specifically for depressive conditions.

Cognitive Theories

Cognitive Therapy (CT)

The cognitive model purports that the way in which individuals construe their experiences influences their emotional, behavioral, and physiological responses (Beck 1964). That is, it is not a specific event that affects individuals' feelings, behaviors, and physiological responses, but rather how individuals process or perceive those events. The cognitive theory of Beck and colleagues (1979) identifies three elements germane to the psychopathology of depression. These components include: 1) negative cognitive set (cognitive triad); 2) negative beliefs, silent assumptions, and automatic thoughts; and 3) cognitive errors or distortions (Beck 1976).

Depressed individuals present with a negative cognitive set (i.e., the cognitive triad), which includes negative views of the self, world, and future (Beck et al. 1979). For example, a depressed woman may consistently view herself as defective, inadequate, or stupid regardless of contrary evidence. This same depressed individual perceives her daily life as a battle in which she is constantly struggling to cope with what she perceives as constant and unrelenting attacks and demands. She perceives her future as hopeless and believes life will forever be a struggle to survive.

This negative cognitive set is a derivative of particular beliefs or schemas that, in turn, have developed from past experiences. Schemas influence the way in which depressed individuals process information. A schema such as "I am inadequate if I don't succeed" would be triggered and influence the processing of such information as when a depressed person perceives a situation as insurmountable.

Silent assumptions or underlying conditional beliefs include beliefs germane to a sense of being approved of or loved by others or a sense of accomplishment (sociotropy, autonomy). Silent assumptions or conditional beliefs influence how depressed people act and feel. For example, when depressed individuals are given a task they may feel overwhelmed and more depressed. However, they are unclear why they feel this way. The increase in their depression may be related to an underlying belief that they are incapable of completing the task. Thus, they silently may be saying to themselves, "If I don't complete this task perfectly then I will be fired." This erroneous assumption is triggered by the core belief or schema, "I am inadequate," which is what is actually fueling the depression.

Underlying assumptions and automatic thoughts about certain events are often distorted or illogical, as evidenced in cognitive errors or distortions in their perceptions. CT focuses on identifying the negative cognitive patterns of automatic thoughts, faulty assumptions or conditional beliefs, and maladaptive schemas or core beliefs. Once patients become aware of their habitual thinking patterns, various techniques are employed to assist them in viewing and coping with the world in a more realistic and adaptive manner that, in turn, both alleviates the depression, and, in theory, should provide some protection from future episodes.

CT is a time-limited, focused, and collaborative process aimed at modifying dysfunctional thinking and maladaptive behavior that create conditions for the development and maintenance of depressive symptoms. The development of CT has rested upon the foundation of the empirical evaluation of efficacy. CT has been shown to be as efficacious as other psychotherapies (e.g., interpersonal, behavioral) and pharmacotherapies in the treatment of nonpsychotic mildly to moderately depressed outpatients (Depression Guideline Panel 1993).

Behavioral Theories

The three major, related behavioral approaches to depression include social learning theory (Ferster 1973), stress management (Lewinsohn 1974), and self-control therapy (Rehm et al. 1979). The following is a brief synopsis of each approach.

One of the first conceptualizations of clinical depression, based on operant learning theory (Ferster 1965, 1973), suggested depression occurred because individuals are unable to engage in enough adaptive behaviors that provide them with positive reinforcement. Thus, the absence of a link between adaptive behaviors and positive reinforcers created the conditions necessary for the experience of depression. The majority of behavioral theories of depression are based on this operant formulation (Fuchs and Rehm 1977; Lewinsohn 1974; Rehm et al. 1979).

Lewinsohn's (1974) model of depression indicates depression is a "consequence of a low rate of response contingent positive reinforcement" and a high rate of response contingent punishing experiences. Lewinsohn's treatment aims at increasing patients' positively reinforced interactions and decreasing their negative or punishing experiences. These goals are accomplished by addressing social skill deficits, lack of responses, contingent positive reinforcers, and cognitive errors or difficulties.

Therapists conduct a thorough assessment or functional analysis of their patients to pinpoint the events associated with a fluctuation of the depressed mood. Often this analysis reveals a social skills deficit or the lack of an adaptive response requiring social skills training. The type of deficit or lack of appropriate response observed dictates the type of intervention provided by the therapist. For example, assertiveness training, communication skills, or modifications of interpersonal style are often taught to patients with social skill deficits or who have never been taught how to effectively communicate with others or behave in an assertive manner. These types of skills are presented to patients through didactic presentations, modeling and coaching by therapists, role playing and rehearsal within the sessions, practicing of skills outside therapy sessions, and through direct application of the new and adaptive skills into patients' daily lives.

Many depressions are associated with a lack of response contingent positive reinforcement. In these cases, therapists assist patients in increasing pleasant activities that will lead to positive reinforcement that will, in turn, assist in improving the depressed mood (e.g., attending an enjoyable movie, spending time with a good friend, a walk in the park). Conversely, unpleasant activities are also decreased in an effort to reduce negative experiences that fuel the dysphoria. These activities are often accomplished by having patients intentionally participate or not participate in specific activities between sessions.

Depression can also be generated and/or fueled by patients' cognitive errors or difficulties (Lewinsohn et al. 1980). Social learning tactics for addressing cognitive difficulties consist of increasing positive thinking (e.g., self-rewarding thoughts, noticing accomplishments) and decreasing negative thinking (e.g., worrying time, thought interruption) (Lewinsohn et al. 1980).

Stress management is another social learning tactic used to combat depression (Lewinsohn et al. 1980). Relaxation training, a common component of stress management training, focuses on teaching patients how to cope with potentially stressful situations in an adaptive manner in order to reduce aversive experiences and prevent the interference of enjoyable activities. Other stress management techniques focus on problem-solving skills, correction of cognitive errors, and self-instruction (Lewinsohn et al. 1980). Behavioral therapists who use components of Lewinsohn's model of depression display an active and directive style with their patients combined with a psychoeducational component.

In contrast, the self-control model suggests depression is associated with an individual's difficulty using self-control behaviors when coping with the delay or loss of reinforcement (Fuchs and Rehm 1977; Rehm et al. 1979). Rehm suggests depression is not only the result of a lack of adaptive behaviors that produce positive reinforcement but is also a consequence of negative self-evaluations, a lack of self-reinforcement, as well as high frequency of self-punishment. Fuchs and Rehm (1977) developed a 6-week treatment program for depression that initially determines the deficit area that will be the focus of treatment. Treatment interventions focus on changing deficits in self-control behaviors by using self-monitoring, self-evaluation, and self-reinforcement techniques (Fuchs and Rehm 1977; Rehm et al. 1979).

Self-monitoring teaches patients how to monitor their moods and activities. This technique helps patients to identify areas in which they need to 1) learn more adaptive coping strategies and 2) recognize the activities that are associated with enjoyment.

Depressed patients engage in negative self-evaluations. Self-control therapy involves identifying patients specific self-evaluation deficit(s). These deficits vary and may involve unrealistic expectations and/or perfectionist standards about themselves addressed in therapy. Other patients may exhibit deficits in the area of self-reinforcement. At these times, therapists assist the patient in learning how to provide themselves with positive reinforcement and/or remove obstacles in the environment that may be blocking positive reinforcement. As with cognitive and other behavioral approaches, self-control therapists are active and directive, often instructing their patients and usually using homework assignments.

Variations of Cognitive and Behavioral Therapies

Cognitive and behavioral therapies have been modified, both singly and in combination, to accommodate different therapy formats (e.g., couples vs. individual), depressive subtypes (chronic vs. nonchronic), and patient populations (e.g., adult vs. adolescents) for the treatment of depression. For example, several forms of couples therapy have been developed that focus on the marital relationship to reduce depressive symptoms and to improve the quality of the relationship. Marital therapies, as in individual therapies, vary in their theoretical focus. That is, some marital therapies place more emphasis on Beck and colleagues' (1979) cognitive model (cognitive marital therapy [CMT], Teichman and Teichman, 1990; enhancing marital intimacy therapy [EMIT], Waring, 1988, 1994), whereas other forms of couples therapy place a greater emphasis on behavioral methods (behavioral marital therapy [BMT], Jacobson et al. 1991; O'Leary and Beach 1990) within the context of the marital relationship.

Similarly, cognitive and behavioral therapies have been adapted to a group format for the treatment of depressive disorders. For example, variations of group CT for the treatment of depression include: 1) Hollon and Shaw's (1979) model that transfers Beck et al.'s (1979) individual CT to a group format (Zettle et al. 1992); 2) Yost and colleagues' (1986) group cognitive behavior therapy (CBT), which incorporates both cognitive and behavioral procedures with a greater emphasis on Beck et al.'s (1979) CT (Beutler et al. 1991); and 3) group coping therapy (Wollersheim et al. 1980), which integrates ingredients of both standard CT (Beck et al. 1979) and Ellis' (1962) rational-emotive therapy (RET). However, group coping therapy reportedly focuses more extensively on emotions as compared with standard CT and RET (Wollersheim and Wilson 1991).

Behavioral therapies that have been tested and modified for the group treatment of depression include: 1) group structured learning therapy (a form of social skills training used with adolescents); 2) group problem-solving therapy, which focuses on teaching geriatric patients problem-solving skills that assist them in coping with stressful life events and continuous daily problems (Arean et al. 1993; Nezu 1986;

Nezu and Perri 1989); and 3) a coping with depression course, which is a cognitive-behavioral group intervention for adults (Lewinsohn et al. 1984) and adolescents, with and without their parents (Clarke and Lewinsohn 1989; Rohde et al. 1994).

Cognitive and behavioral orientations have been combined to address different variations of depression such as chronic depressions (McCullough 1991) and bipolar disorder in conjunction with medication management (Basco and Rush 1996).

Cognitive and behavioral treatments of depression also have been adapted to different patient populations. For example, standard CT has been modified for the individual treatment of depressed adolescents (Wilkes et al. 1994) and religious depressed patients (Propst et al. 1992). Behavioral therapy has been modified for the geriatric population and their caregivers (Gallagher and Thompson 1982; Gallagher-Thompson and Steffen 1994). In addition, problem-solving therapy has been varied for the treatment of depression in primary care patients (Mynors-Wallis et al. 1995), whereas self-control therapy has been incorporated into a standard psychiatric day treatment program (van den Hout et al. 1995). Regardless of the type of depression, treatment format, patient age, or treatment setting, several of the aims of cognitive and/or behavioral therapies, alone or with pharmacotherapy, remain the same.

Aims of Cognitive, Behavioral, and Pharmacotherapies

Symptom Resolution

The first phase of treatment for depression focuses on the reduction and amelioration of depressive symptoms. Although reduction of symptoms is required, remission of depressive symptoms is recommended and preferred, because a better prognosis is associated with full symptom remission than simply with a reduction in depressive symptoms (Rush and Trivedi 1995).

Psychosocial Restoration

Psychosocial restoration is often attained during acute phase treatment but may proceed into continuation phase treatment. By definition, major depressive disorders significantly impair patients' psychosocial and/or occupational functioning. Mintz and colleagues (1992) investigated the effects of treatments (psychotherapy and antidepressant medications) of depression and the functional capacity to work. Fifty-five percent of depressed outpatients reported significant functional work impairment during an acute depressive episode. Work impairment was classified into two categories: 1) behavioral or functional impairment as characterized by absenteeism, lack of productivity, and interpersonal problems, and 2) affective impairment as manifested by feelings of inadequacy, distress, and lack of interest. Results indicated that functional and affective impairment differed in that functional work impairment was worse in patients with more severe depressive symptoms, whereas affective impairment was prevalent in mild, moderate, and severe depressive episodes. Improved work restoration was significantly better for patients whose depressive symptoms had remitted. For patients whose symptoms had not remitted at the time of the assessment, results indicated better work outcomes occurred steadily over time as the duration of treatment increased from 4 to 6 months. The delay in recovery of functional capacity is similar to the findings on social adjustment in depression. For example, one report suggested that it takes approximately 6 to 8 months for the effects of interpersonal psychotherapy to effect improvement in social adjustment (Weissman et al. 1974).

Relapse Prevention

Continuation phase treatment aims at relapse prevention. During the continuation phase, patients use psychotherapeutic skills (e.g., symptom monitoring, problem-solving, cognitive restructuring) acquired during acute phase treatment to identify symptom breakthroughs and to prevent a relapse of a full-blown depressive episode. Health care providers also monitor patients' symptoms and functioning during the continuation phase to sustain or promote full psychosocial restoration, as well as to prevent a relapse. When patients, therapists, and/or prescribing physicians notice symptom breakthroughs or incomplete psychosocial restoration, therapy sessions and/or medication reevaluations may be temporarily increased to resolve these problems (Depression Guideline Panel 1993).

Recurrence Prevention

Maintenance phase treatment, whether with psychotherapy, medication, or a combination, aims at recurrence prevention. The frequency of psychotherapy visits during maintenance phase treatment varies but usually occurs once every 1 to 3 months depending upon patients clinical presentation, type of treatment, and therapists (Beck et al. 1979). Patients on maintenance medications generally see their prescribing physician every 2 to 3 months for medication management (Depression Guideline Panel 1993).

Recurrence prevention, regardless of the type of treatment, focuses on monitoring depressive symptoms, maintenance of unimpaired psychosocial functioning, treatment adherence to medication and/or psychotherapy visits and assignments, and reinforcement of patient education regarding course of the illness and treatment. When breakthrough symptoms and/or psychosocial difficulties are identified, treatment regimens are modified to prevent a recurrence of a full-blown depressive episode.

Adherence

Adherence to treatment, whether medication, psychotherapy, or a combination, is a concern that must be addressed in all phases of treatment. A review of the treatment adherence literature on mood disorders indicated a high prevalence of nonadherence to both psychotherapy and pharmacotherapy (Basco and Rush 1995; Persons et al. 1988). Persons and colleagues (1988) reported a 50% dropout rate of psychiatric outpatients receiving psychotherapy in private practices versus a 0%–31% dropout rate for psychiatric patients in clinical research protocols. Premature termination of antidepressant medication in patients with mood disorders, receiving pharmacotherapy alone or in conjunction with psychotherapy, range from 38% to 60% in psychiatric settings (Jacob et al. 1984; Overall et al. 1987; Park and Lipman 1964; Pugh 1983), as compared with 68% in general practice settings (Johnson 1981; see Basco & Rush 1995 for review). Studies assessing nonadherence to treatment in terms of missed appointments reported that 11%–12% of patients with mood disorders were likely to not keep their clinic appointment (Connelly 1984; Connelly et al. 1982; Kucera-Bozarth et al. 1982).

Treatment adherence has been estimated to vary from 4% to 90% in patients with mood disorders, depending upon what adherence measures (e.g., appointment attendance, medication blood levels, homework assignments) are being used to assess treatment adherence (Depression Guideline Panel 1993). These reports highlight the importance of addressing adherence in all patients who are receiving treatment for mood disorders.

If the issue of treatment adherence is ignored and patients are not consistent with the prescribed medical or psychological regimens, then lack of adherence to treatment will not only be misconstrued as a treatment failure, but can also lead to increased risk of relapse (Coppen et al. 1978; Kragh-Sorensen et al. 1976; Suppes et al. 1991), poor symptom control, unnecessary patient suffering, impaired psychosocial functioning, an increased need for emergency and inpatient services, and increased financial costs for patients and society (Depression Guideline Panel 1993; Greenberg et al. 1993; Lane and McDonald 1994; Meichenbaum and Turk 1987; Mintz et al. 1992).

No single diagnostic, demographic, or treatment related variable consistently predicts poor adherence to treatment (see Basco and Rush [1995] for review). However, the most reliable predictor of poor treatment adherence is a current comorbid psychiatric disorder, particularly substance use (Aagaard and Vestergaard 1980) and personality disorders (Depression Guideline Panel 1993). Specific psychiatric symptoms, such as endogenous and melancholic features (Last et al. 1985), psychotic symptoms (Wilson and Enoch 1967), grandiosity

(Lenzi et al. 1989), and hostility (Pugh 1983) have also been reported to reduce treatment adherence in patients with mood disorders.

The process and forms of treatments have also been associated with low treatment adherence. For example, the patient-clinician relationship (Connelly et al. 1982; Gitlin et al. 1989; Johnson 1981), the side effects of medications (Gitlin et al. 1989; Johnson 1973, 1981), the general idea of having to take medication (Jamison et al. 1979), as well as some pragmatic issues such as the time and transportation required to attend treatment appointments (Simons et al. 1984) contribute to poor treatment adherence.

Several investigations have reported that patient and family education regarding the diagnosis, course of illness, and its treatment improve adherence (Altamura and Mauri 1985; Anderson et al. 1986; Myers and Calvert 1984; Peet and Harvey 1991; Seltzer et al. 1980; Van Gent and Zwart 1991; Youssel 1983). Common elements of these educational groups seem to include didactics; written information on the illness and treatment; opportunity to discuss the illness and treatment regimen; and a forum to discuss, share, and normalize the difficulties commonly associated with adhering to a prescribed treatment regimen.

Psychosocial treatments, such as cognitive and behavior therapies alone or in combination with pharmacotherapy, have also been found to facilitate treatment adherence in patients with mood disorders (see Basco and Rush [1995] for a review; Meichenbaum and Turk 1987). Psychotherapeutic interventions not only focus on educating the patients and, when appropriate, families and significant others, on the diagnosis, course of illness, and the treatment, but also address adherence problems directly, assist patients with developing strategies to facilitate treatment adherence (e.g., complying with therapy assignments, behavioral experiments, or taking medications), provide emotional support, teach patients how to identify the early warning signs of relapse, recurrence , or symptom breakthroughs, and assist patients in coping with psychosocial, occupational, and interpersonal problems (Cochran 1984; Davenport et al. 1977; Powell et al. 1977; Schwarcz and Silbergeld 1983; Shakir et al. 1979; Wulsin et al. 1988).

Evidence for the Efficacy of CT

Acute Phase Treatment

Table 6–1 summarizes the studies of acute phase treatment for depression with CT that were included in the Depression Guideline Panel's (1993) meta-analysis. The panel used the confidence profile method (CPM) (Eddy et al. 1990; Hasselblad and Eddy 1992) to analyze the studies that met specified inclusion criteria. Studies on acute phase CT reported in peer-reviewed journals (with data for the intent-to-treat [ITT] samples) were included in the analyses. These studies involved randomized controlled trial (RCT) methodology, patients diagnosed by some specified diagnostic system (e.g., research diagnostic criteria [RDC; Endicott and Spitzer 1978] or DSM-III-R [American Psychiatric Association 1987]), and a standard depression symptom severity outcome measure (e.g., Hamilton Rating Scale for Depression [HRSD; Hamilton 1960, 1968], Clinician Global Impression [CGI; Guy 1976], Beck Depression Inventory [BDI; Beck et al. 1961]). Table 6–1 presents the overall efficacy for each type of therapy in the first row and then compares each therapy to other conditions (e.g., therapy vs. wait list) in the second and subsequent rows.

TABLE 6–1

Meta-analyses of cognitive and behavioral psychotherapy trials in outpatients with major depressive disorder

	BT alone[a]			CT alone		
Condition	%	SD	No. of cells	%	SD	No. of cells
Overall efficacy	55.3	9.3	10	46.6	6.9	12
Therapy vs. wait list	17.1	34.0	5	30.1	22.0	2
Therapy vs. placebo	NA	NA	NA	9.4	8.3	1
Therapy vs. other therapy	9.1	19.9	6	−4.4	16.9	6
Therapy vs. drug alone	23.9	11.6	2	15.3	26.1	3

Note. *Both are ITT samples with adult and geriatric patient studies combined.*
[a] *Includes one cell with behavioral therapy plus placebo (Hersen et al. 1984).*
Source. *Adapted from Depression Guideline Panel (1993).*

Altogether, 22 studies from 1966 through 1990 investigated the efficacy of acute phase CT for major depression (Beck et al. 1985; Blackburn et al. 1981; Covi and Lipman 1987; de Jong et al. 1986; Elkin et al. 1989; Gallagher and Thompson 1982; Hogg and Deffenbacher 1988; Murphy et al. 1984; Neimeyer and Feixas 1990; Neimeyer and Weiss 1990; Neimeyer et al. 1985; O'Leary and Beach 1990; Pecheur and Edwards 1984; Ross and Scott 1985; Rush and Watkins 1981; Rush et al. 1977; Scott and Stradling 1990 [two trials]; Selmi et al. 1990; Steuer et al. 1984; Thompson et al. 1987; Turner and Wehl 1984). Of the 22 studies, 12 met the meta-analytic inclusion criteria. The CPM analysis indicated an overall efficacy of 46.6% response rate for acute phase CT with outpatients, using a 50% reduction in the initial symptom severity rating scale (e.g., BDI), or a CGI score of 1 or 2. The only inpatient study of CT (de Jong et al. 1986) available for CPM analysis reported a 58.3% response rate to treatment (Depression Guideline Panel 1993).

Efficacy studies using acute phase CT with geriatric patients have also been reported to be efficacious (51.3%) in the treatment of depressive disorders (Depression Guideline Panel 1993; Gallagher and Thompson 1982; Gallagher-Thompson and Steffen 1994; Gallagher-Thompson et al. 1990; Steuer et al. 1984; Thompson and Gallagher 1984; Thompson et al. 1987). However, for the purposes of the meta-analysis, all acute phase treatment studies of CT with older adults were combined with similar studies that assessed other adult samples (18 to 65 years of age). This method does not imply that the Depression Guideline Panel (1993) was insensitive to the unique issues that must be addressed in the cognitive treatment plans for older adult samples, but rather the number of geriatric studies were few and there were no data to suggest significant differences between geriatric and younger adult samples.

Several significant CT treatment studies for depression that either did not meet the inclusion criteria or were published following the review warrant discussion. The Edinburgh primary care depression study was a prospective RCT that compared amitriptyline (AMI) as administered by a psychiatrist, cognitive behavior therapy (CT) provided by a clinical psychologist (CT), counseling conducted by a social worker (COUNSEL), and routine care provided by a general practitioner (GP) (Scott and Freeman 1992). The study included 14 primary care practices that received referrals from 37 general practitioners. One hundred and twenty-one patients with major depression according to DSM-III (American Psychiatric Association 1980) criteria were randomly assigned to one of the four treatment cells: AMI = 31, CT = 30, COUNSEL = 30, and GP = 30. The results, using data provided from the article and calculating the response rate based on the ITT sample (with response defined as an HRSD score <7), revealed the following response rates after 16 weeks of treatment: AMI = 48.8% (15/31), CT = 40.0% (12/30), COUNSEL = 70.0% (21/30), and GP = 46.7% (14/30). Although the ITT efficacy rates are lower than the response rates based on completer samples (which would be expected), the response rates for each treatment, regardless of the type of analyses used, all appear to significantly reduce depressive symptoms. Response rates for the completer samples were AMI = 58% (15/26); CT = 41% (12/29); COUNSEL = 72% (21/29), and GP = 48% (14/29). However, the counseling by a social worker was significantly better in reducing depressive symptoms when compared with other treatments (Scott and Freeman 1992). In terms of patient preferences with treatment, patients in the counseling condition rated this form of treatment more acceptable and helpful as compared with patient ratings of the other treatment conditions. Interestingly, this investigation also revealed that specialist treatments required four times more therapist contact and cost twice as much as routine general practitioner care, which suggested that the advantages of specialist care as compared with general practitioner care were small. This study highlights the need for future studies to address how health care professionals can provide the most acceptable and effective treatments to patients, while reducing unnecessary health care costs.

Teichman and Teichman (1990) developed CMT as an integration of traditional CT and marital therapy that focuses on systemic issues to treat depression. The efficacy of CMT was compared with individual CT and to no treatment (NT, or waiting list control group) in outpatients with major depression or dysthymia (Teichman et al. 1995). Fifty-six patients were assigned to the following conditions: CMT = 18, CT = 19, and NT = 19. A BDI score of 10 was used to define response. Based on the response criteria and our ITT calculations, the

CMT group evidenced more treatment responders (55.6% or 10/18) than the CT (10.6% or 2/19) or NT (10.6% or 2/19) groups. However, at 6-month follow-up our ITT calculations revealed a loss of treatment effects in the CMT condition (38.9% or 7/18) and an increase in treatment effects in the CT condition (26.3% or 5/19) (Y. Teichman, personal communication, February 5, 1996). These findings were consistent with the completer analyses reported elsewhere (Teichman et al. 1995). The low response rates in the CT cell were inconsistent with previous studies, which bring into question the application of the CT treatment in this study. However, these results provide support for a new form of CMT that warrants further investigation. Perhaps an emphasis on relapse prevention might be considered in future investigations of CMT in the treatment of depression in an effort to reduce the loss of treatment effects.

Waring (1988) developed EMIT as a brief, structured, cognitively oriented therapy that focuses on facilitating patients self-disclosure of personal constructs to their spouses in order to reduce depressive symptoms and enhance marital intimacy and adjustment. In a pilot study, the EMIT ($n = 5$ couples) group was compared with a waiting list control group ($n = 4$ couples) for 10 weeks in the treatment of depressed married women (Waring 1994; Waring et al. 1995). The results indicated that EMIT alone significantly reduced depressive symptomatology, as assessed by the pre- and posttreatment scores on the HRSD and the BDI, when compared with the control condition. A serious limitation to this study was the small sample size. However, further studies to compare EMIT to both a control condition and established efficacious treatments for depression, such as standard CT, interpersonal psychotherapy (IPT; Klerman et al. 1984), BMT, or CMT are warranted.

Many psychotherapies for depression have been modified and applied to a group format. Beutler and colleagues (1991) compared group cognitive behavior therapy (CT: modification of Beck et al.'s [1979] protocol), focused expressive psychotherapy (FEP or gestalt-based group therapy), and a supportive, self-directed therapy (S/SD). Eighty-one outpatients with major depressive disorder were entered into one of the three treatment conditions (CT = 29; FEP = 30, S/SD = 22) (L. E. Beutler, personal communication, March 4, 1996). Sixty-three patients comprised the final sample with 21 patients in CT, 22 patients in FEP, and 20 patients in S/SD. Overall, the final sample indicated that all treatments provided approximately equivalent and positive effects as evidenced by a HRSD score ≤10 in 58% of all subjects. A trend in the treatment main effects was noted to be slightly in favor of CT.

However, the main focus of this study was on predictors of differential response to the three treatment conditions based on patient characteristics, such as coping style (externalization) and resistance potential. Patients defined as having externalizing coping styles were described as having difficulty controlling stress, problems with irritability, poor impulse control, and a tendency to place blame on others. Resistance potential was characterized by patients needing control and having a tendency to be socially defensive and anxious.

Results revealed that patient characteristics interacted with treatments and should be considered by clinicians when recommending a specific form of therapy for a patient. Specifically, the results indicated that depressed patients who used a coping style of externalization, as compared with those who did not, responded better to CT. In contrast, nonexternalizing patients responded better to S/SD. Resistant patients improved most in the S/SD group, as compared with the CT and FEP groups. In contrast, less resistant patients showed a better response to CT than to S/SD.

The main treatment effects of this study were consistent with those of most other psychotherapy efficacy studies and provided support for using group treatments as a viable option for the treatment of depression. In addition, this study suggested that patient characteristics influence treatment outcomes and as a result require further study and consideration by clinicians during treatment planning (i.e., matching type of therapy with the type of patient may well substantially improve overall outcome).

In a comparison of individual and group CT in outpatients with depression, Zettle and colleagues (1992) reported that both groups evidenced significant improvement in depressive symptomatology as indicated by a significant reduction in posttreatment BDI and HRSD scores. However, no significant differences were noted between groups on depression outcome measures. Response rates by groups using an

ITT calculation were as follows: 64% (9 of 14, including dropouts) for individual CT, and 60% (9 of 15, including dropouts) for group CT (R. D. Zettle, personnel communication, February 16, 1996). Whereas both groups evidenced improvement from pre- to posttreatment on the BDI, only the patients in group CT showed a significant reduction on the BDI from posttreatment to 2-month follow-up.[1]

Wollersheim and Wilson (1991) conducted an investigation that assessed group treatment of unipolar depression over a 10-week period by comparing four treatments: coping therapy, supportive therapy, bibliotherapy, and delayed treatment. Coping therapy, a form of cognitive behavioral therapy, is similar to the therapeutic modalities of Ellis (1962) and Beck et al. (1979), but it differs in that it "focuses more extensively on emotions" (Wollersheim and Wilson 1991). This investigation revealed improvements in depression based on a significant reduction in BDI scores from pre- to posttreatment in all three active treatments. Response rates based on ITT samples, and a BDI score of ≤ 10 to define response, revealed the following treatment efficacies: 38% in the coping group, 13% in the supportive group, 50% in the bibliotherapy group, and 13% in the delayed treatment condition. Although depressive symptoms were reduced in all active treatments, the results did not support the hypothesis that either coping or supportive therapy was more efficacious than bibliotherapy or a control condition, but given the small sample size (N = 32 with 8 subjects in each group), the study may fail to discriminate between treatment conditions.

Few treatment outcome studies of depression have addressed religious issues or orientations with patients and/or therapists. Propst and colleagues (1992) conducted a unique clinical trial that assessed the efficacy of religious and nonreligious cognitive-behavioral therapy for the treatment of depression in religious patients. Patients were randomly assigned to one of six groups: religious cognitive-behavioral therapy–nonreligious therapist (ReCT-NT), religious cognitive-behavioral therapy–religious therapist (ReCT-RT), nonreligious (standard) cognitive-behavioral therapy–religious therapist (NReCT-RT), nonreligious (standard) cognitive-behavioral therapy–nonreligious

---

1. A limitation of this investigation was that it included only females.

therapist (NReCT-NT), a pastoral counseling treatment with only religious therapists (PCT), or a waiting list condition (WLC). Without assessing for therapist effects, the ReCT groups reported significant reduction of depressive symptoms (BDI <10) as compared with the WLC group. However, a nonsignificant trend of lower BDI scores was exhibited in the NReCT and PCT conditions when compared with the WLC condition. Using the reliable change index as a measure of clinically significant differences, the proportion of patients in each group that evidenced a clinically meaningful change from pre- to post-treatment was 80% for PCT and 68% for ReCT, as compared with 27% for the WLC. When treatment and therapist effects were both analyzed, results indicated an interaction that suggested a difference between religious and nonreligious therapists, with the nonreligious therapists performing better in the ReCT condition than in the NReCT condition. Overall, religious patients who received ReCT reported a greater reduction in depressive symptoms than did religious patients in the standard CT condition regardless of religious status of the therapist. This study provides a limited amount of support for the efficacy of religious CT in a small subsample of religious patients — a finding consistent with the notion of matching therapy and patient to improve outcome. A significant limitation of this study was all therapists were graduate students in training and had little therapy experience (e.g., "at least one prior practicum") and no previous training in CT.

Little information is known about the predictors of response or nonresponse to CT for depression (Sotsky et al. 1991). The Depression Guideline Panel (1993) review indicated that CT studies yielded mixed results regarding its treatment of major depression with melancholic features, but strong evidence to support the treatment of depression with melancholic features with pharmacotherapy. Other psychobiological correlates reportedly related to poorer response to CT are unemployment, abnormal electroencephalographic sleep profiles (Thase et al. 1993), marital status (single vs. married), and higher pretreatment symptom severity scores (e.g., BDI) (Jarrett et al. 1991; Thase et al. 1993).

Patients with comorbid conditions, such as personality disorders, have also been reported to be less responsive or slower to respond to

CT (Depression Guideline Panel 1993; Fennell and Teasdale 1982; Frank et al. 1987; Scott 1992), whereas patients without personality disorders have been reported to have a better response to CT (Pilkonis and Frank 1988). Other reports on the predictors of response to CT indicated that patients with better emotional health and social adjustment may respond better in CT (Rounsaville et al. 1981), whereas a poorer response to CT has been noted in patients with persistent marital discord or severe interpersonal problems (Robins and Hayes 1993).

The experience of the therapist has also been associated with response to CT for depression. That is, therapists with more experience (four or more years) who exhibit a high level of competence (Burns and Nolen-Hoeksema 1992), as well as those who adhere to the cognitive model, tend to have better patient outcomes (DeRubeis and Feeley 1990).

A review CT in chronically depressed outpatients indicated that greater chronicity was associated with slower and less complete responses to CT (see Markowitz [1994] for review; Thase et al. 1993, 1994). Markowitz's (1994) review of seven studies reported a 41% response rate to CT in chronically depressed patients. These findings should be interpreted cautiously because they are based on a small number of studies with small sample sizes, varying lengths of treatment, inclusion of both inpatient and outpatient studies, and a variety of forms of CT.

The use of CT in children and adolescents is currently under development and empirical scrutiny. Wilkes and colleagues (1994) developed a treatment manual for depressed adolescents. Pilot data on this treatment intervention look promising, but no RCTs of CT in depressed juveniles have been reported (Belsher et al. 1995).

Continuation Phase Treatment

Continuation phase treatment aims to reduce the risk of relapse following acute phase treatment. No RCTs of CT for depression have been reported. Naturalistic follow-up studies suggest that a significant portion of patients (e.g., 12%–50%) with residual symptoms following acute phase treatment experience a relapse within 6–12 months

(Blackburn, et al. 1986; Evans et al. 1992; Kovacs et al. 1981; Thase et al. 1992). These findings suggest that continuation phase CT may be indicated especially for patients who exhibit lingering depressive symptoms or incomplete interepisode remission following acute phase treatment.

Two open studies that provided continuation phase CT suggest that it may improve outcomes and reduce relapse rates (e.g., 12%–20%) (Blackburn et al. 1981; Jarrett et al. 1992), though no randomized control groups were used.

A continuation phase study of patients who had been successfully treated with pharmacotherapy, who were then randomized either to CT or clinical management (CM) for residual depressive symptoms, indicated that patients who received CT had a lower rate of relapse (15%) than those who received CM at 2- (35%) and 4-year (70%) follow-ups (Fava et al. 1994; 1996). Whether continuation phase treatment is called for is unclear. However, preliminary data clearly support further empirical study.

Maintenance Phase Treatment

Maintenance phase treatment focuses on preventing a recurrence of a new depressive episode. To date, there are no randomized controlled maintenance phase trials with CT for the treatment of depression. However, CT may be an alternative form of treatment to be considered during maintenance phase treatment with individuals who have recurrent depression and have previously responded to medication plus psychotherapy, but are currently unable to continue pharmacotherapy (e.g., women trying to become pregnant; surgery) (Depression Guideline Panel 1993).

Evidence for the Efficacy of Behavior Therapy (BT)

Acute Phase Treatment

Table 6–1 also reviews reports on the efficacy of BT as defined by RCTs, use of a valid diagnostic classification system of major depressive disorder (e.g., RDC or DSM-III-R), ITT samples, and categorical out-come measures (e.g., BDI) when available (Brown and Lewinsohn 1984; Gallagher and Thompson 1982; Hersen et al. 1984; Kornblith et al. 1983; McLean and Hakstian 1979; Nezu 1986; Nezu and Perri 1989; Rabin et al. 1984; Rehm et al. 1981; Roth et al. 1982; Rude 1986; Teri and Lewinsohn 1986; Thompson et al. 1987; Usaf and Kavanagh 1990). The analyses combined adult and geriatric samples. Overall efficacy was 55.3% for BT, which was more effective than wait list controls (see Table 6–1).

Several studies that did not meet the meta-analytic inclusion criteria or were published following the report are important to consider when evaluating the treatment of depression. Mynors-Wallis and colleagues (1995) conducted a 12-week acute phase randomized controlled comparison of problem-solving therapy (PST), amitriptyline (AMI), and placebo plus clinical management (PLAC) for the treatment of major depression in a primary care setting. Both PST and AMI were equivalently effective and both exceeded the effects of PLAC in reducing depressive symptoms. Remission rates were calculated based on a BDI score of ≤ 8 and for subjects who received adequate exposure to treatment as defined by attendance of four or more treatment sessions. The remission rates by treatment condition were: 57% for PST group ($n = 30$), 36% for the AMI group ($n = 31$), and 30% for the PLAC group ($n = 30$).

Jacobson and colleagues (1991) conducted an acute phase treatment study comparing CT, BMT, and the combination of both in the treatment of married women with depression. Results revealed that all three treatment modalities were effective in reducing depressive symptoms. When couples were split into maritally distressed versus nondistressed groups, the nondistressed couples evidenced a significantly better response to CT as compared with BMT; whereas, the maritally distressed couples responded equally to both CT and BMT. Combination treatment did not appear more effective than either CT or BMT. An estimation of response rates (weighted average) by treatment cell indicated that 67%–83% of CT subjects responded to treatment, 48%–78% of subjects responded to BMT, and 57% of the subjects receiving the combination responded to treatment. Although this study supports several forms of psychotherapy in the treatment of certain subsamples of individuals with depression, these results should be interpreted cautiously because this investigation did not include a control condition.

Another study comparing the treatment of depression in couples with and without marital discord, examined the comparative efficacy of CT, BMT, and a waiting list control (WLC) in married women with depression. Preliminary findings of this study were previously reported with an incomplete sample (O'Leary and Beach 1990). The final report indicated that 45 couples were randomly assigned to either CT ($n = 15$), BMT ($n = 15$), or WLC ($n = 15$). At the end of 15 weeks of outpatient treatment, both CT and BMT significantly reduced depressive symptomatology more than WLC. No significant differences were reported between the two treatment cells. However, wives in BMT reported better marital adjustment following treatment as compared with CT or the WLC. These differences are not surprising given that BMT specifically focuses on enhancing the marital relationship, whereas CT does not. An ITT analysis of this study indicated equivalent response rates in the treatment conditions (46.6%) as compared with the WLC (13.3%) based on a BDI score <10 (S. R. H. Beach, personal communication, February 19, 1996).

With respect to overall treatment effects and improved marital adjustment following BMT for the treatment of married women with depression, the results of this study are consistent with Jacobson et al.'s (1991) report (Beach and O'Leary 1992). However, these two studies reported contradictory findings with regard to CT's impact on spouses' adjustment or satisfaction with their marriages following treatment. Thus, it seems clear that additional empirical investigations are needed prior to concluding that CT does or does not improve marital satisfaction or adjustment in depressed spouses who report marital discord. A study on group psychotherapies for the treatment of depression compared three forms of self-control therapy (behavioral, cognitive, and a combination of cognitive and behavioral components) for the treatment of major depression in female volunteers (Rabin et al. 1984). Ninety-eight subjects were randomized to one of the three groups and received 10 weeks of structured group therapy. The specific number of subjects per cell was not reported; however, no differences were noted between groups. All treatments were equally effective in reducing depressive symptomatology as measured by a reduction in BDI scores. The results also revealed a significant reduction in symptoms in the first 3 to 4 weeks of treatment.

Several limitations are evident in this study. First, no control condition was used. Second, only one measure of depressive symptomatology (BDI) was employed, which limits the generalizability of the study given the BDI's narrow focus on depressive symptoms (e.g., absence questions that assess an increase in appetite or sleep). However, the comparative effects of treatment rendered by this study are consistent with the literature.

Arean and colleagues (1993) conducted an RCT that compared the efficacy of problem-solving group therapy (PST) ($n = 28$), reminiscence group therapy (RT) ($n = 27$), and waiting list control (WLC) ($n = 20$) in a sample of geriatric patients ($N = 75$) with major depressive disorder. Response to treatment was assessed by significant changes in HRSD and BDI scores prior to and following the 12-week trial. Results indicated that PST and RT were equal, and each was significantly more effective than WLC in reducing the severity of depressive symptoms. The proportion of subjects assigned to each cell who did not meet posttreatment criteria for a major depressive disorder was used to calculate response rates. A significantly greater percentage of subjects in the PST group (61%) did not endorse a depressive syndrome as compared with the RT (30%) and WLC groups (10%). This study supports the overall efficacy of PST in the treatment of late-life depression in that following treatment, 64% *of all completers* were classified as improved or in remission. These response rates are consistent with other investigations of psychotherapy for depression in the elderly (Beutler et al. 1987; Thompson et al. 1987).

Gallagher-Thompson and Steffen (1994) assessed the comparative effects of CT and brief psychodynamic psychotherapy (BPD) with depressed family caregivers of the elderly. Sixty-six depressed outpatient caregivers were randomly assigned to 20 sessions of one of the two individual treatment conditions. Response rates were evaluated by the presence of a depressive syndrome according to RDC. Overall, 71% of all patients responded to treatment and no significant differences were reported between CT (77% remission) and BPD (62% remission) (ITT samples). Results also indicated that patients who had been caregivers for a longer period of time (>44 months) responded better to CT, whereas patients who had been caregivers for a shorter period of time evidenced a better response to BPD. This study supports the efficacy of CT and BPD and highlights the importance of considering specific patient characteristics in the treatment planning of caregivers with depression.

The work of Shapiro and colleagues (1994) compared individual CT, with an emphasis on behavioral components, with individual psychodynamic-interpersonal psychotherapy (PI) in the treatment of 117 outpatients with depression. The two treatments were conducted for either 8 or 16 weeks, resulting in four treatment conditions (i.e., 8 weeks CT, 16 weeks CT, 8 weeks PI, and 16 weeks PI). Patients were randomly assigned to one of these four treatment conditions stratified by severity of depression (e.g., mild, moderate, and severe).

CT and PI were equally effective in the treatment of depression, regardless of depressive severity or length of treatment. However, a slight benefit was noted for CT as evidenced by the BDI. Given that the BDI was developed based on the CT model of depression, it is not surprising that it evidenced a slight advantage to PI in the treatment of depression. However, this finding does not support a significant advantage of CT over PI, but rather should be considered cautiously.

An evaluation of the treatment cells using an ITT sample revealed the following response rates based on a posttreatment BDI scores of <9: 8 weeks CT had a 42.4% response rate, 16 weeks CT had a 50.0% response rate, 8 weeks PI had a 32.4% response rate, and 16 weeks PI had a 44.1% response rate (D. A. Shapiro and M. Barkham, personal communication, February 12, 1996). As expected, the ITT sample response rates were somewhat lower than the completer response rates as noted in Shapiro et al. (1994). Further comparative studies of CT and PI for the treatment of depression and inclusion of this study's results in future meta-analyses should be considered.

The work of van den Hout and colleagues (1995) assessed the efficacy of a self-control program in a psychiatric day treatment center. Twenty-five patients diagnosed with depression were randomly assigned to either standard day treatment or standard day treatment plus self-control therapy for 12 weeks. Following treatment, patients in the combination treatment evidenced more improvement in depression, self-esteem, self-control, and a greater potential to enjoy pleasant events as compared with the standard treatment group. However, at the 13-week follow-up, between-group differences were no longer significant, except on self-control. The follow-up results provide support for evaluating the efficacy of standard day treatment plus self-control therapy during the continuation and maintenance phases to prevent the loss of treatment gains.

There are no clear indicators that predict response or nonresponse to BT, although endogenous forms of depression may do less well (Thompson and Gallagher 1984). Older patients with mild and moderate depressions (compared with more severe depressions) have been reported to respond more quickly to BT, CT, and BPD (Thompson and Gallagher 1984). In contrast, Thase and colleagues (1991) reported no differences in the response of endogenous versus nonendogenous depressions to CBT. The mixed findings in the literature prevent any firm conclusions on which variables consistently predict a response to BT.

Reed (1994) evaluated the efficacy of structured learning therapy (SLT), a form of social skills training, in the group treatment of depression in adolescents. The results indicated that SLT consistently reduced depressive symptoms in males as compared with a control group. However, female subjects did not report a significant reduction in depressive symptoms when compared with control subjects.

Rohde et al. (1994) compared two forms of group CBT (with an emphasis on behavioral techniques) (adolescents only and adolescents and parent groups) and a waiting list control group with two samples of adolescents, ages 14 to 18, who met criteria for major depressive disorder (by DSM-III and DSM-III-R, respectively). Outcome measures to monitor depressive symptoms included the BDI and the Center for Epidemiologic Studies-Depression Scale (CES-D; Radloff 1977) for samples 1 and 2, and the HRSD for sample 2. Comparison of the experimental and control conditions in sample 1 indicated that the two CBT group treatments were significantly better in reducing depressive symptoms than the waiting list control group using the BDI and CES-D. Results for sample 2 revealed that the two active treatment conditions were superior to waiting list control group in reducing depressive symptoms in a subset of subjects with a high severity of depression on the BDI, HRSD, and CES-D. However, no significant differences were found in the sample 2 group (subjects with low severity depression) as compared with the control condition. Contrary to the authors' hypothesis, an accentuated treatment effect in adolescents with more severe depression was evidenced only in one of the two samples.

Lewinsohn et al. (1990) conducted a school-based RCT with adolescents, ages 14 to 18, who met criteria (DSM-III or RDC) for major depressive disorder. The CBT intervention has a behavioral emphasis and was adapted for adolescents. The CBT intervention consisted of a 7-week psychoeducational course aimed at reducing depressive symptomatology and improving psychosocial functioning (Clarke and Lewinsohn 1989). The three comparison groups consisted of: 1) group CBT with adolescents only, 2) group CBT with adolescents and parents, and 3) a waiting list control group (WLC). Severity of depression was measured using the BDI and CES-D. Both CBT groups were superior to WLC in reducing depressive symptoms on both symptom severity measures.

Continuation and Maintenance Phase Treatment

There are no RCTs of BT alone that have assessed the efficacy and utility of continuing BT following a response to acute phase treatment to prevent relapse. Similarly, there are no RCTs that have evaluated the efficacy and utility of BT alone in the prevention of a recurrence of depression during the maintenance phase. Whether continuation and maintenance phase treatments with BT for depression are called for has yet to be determined.

Evidence for Efficacy of Combination Therapy

Acute Phase Treatment

Table 6–2 summarizes the RCTs for combined treatment using medication and a time-limited form of psychotherapy. The overall efficacy

TABLE 6–2

Meta-analyses of combined treatment in outpatients with major depressive disorder

Condition	BT plus medication			CT plus medication		
	%	SD	No. of cells	%	SD	No. of cells
Combination efficacy	34.6	10.9	2	53.7	17.3	5
Combination vs. wait list or placebo	NA	NA	NA	NA	NA	NA
Combination vs. therapy alone[a]	−7.4	22.3	2	6.4	15.3	6
Combination vs. other therapy alone[b]	−2.2	11.5	1	35.4	9.4	1
Combination vs. drug alone	6.2	11.4	1	39.4	32.9	2

Note. *Both BT and CT combinations are ITT samples.*

[a] *Indicated therapy plus medication versus therapy alone (e.g., BT plus medication vs. BT alone).*

[b] *Therapy plus medication was compared with a different form of psychotherapy alone.*

Source. *Adapted from Depression Guideline Panel (1993).*

for BT plus medication was 34.6% (2 studies); the combination of CT plus medication was 53.7% (5 studies) (Depression Guideline Panel 1993). Studies comparing psychotherapy alone to the combination have generally indicated that combined treatment modalities are equivalent in the treatment of mild to moderate depressive disorders (Beck et al. 1985; Covi and Lipman 1987; Hersen et al. 1984; Murphy et al. 1984; Roth et al. 1982; Rush and Watkins 1981). Overall, combination treatments for the treatment of major depressive disorder appear roughly equivalent to pharmacotherapy alone and to psychotherapy alone (Depression Guideline Panel 1993).

A pivotal study that did not meet inclusion or exclusion criteria for the Depression Guideline Panel's meta-analysis on combination treatment for depression was conducted by Blackburn and colleagues (1981). Patients were referred to the study from a general practice setting ($n = 39$) and a psychiatric outpatient clinic ($n = 49$). All subjects were randomly assigned to one of the three treatment conditions. Comparison groups were CT alone, pharmacotherapy alone, and CT plus medication. CT was minimally more effective when compared with pharmacotherapy alone in general practice patients. The combination treatment accounted for the largest degree of improvement in depression with the general practice patient sample. Treatment effects in general practice settings showed a greater response to CT alone or in combination with antidepressants as compared with drugs alone. There were no significant differences noted among the three treatment conditions for the psychiatric outpatient sample. However, the data did reveal a trend that favored the combination treatment for this group. These findings suggest differential treatment effects may be due to chronicity, severity, or prior treatment failure (general practice vs. psychiatric outpatient clinics) that may be associated or perhaps accounted for by the type of treatment setting.

Several studies of combination treatment in depression have been reported since the Depression Guideline Panel (1993) report. Hollon and colleagues (1992a) compared the efficacy of CT and pharmacotherapy for depression singly and in combination in 107 depressed outpatients over 12 weeks. The study groups were: 1) imipramine hydrochloride alone (drug), 2) CT alone, and 3) combination of CT plus drug. Response was defined by a BDI score <10 or a HRSD score <7. The results indicated that CT (44% response), drug (40% response), and the combination treatment (48% response) did not differ in terms of overall efficacy based on BDI scores (ITT samples). The study supports the equivalent efficacy of both pharmacotherapy and psychotherapy even in the outpatients with more severe depression and does not maintain significantly greater efficacy for combined treatment. However, in the absence of comparable control conditions (e.g., placebo control), results must be interpreted with caution.

Wilson and colleagues (1995) examined the long-term effects of CT and lithium therapy on depression in the elderly. The study included three phases: acute, continuation, and maintenance. The acute phase consisted of a treatment as usual group and treatment as usual plus CT. Once patients achieved a HRSD ≤17, they were entered into a 6-month continuation phase treatment. At the conclusion of continuation treatment, patients with a HRSD ≤17 were entered into the 12-month maintenance phase. Maintenance treatment included discontinuation of antidepressant medications. Patients were then entered into a double-blind, placebo-controlled, lithium carbonate therapy. Patients in the treatment as usual plus CT condition received booster CT sessions every 6 months during the maintenance phase. The results indicated that patients receiving treatment as usual plus CT evidenced fewer depressive symptoms following both acute and continuation treatment as compared with the treatment as usual group. No significant treatment effects were noted between the lithium and placebo-control groups during maintenance treatment.

Table 6–3 provides suggestions as to when and under what conditions combination treatment might be preferable (Depression Guideline Panel 1993). No RCTs have been conducted that specifically evaluate these recommendations for when this combined approach might be preferentially effective.

Continuation and Maintenance Phase Treatment

There are no RCTs that compare combination treatment during either continuation or maintenance phases of treatment for depression.

Cognitive, Behavioral, and Combination Posttreatment Outcomes

Post–acute phase treatment outcomes have largely been evaluated naturalistically. The lack of controlled follow-up studies prevent any firm conclusions regarding posttreatment outcomes for the treatment of depression. However, naturalistic studies do provide some preliminary findings worth considering, albeit cautiously.

Posttreatment outcomes (naturalistic) following CT are mixed. There appears to be a trend for CT patients to report fewer depressive symptoms at 1- and 2-year follow-up as compared with pharmacotherapy or wait-list control groups (see Depression Guideline Panel [1993] and Hollon et al. [1992b] for more detailed reviews) (Beck et al. 1985;

TABLE 6–3

Considerations for combined treatment

A. Consider combined treatment as an initial option more strongly if
    (1) history reveals a partial response to a full trial of either treatment alone.
    (2) current episode of major depression is longer than 2 years.
    (3) patient has a history of two or more episodes with poor interepisode recovery.
    (4) significant psychosocial difficulties are present that interfere with adherence *and* indications for medication are present.
    (5) patient requests it.
B. Add medication to psychotherapy if patient shows poor response to psychotherapy alone after 6 weeks or only a partial response after 12 weeks; if no response at all to psychotherapy, it may be discontinued and clinical management provided.
C. Add psychotherapy to medication (if medication has been used optimally) if
    (1) patient shows partial response to medication and residual symptoms are largely psychological (e.g., low self-esteem).
    (2) patient shows partial or complete response to medication and psychosocial problems remain significant.
    (3) patient has difficulty with adherence.

Source. *Adapted from Depression Guideline Panel (1993), Vol 2, p 90.*

Blackburn et al. 1986; Evans et al. 1992; Gallagher and Thompson 1982; Gallagher-Thompson et al. 1990; Kovacs et al. 1981; O'Leary and Beach 1990; Ross and Scott 1985; Scott and Stradling 1990; Shea et al. 1992; Simons et al. 1986). No differences were reported between groups (CT, IPT, pharmacotherapy alone, and placebo coupled with clinical management) on the proportion of self-reported depressive symptoms in the NIMH Collaborative Study (Elkin et al. 1989) at 18-month follow-up (Shea et al. 1992).

Naturalistic post–acute phase treatment outcome studies following BT also reveal mixed results, although fewer such studies are available for BT as compared with CT (Brown and Lewinsohn 1984; Gallagher and Thompson 1982; Gallagher-Thompson et al. 1990; McLean and Hakstian 1990) (see Depression Guideline Panel [1993] for more detailed review). A more recent study, not included in the Depression Guideline Panel report, revealed that at 1-year follow-up, treatment responders (contacted by mail) reported that 8 and 16 weeks of CBT and 16 weeks of psychodynamic-interpersonal therapy (PI) were more efficacious than 8 weeks of PI in the maintenance of treatment gains (i.e., fewer self-reported depressive symptoms) (Shapiro et al. 1995).

Two uncontrolled studies have investigated the effects of acute phase treatment of depression using BMT at 1-year follow-up (Beach and O'Leary 1992; Jacobson et al. 1993). No significant differences were found between BMT and CT groups (S. R. H. Beach, personal communication, February 19, 1996; Beach and O'Leary 1992), or BMT, individual CT, or standard CT (Jacobson et al. 1993).

Results of naturalistic follow-up studies of responders to the combination of medication and psychotherapy for acute phase treatment also revealed mixed findings (Beck et al. 1985; Blackburn et al. 1986; Evans et al. 1992; Simons et al. 1986) (see Hollon et al. [1992a, 1993] and Scott [1996] for more detailed discussion of follow-up and relapse rates in treatment responders).

Without comparable and replicable RCTs of the post–acute phase treatment effects of cognitive and behavioral treatments, with and without pharmacotherapy, we cannot conclude whether treatment gains are maintained once treatment is discontinued. Although costly, future research must determine which treatments for depression not only reduce acute phase symptoms but also produce enduring treatment effects.

Discussion and Future Research Considerations

This chapter focuses on a review of randomized controlled efficacy trials on cognitive and behavioral psychotherapies, with and without pharmacotherapy, for the treatment of depression. In general, efficacy studies focus on comparing highly controlled and specified treatments (e.g., manualized psychotherapies) that specifically address a particular domain (e.g., depressive symptoms; disability), as compared with other forms of treatments (e.g., CT versus IPT or bibliotherapy), or control conditions (e.g., wait list control). That is, does the manualized treatment really work under highly controlled research conditions, with highly trained and monitored providers who are treating research patients? It is clear from this review that cognitive, behavioral, and combination treatments are efficacious for major depressive disorder in RCTs (i.e., in research environments). There is considerable value in the information generated from efficacy studies and a high degree of internal validity.

However, there are a number of methodological problems with the existing efficacy studies. Specifically, there is a strong need for nonspecific treatment controls (e.g., pill placebo). It has been established that cognitive and behavior therapies are more efficacious in the treatment of depressive disorders as compared with wait list controls. However, studies are needed that compare efficacious psychotherapies to active contract groups such as bibliotherapy or supportive counseling. Furthermore, studies need to define for which populations psychotherapies are equivalent, better, or worse than active control conditions.

There is also a strong need for *controlled* posttreatment outcome studies. There are plenty of naturalistic follow-up studies that suggest treatment effects of CT may last and, perhaps, even provide protection against relapse. However, there is no conclusive evidence to support these hopes.

Furthermore, what is the role of CT or BT following response to pharmacotherapy in patients who report residual symptoms? Fava and colleagues (1996) developed a unique seminaturalistic 4-year follow-up study that assessed the relapse rates of patients who had been successfully treated with pharmacotherapy. Specifically, following acute phase treatment patients were randomly assigned to 10 sessions of CT or standard clinical management (CM) for residual symptoms. Simultaneously, both groups were tapered and discontinued from antidepressant medications. Results indicated that relapse rates in the CT group (35%) were significantly lower than in the CM group (70%) at 4-year follow-up. These findings are consistent with the hypothesis that CT may provide a protective effect against subsequent depressive episodes (Hollon et al. 1993). These results have treatment implications that require further testing, such as, should patients with residual symptoms following response to pharmacotherapy be prescribed brief courses of CT to reduce their risk of relapse? In theory, residual symptoms may be cognitive (negative self-esteem; hopelessness) in nature, an idea which suggests that they might preferentially respond to psychotherapy. Thus, the question remains, should CT or BT be used to treat residual symptoms, which could possibly reduce the risk of relapse or recurrence?

From a more global perspective, where in the treatment package or algorithm are CT, BT, or combination treatment to be recommended? As a first line treatment? If yes, with what types of depressions? After pharmacotherapy? At the continuation and maintenance phases of treatment? Research is needed to answer these kinds of questions.

Although the literature supports the efficacy of cognitive and behavioral therapies with and without pharmacotherapy in some patients with depressive disorders, it is unclear which pretreatment variables are useful in predicting positive and negative outcomes (Hollon 1990; Wright and Thase 1992). Jarrett and colleagues (1991) summarized the problem quite clearly when they stated that we need to know "Which depressions respond best to what treatments under what conditions?" (Jarrett et al. 1991, p. 245). Further, they reported preliminary findings suggesting that patients with more severe depressions and greater dysfunctional attitudes exhibited a poorer response to CT (Jarrett et al. 1991). Thase and colleagues (1993) also conducted a study assessing differential predictors of response to CT (Thase et al. 1993) to find that unemployment, more severe depressive symptoms prior to treatment, and abnormal electroencephalographic sleep profiles were associated with nonresponse to CT. Poor response to CT was also noted in men with chronic depressions; a trend of poorer response to CT was reported in women who endorsed more dysfunctional attitudes.

Future studies must be designed to prospectively identify clinical and psychobiological pretreatment variables as outcome predictors for cognitive, behavioral, and combination treatments. These studies would allow us to match treatments to specific patients, thereby reducing the need for repeated empirical treatment trials.

Moreover, the role of CT or BT for patients who fail to respond to a specific pharmacotherapy or another psychotherapy has not been evaluated. For example, following failure to the first adequate trial of an antidepressant medication, would patients respond better to a course of psychotherapy or to a new or different antidepressant medication? Alternatively, if patients fail to respond to an adequate course of a specified psychotherapy, should they be switched to a different form of psychotherapy or pharmacotherapy? Furthermore, how do patients who are unable to tolerate or participate in pharmacotherapy (e.g., pregnant women) respond to psychotherapy? For partial responders to medication, does psychotherapy convert these patients to remitted status? Does the nature of residual symptoms in medication partial responders predict response to psychotherapy (e.g., do cognitive residua respond better than vegetative residua)?

The role of combined cognitive or behavioral psychotherapies with pharmacotherapy is not well established. Does combination treatment increase the *thoroughness-of-response* as compared with CT, BT, or pharmacotherapy alone? Does combination treatment preferentially affect a wider domain of outcomes (e.g., symptoms and psychosocial disability)? Does combination treatment hasten the *time-to-response*? Do patients who respond symptomatically to the combination experience faster restoration of psychosocial functioning (e.g., fewer days lost from work), as compared with those treatment responders who receive CT, BT, or pharmacotherapy alone?

One of the challenges scientists and practitioners face is transferring and implementing findings from efficacy trials to routine clinical practice, while simultaneously testing their clinical effectiveness (Rush, in press a,b). Although CT, BT, and combination treatments are efficacious, there are little data to support the effectiveness of these treatments in such settings. That is, efficacy of RCTs under research conditions do not necessarily imply effectiveness in general practice (Depression Guideline Panel 1993; Persons et al. 1988). Effectiveness studies assess the external validity of a treatment, as compared with efficacy studies, which focus more on issues related to the internal validity of a procedure.

Mynors-Wallis and colleagues (1995) developed a hybrid study design to address both effectiveness and efficacy issues. Treatment occurred in routine practice, but it was presented by research methods and provided by trained general practitioners. Given the current changes in mental health care and the demands of managed care companies to justify treatments, it is essential that more hybrid studies be conducted to evaluate both efficacy and effectiveness. However, this can only be accomplished if scientists, treatment providers of all disciplines, patients, mental health service systems, policy makers in the private and public sectors, and managed care companies all work collaboratively to determine the preferred treatments for specific depressive disorders across multiple settings (e.g., private practice, community mental health clinics, inpatient settings) and providers (e.g., psychiatrists, psychologists).

References

Aagaard J, Vestergaard P: Predictors of outcome in prophylactic lithium treatment: a 2-year prospective study. J Affective Disord 18:259–266, 1980

Altamura AC, Mauri M: Plasma concentrations, information and therapy adherence during long-term treatment with antidepressants. Br J Clin Pharmacol 20:714–716, 1985

American Psychiatric Association: Diagnostic and Statistical Manual of Mental Disorders, 3rd Edition. Washington, DC, American Psychiatric Association, 1980

American Psychiatric Association: Diagnostic and Statistical Manual of Mental Disorders, 3rd Edition, Revised. Washington, DC, American Psychiatric Association, 1987

Anderson CM, Griffin S, Rossi A, et al: A comparative study of the impact of education vs. process groups for families of patients with affective disorders. Fam Process 25:185–205, 1986

Arean PA, Perri MG, Nezu AM, et al: Comparative effectiveness of social problem-solving therapy and reminiscence therapy as treatments for depression in older adults. J Consult Clin Psychol 61:1003–1010, 1993

Basco MR, Rush AJ: Compliance with pharmacotherapy in mood disorders. Psychiatric Annals 25:78–82, 1995

Basco MR, Rush AJ: Cognitive-Behavioral Therapy for Bipolar Disorder. New York, Guilford, 1996

Beach SRH, O'Leary KD: Treating depression in the context of marital discord: outcome and predictors of response of marital therapy versus cognitive therapy. Behavior Therapy 23:507–528, 1992

Beck AT: Thinking and depression: 2. theory and therapy. Arch Gen Psychiatry 10:561–571, 1964

Beck AT: Cognitive Therapy and the Emotional Disorders. New York, International Universities Press, 1976

Beck AT, Ward CH, Mendelson M, et al: An inventory for measuring depression. Arch Gen Psychiatry 4:561–571, 1961

Beck AT, Rush AJ, Shaw BF, et al: Cognitive Therapy of Depression. New York, Guilford, 1979

Beck AT, Hollon SD, Young JE, et al: Treatment of depression with cognitive therapy and amitriptyline. Arch Gen Psychiatry 42:142–148, 1985

Belsher G, Wilkes TCR, Rush AJ: An open, multisite pilot study of cognitive therapy for depressed adolescents. J Psychother Pract Res 4:52–66, 1995

Beutler LE, Scogin F, Kirkish P, et al: Group cognitive therapy and alprazolam in the treatment of depression in older adults. J Consult Clin Psychol 55:550–556, 1987

Beutler LE, Engle D, Mohr D, et al: Predictors of differential response to cognitive, experiential, and self-directed psychotherapeutic procedures. J Consult Clin Psychol 59:333–340, 1991

Blackburn IM, Bishop S, Glen AIM, et al: The efficacy of cognitive therapy in depression: a treatment trial using cognitive therapy and pharmacotherapy, each alone and in combination. Br J Psychiatry 139:181–189, 1981

Blackburn IM, Eunson KM, Bishop S: A two-year naturalistic follow-up of depressed patients treated with cognitive therapy, pharmacotherapy and a combination of both. J Affective Disord 10:67–75, 1986

Brown GW, Harris T: Social Origins of Depressions: A Study of Psychiatric Disorders in Women. London, Tavistock Press, 1978

Brown RA, Lewinsohn PM: A psychoeducational approach to the treatment of depression: comparison of group, individual, and minimal contact procedures. J Consult Clin Psychol 52:774–783, 1984

Brown GW, Lemyre L, Bifulco A, et al: Social factors and recovery from anxiety and depressive disorders: a test of specificity. Br J Psychiatry 161:44–54, 1992

Burns DD, Nolen-Hoeksema S. Therapeutic empathy and recovery from depression in cognitive-behavioral therapy: a structural equation model. J Consult Clin Psychol 60:441–449, 1992

Clarke GN, Lewinsohn PM: The coping with depression course: a group psychoeducational intervention for unipolar depression. Behavior Change 6:54–69, 1989

Cochran SD: Preventing medical noncompliance in the outpatient treatment of bipolar affective disorders. J Consult Clin Psychol 52:873–878, 1984

Connelly CE: Compliance with outpatient lithium therapy. Perspect Psychiatr Care 22:44–50, 1984

Connelly CE, Davenport YB, Nurnberger JI: Adherence to treatment regimen in a lithium carbonate clinic. Arch Gen Psychiatry 39:585–588, 1982

Coppen A, Ghose K, Montgomery S, et al: Amitriptyline plasma-concentration and clinical effect: a World Health Organization collaborative study. Lancet 1:63–66, 1978

Covi L, Lipman RS: Cognitive behavioral group psychotherapy combined with imipramine in major depression. Psychopharmacol Bull 23:173–176, 1987

Davenport YB, Ebert MH, Adland ML, et al: Couples group therapy as an adjunct to lithium maintenance of the manic patient. Am J Orthopsychiatry 47:495–502, 1977

de Jong R, Treiber R, Henrich G: Effectiveness of two psychological treatments for inpatients with severe and chronic depressions. Cognitive Therapy and Research 10: 645–663, 1986

Depression Guideline Panel: Clinical Practice Guideline, Number 5. Depression in Primary Care. Vol 2. Treatment of Major Depression. Rockville, MD, U.S. Department of Health and Human Services, Public Health Service, Agency for Health Care Policy and Research, AHCPR Publication No. 93-0551, 1993

DeRubeis RJ, Feeley M: Determinants of change in cognitive therapy for depression. Cognitive Therapy and Research 14:469–482, 1990

Eddy DM, Hasselblad V, Schacter R: A Bayesian method for synthesizing evidence: the confidence profile method. Int J Technol Assess Health Care 6:31–35, 1990

Elkin I, Shea TM, Watkins JT, et al: National Institute of Mental Health Treatment of Depression Collaborative Research Program: general effectiveness of treatments. Arch Gen Psychiatry 46:971–982, 1989

Ellis A: Reason and Emotion in Psychotherapy. New York, Lyle Stuart, 1962

Endicott J, Spitzer RL: A diagnostic interview: the schedule for affective disorders and schizophrenia. Arch Gen Psychiatry 35:837–844, 1978

Evans MD, Hollon SD, DeRubeis RJ, et al: Differential relapse following cognitive therapy and pharmacotherapy for depression. Arch Gen Psychiatry 49:802–808, 1992

Fava, GA, Grandi S, Zielezny M, et al: Cognitive behavioral treatment of residual symptoms in primary major depressive disorder. Am J Psychiatry 151:1295–1299, 1994

Fava GA, Grandi S, Zielezny M, et al: Four-year outcome for cognitive behavioral treatment of residual symptoms in major depression. Am J Psychiatry 153:945–947, 1996

Fennell MJV, Teasdale JD: Cognitive therapy with chronic, drug-refractory depressed outpatients: a note of caution. Cognitive Therapy and Research 6:455–460, 1982

Ferster CB: Classification of behavioral pathology, in Research in Behavior Modification: New Development and Implications. Edited by Krasner L, Bandura A, Ullman LP. New York, Holt, Rinehart & Winston, 1965, pp 6–26

Ferster CB: A functional analysis of depression. Am Psychol 28:857–870, 1973

Frank E, Kupfer DJ, Jacob M, et al: Personality features and response to acute treatment in recurrent depression. J Personal Disord 1:14–26, 1987

Frasure-Smith N, Lespérance F, Talajic M: Depression following myocardial infarction: impact on 6-month survival. JAMA 270:1819–1825, 1994

Frasure-Smith N, Lespérance F, Talajic M: Depression and 18-month prognosis after myocardial infarction. Circulation 91:999–1005, 1995

Fuchs, CZ, Rehm LP: A self-control behavior therapy program for depression. J Consult Clin Psychol 45:206–215, 1977

Gallagher DE, Thompson LW: Treatment of major depressive disorder in older adult outpatients with brief psychotherapies. Psychotherapy: Theory, Research and Practice 19: 482–490, 1982

Gallagher-Thompson D, Hanley-Peterson P, Thompson LW: Maintenance of gains versus relapse following brief psychotherapy for depression. J Consult Clin Psychol 58:371–374, 1990

Gallagher-Thompson D, Steffen AM: Comparative effects of cognitive-behavioral and brief psychodynamic psychotherapies for depressed family caregivers. J Consult Clin Psychol 62:543–549, 1994

Giles DE, Jarrett RB, Biggs MM, et al: Clinical predictors of recurrence in depression. Am J Psychiatry 146:764–767, 1989

Gitlin MJ, Cochran SD, Jamison KR: Maintenance lithium treatment: side effects and compliance. J Clin Psychiatry 950:127–131, 1989

Greenberg PE, Stiglin LE, Finkelstein SN, et al: The economic burden of depression in 1990. J Clin Psychiatry 54:405–418, 1993

Guy W: ECDEU Assessment Manual for Psychopharmacology. Washington, DC, U.S. Department of Health, Education, and Welfare, 1976

Hagnell O, Lanke J, Rorsman B, et al: Are we entering an age of melancholy? Depressive illnesses in a prospective epidemiologic study over 25 years: the Lundby Study, Sweden. Psychol Med 13:279–289, 1982

Hamilton M: A rating scale for depression. J Neurol Neurosurg Psychiatry 23:56–62, 1960

Hamilton M: Development of a rating scale for primary depressive illness. British Journal of Social and Clinical Psychology 6:278–296, 1968

Harpin RF, Liberman RP, Marks I, et al: Cognitive-behavior therapy for chronically depressed patients: a controlled pilot study. J Nerv Ment Dis 170: 295–301, 1982

Hasselblad V, Eddy DM: FAST*PRO Software for Meta-Analysis by the Confidence Profile Method. New York, Academic Press, 1992

Hersen M, Bellack AS, Himmelhoch JM, et al: Effects of social skills training, amitriptyline, and psychotherapy in unipolar depressed women. Behavior Therapy 15:21–40, 1984

Hoberman HM, Lewinsohn PM, Tilson M: Group treatment of depression: individual predictors of outcome. J Consult Clin Psychol 56:393–398, 1988

Hogg JA, Deffenbacher JL: A comparison of cognitive and interpersonal-process group therapies in the treatment of depression among college students. Journal of Counseling Psychology 35:304–310, 1988

Hollon SD: Cognitive therapy and pharmacotherapy for depression. Psychiatric Annals 20:249–258, 1990

Hollon SD, Shaw BF: Group cognitive therapy for depressed patients, in Cognitive Therapy of Depression. Edited by Beck AT, Rush AJ, Shaw BF, et al. New York, Guilford, 1979, pp 328–353

Hollon SD, DeRubeis R, Evans M, et al: Cognitive therapy and pharmacotherapy for depression: singly and in combination. Arch Gen Psychiatry 49:774–781, 1992a

Hollon SD, DeRubeis RJ, Seligman MEP: Cognitive therapy and the prevention of depression. Applied and Preventive Psychology 1:89–95, 1992b

Hollon SD, Shelton RC, Davis DD: Cognitive therapy for depression: conceptual issues and clinical efficacy. Special section: recent developments in cognitive and constructivist psychotherapies. J Consult Clin Psychol 61:270–275, 1993

Howland RH: Pharmacotherapy of dysthymia: a review. J Clin Psychopharmacol 11:83–92, 1991

Jacob M, Turner L, Kupfer DJ, et al: Attrition in maintenance therapy for recurrent depression. J Affective Disord 6:181–189, 1984

Jacobson NS, Dobson K, Fruzzetti AE, et al: Marital therapy as a treatment for depression. J Consult Clin Psychol 59:547–557, 1991

Jacobson NS, Fruzzetti AE, Dobson K, et al: Couple therapy as a treatment for depression: II. The effects of relationship quality and therapy on depressive relapse. J Consult Clin Psychol 61:516–519, 1993

Jamison KR, Gerner, RH, Goodwin FK: Patient and physician attitudes toward lithium. Arch Gen Psychiatry 36:866–869, 1979

Jarrett RB, Eaves GG, Grannemann BD, et al: Clinical, cognitive, and demographic predictors of response to cognitive therapy for depression: a preliminary report. Psychiatry Res 37:245–260, 1991

Jarrett RB, Ramanan J, Eaves GG, et al: How prophylactic is cognitive therapy in treating depressed outpatients? Paper presentation at the World Congress of Cognitive Therapy, Toronto, Ontario, June 17–21, 1992

Johnson DAW: Treatment of depression in general practice. BMJ 2:18–20, 1973

Johnson DAW: Depression: treatment compliance in general practice. Acta Psychiatr Scand 290(suppl):447–453, 1981

Klerman GL: Age and clinical depression: today's youth in the twenty-first century. J Gerontol 31:318–323, 1976

Klerman GL, Weissman MM, Rounsaville BJ, et al: Interpersonal Psychotherapy of Depression. New York, Basic Books, 1984

Kornblith SJ, Rehm LP, O'Hara MW, et al: The contribution of self-reinforcement training and behavioral assignments to the efficacy of self-control therapy for depression. Cognitive Therapy and Research 7:499–528, 1983

Kovacs M, Rush AJ, Beck AT, et al: Depressed outpatients treated with cognitive therapy or pharmacotherapy: a one-year follow-up. Arch Gen Psychiatry 38:33–41, 1981

Kragh-Sorensen P, Hvidberg EF, Hansen CE, et al: Therapeutic control of plasma concentrations and long-term effect of nortriptyline in recurrent affective disorders. Pharmakopsychiatrie Neuro-Psychopharmakologie 9:178–182, 1976

Kucera-Bozarth K, Beck NC, Lyss L: Compliance with lithium regimens. J Psychosoc Nurs Ment Health Serv 20:11–15, 1982

Kupfer DJ: Long-term treatment of depression. J Clin Psychiatry 52(suppl):28–34, 1991

Lane R, McDonald G: Reducing the economic burden of depression. Int Clin Psychopharmacol 9:229–243, 1994

Last CG, Thase ME, Hersen M, et al: Patterns of attrition for psychosocial and pharmacologic treatments of depression. J Clin Psychiatry 46:361–366, 1985

Lavori P, Klerman G, Keller M, et al: Age-period-cohort analysis of secular trends in onset of major depression: findings in siblings of patients with major affective disorder. J Psychiatr Res 21:23–35, 1987

Lavori PW, Warshaw M, Klerman G, et al: Secular trends in lifetime onset of MDD stratified by selected sociodemographic risk factors. J Psychiatr Res 27:95–109, 1993

Lavori PW, Keller MB, Mueller TI, et al: Recurrence after recovery in unipolar MDD: an observational follow-up study of clinical predictors and somatic treatment as a mediating force. International Journal of Methods in Psychiatric Research 4:211–229, 1994

Lenzi A, Lazzerini F, Placidi GF, et al: Predictors of compliance with lithium and carbamazepine regimens in the long-term treatment of recurrent mood and related psychotic disorders. Pharmacopsychiatry 22:34–37, 1989

Lewinsohn PM: A behavioral approach to depression, in The Psychology of Depression: Contemporary Theory and Research. Edited by Friedman RM, Katz MM. Washington, DC, Winston/Wiley, 1974, pp 157–178

Lewinsohn PM, Sullivan JM, Grosscup SJ: Changing reinforcing events: an approach to the treatment of depression. Psychotherapy: Theory, Research and Practice 17:322–334, 1980

Lewinsohn PM, Antonuccio DA, Steinmetz J, et al: The Coping With Depression Course: A Psychoeducational Intervention for Unipolar Depression. Eugene, OR, Castalia Press, 1984

Lewinsohn P, Clarke GN, Hops H, et al: Cognitive-behavioral treatment for depressed adolescents. Behavior Therapy 21:385–401, 1990

Markowitz JC: Psychotherapy of dysthymia. Am J Psychiatry 151:1114–1121, 1994

Mason BJ, Markowitz JC, Klerman GL: Interpersonal psychotherapy for dysthymic disorders, in New Applications of Interpersonal Therapy. Edited by Klerman GL, Weissman MM. Washington, DC, American Psychiatric Press, 1993, pp 225–264

McCullough JP: Psychotherapy for dysthymia: a naturalistic study of ten patients. J Nerv Ment Dis 179:734–740, 1991

McLean PD, Hakstian AR: Clinical depression: comparative efficacy of outpatient treatments. J Consult Clin Psychol 47:818–836, 1979

McLean PD, Hakstian AR: Relative endurance of unipolar depression treatment effects: longitudinal follow-up. J Consult Clin Psychol 58:482–488, 1990

Meichenbaum D, Turk D: Treatment Adherence. New York, Plenum, 1987

Mercier MA, Stewart JW, Quitkin FM: A pilot sequential study of cognitive therapy and pharmacotherapy of atypical depression. J Clin Psychiatry 53:166–170, 1992

Meyers JK, Weissman MM, Tischler GL, et al: Six-month prevalence of psychiatric disorders in three communities: 1980 to 1982. Arch Gen Psychiatry 41:959–967, 1984

Miller IW, Norman WH, Keitner GI: Treatment response of high cognitive dysfunction depressed inpatients. Compr Psychiatry 30:62–71, 1990

Mintz J, Mintz LI, Arruda MJ, et al: Treatments of depression and the functional capacity to work. Arch Gen Psychiatry 49:761–768, 1992

Murphy GE, Simons AD, Wetzel RD, et al: Cognitive therapy and nortriptyline, singly and together, in the treatment of depression. Arch Gen Psychiatry 41:33–41, 1984

Myers ED, Calvert EJ: Information, compliance and side-effects: a study of patients on antidepressant medication. Br J Clin Pharmacol 17:21–25, 1984

Mynors-Wallis LM, Gath DH, Lloyd-Thomas AR, et al: Randomized controlled trial comparing problem solving treatment with amitriptyline and placebo for major depression in primary care. BMJ 310:441–445, 1995

Neimeyer RA, Feixas G: The role of homework and skill acquisition in the outcome of group cognitive therapy for depression. Behavior Therapy 21:281–292, 1990

Neimeyer RA, Weiss ME: Cognitive and symptomatic predictors of outcome of group therapies for depression. Journal of Cognitive Psychotherapy: An International Quarterly 4:23–32, 1990

Neimeyer RA, Heath A, Strauss J: Personal reconstruction during group cognitive therapy of depression, in Anticipating Personal Construct Psychology. Edited by Epting F, Landfield AW. Lincoln, NE University of Nebraska Press, 1985, pp 180–195

Nezu AM: Efficacy of a social problem-solving therapy for unipolar depression. J Consult Clin Psychol 54:196–202, 1986

Nezu AM, Perri MG: Social problem-solving therapy for unipolar depression: an initial dismantling investigation. J Consult Clin Psychol 57:408–413, 1989

O'Leary KD, Beach SRH: Marital therapy: a viable treatment for depression and marital discord. Am J Psychiatry 147:183–186, 1990

Overall JE, Donachie ND, Faillace LA: Implications of restrictive diagnosis for compliance to antidepressant drug therapy: alprazolam versus imipramine. J Clin Psychiatry 48:51–54, 1987

Park LC, Lipman RS: A comparison of patient dosage deviation reports with pill counts. Psychopharmacology 6:299–302, 1964

Paykel ES, Cooper Z, Ramana R, et al: Life events, social support and marital relationships in the outcome of severe depression. Psychol Med 26:121–133, 1996

Pecheur DR, Edwards KJ: A comparison of secular and religious versions of cognitive therapy with depressed Christian college students. Journal of Psychology and Theology 12:45–54, 1984

Peet M, Harvey NS: Lithium maintenance: 1. a standard education program for patients. Br J Psychiatry 158:197–200, 1991

Persons JB, Burns DD, Perloff JM, et al: Predictors of dropout and outcome in cognitive therapy for depression in a private practice setting. Cognitive Therapy and Research 12:557–575, 1988

Pilkonis PA, Frank E: Personality pathology in recurrent depression: nature, prevalence, and relationship to treatment response. Am J Psychiatry 145:435–441, 1988

Post RM: Transduction of psychosocial stress into the neurobiology of recurrent affective disorder. Am J Psychiatry 149:999–1010, 1992

Powell BJ, Othmer E, Sinkhorn C: Pharmacological aftercare for homogeneous groups of patients. Hosp Community Psychiatry 28:125–127, 1977

Propst LR, Ostrom R, Watkins P, et al: Comparative efficacy of religious and nonreligious cognitive-behavioral therapy for the treatment of clinical depression in religious individuals. J Consult Clin Psychol 60:94–103, 1992

Pugh R: An association between hostility and poor adherence to treatment in patients suffering from depression. Br J Med Psychol 56:205–208, 1983

Rabin AS, Kaslow NJ, Rehm LP: Changes in symptoms of depression during the course of therapy. Cognitive Therapy and Research 8:479–488, 1984

Radloff LS: The CES-D scale: A self-report depression scale for research in the general population. Applied Psychological Measurement 1:385–401, 1977

Reed MK: Social skills training to reduce depression in adolescents. Adolescence 29:293–302, 1994

Regier DA, Narrow WE, Rae DS, et al: The defacto US mental and addictive disorders service system: epidemiologic catchment area prospective 1-year prevalence rates of disorders and services. Arch Gen Psychiatry 50:85–94, 1993

Rehm LP, Fuchs CZ, Roth DM, et al: A comparison of self-control and assertion skills treatment of depression. Behavior Therapy 10:429–442, 1979

Rehm LP, Kornblith SJ, O'Hara MW, et al: An evaluation of major components in a self-control behavior therapy program for depression. Behav Modif 5:459–489, 1981

Robins CJ, Hayes AM: An appraisal of cognitive therapy. J Consult Clin Psychol 61:205–214, 1993

Robins LN, Helzer JE, Weissman MM, et al: Lifetime prevalence of specific psychiatric disorders in three sites. Arch Gen Psychiatry 41:949–958, 1984

Rodgers B: Models of stress, vulnerability and affective disorder. J Affective Disord 21:1–13, 1991

Rohde P, Lewinsohn PM, Seeley JR: Response of depressed adolescents to cognitive-behavioral treatment: do differences in initial severity clarify the comparison of treatments? J Consult Clin Psychol 62:851–854, 1994

Ross M, Scott M: An evaluation of the effectiveness of individual and group cognitive therapy in the treatment of depressed patients in an inner city health centre. J R Coll Gen Pract 35:239–242, 1985

Roth D, Bielski R, Jones M, et al: A comparison of self-control therapy and combined self-control therapy and antidepressant medication in the treatment of depression. Behavior Therapy 13:133–144, 1982

Rounsaville BJ, Weissman MM, Prusoff BA: Psychotherapy with depressed outpatients: patient and process variables as predictors of outcome. Br J Psychiatry 138:67–74, 1981

Rovner BW, German PS, Brant LJ, et al: Depression and mortality in nursing homes. JAMA 265:993–996, 1991

Rude SS: Relative benefits of assertion or cognitive self-control treatment for depression as a function of proficiency in each domain. J Consult Clin Psychol 54:390–394, 1986

Rush AJ: Linking efficacy and effectiveness research in the evaluation of psychotherapies, in The Cost-Effectiveness of Psychotherapy: A Guide for Practitioners, Researchers, and Policy Makers. Edited by Miller N, Macgruder K. New York, Oxford University Press, in press a

Rush AJ: Psychotherapy for major mood disorders: from efficacy to effectiveness, in The Cost-Effectiveness of Psychotherapy: A Guide for Practitioners, Researchers, and Policy Makers. Edited by Miller N, Macgruder K. New York, Oxford University Press, in press b

Rush AJ, Trivedi MH: Treating depression to remission. Psychiatric Annals 25:704–705, 1995

Rush AJ, Watkins JT: Group versus individual cognitive therapy: a pilot study. Cognitive Therapy and Research 5:95–103, 1981

Rush AJ, Beck AT, Kovacs M, et al: Comparative efficacy of cognitive therapy and pharmacotherapy in the treatment of depressed outpatients. Cognitive Therapy and Research 1:17–37, 1977

Rush AJ, Hollon S, Beck AT, et al: Depression: must pharmacotherapy fail for cognitive therapy to succeed? Cognitive Therapy and Research 2:199–206, 1978

Schwarcz G, Silbergeld S: Serum lithium spot checks to evaluate medication compliance. J Clin Psychopharmacol 3:356–358, 1983

Scott AI, Freeman CP: Edinburgh primary care depression study: treatment outcome, patient satisfaction, and cost after 16 weeks. BMJ 304:883–887, 1992

Scott J: Chronic depression: can cognitive therapy succeed when other treatments fail? Behavioural Psychotherapy 20:25–36, 1992

Scott J: Cognitive therapy of affective disorders: a review. J Affective Disord 37:1–11, 1996

Scott MJ, Stradling SG: Group cognitive therapy for depression produces clinically significant reliable change in community-based settings. Behavioural Psychotherapy 18:1–19, 1990

Selmi PM, Klein MH, Greist JH, et al: Computer-administered cognitive-behavioral therapy for depression. Am J Psychiatry 147:51–56, 1990

Seltzer A, Roncari I, Garfinkel P: Effect of patient education on medication compliance. Can J Psychiatry 25:638–645, 1980

Shakir SA, Volkmar FR, Bacon S: Group psychotherapy as an adjunct to lithium maintenance. Am J Psychiatry 136:455–456, 1979

Shapiro DA, Barkham M, Rees A, et al: Effects of treatment duration and severity of depression on the effectiveness of cognitive-behavioral and psychodynamic-interpersonal psychotherapy. J Consult Clin Psychol 62:522–534, 1994

Shapiro DA, Rees A, Barkham M, et al: Effects of treatment duration and severity of depression on the maintenance of gains after cognitive-behavioral and psychodynamic-interpersonal psychotherapy. J Consult Clin Psychol 63:378–387, 1995

Shea MT, Elkin I, Imber SD, et al: Course of depressive symptoms over follow-up: findings from the NIMH Treatment of Depression Collaborative Research Program. Arch Gen Psychiatry 49:782–787, 1992

Simons AD, Garfield SL, Murphy GE: The process of change in cognitive therapy and pharmacotherapy for depression. Arch Gen Psychiatry 41:45–51, 1984

Simons AD, Murphy GE, Levine JL, et al: Cognitive therapy and pharmacotherapy for depression: sustained improvement over one year. Arch Gen Psychiatry 43:43–48, 1986

Sotsky SM, Glass DR, Shea MT, et al: Patient predictors of response to psychotherapy and pharmacotherapy: findings in the NIMH Treatment of Depression Collaborative Research Program. Am J Psychiatry 148:997–1008, 1991

Steuer JL, Mintz J, Hammen CL, et al: Cognitive-behavioral and psychodynamic group psychotherapy in treatment of geriatric depression. J Consult Clin Psychol 52:180–189, 1984

Stewart JW, Mercier MA, Agosti V, et al: Imipramine is effective after unsuccessful cognitive therapy and imipramine in depressed outpatients. J Clin Psychopharmacol 13:114–119, 1993

Suppes T, Baldessarini RJ, Faedda GL, et al: Risk of recurrence following discontinuation of lithium treatment in bipolar disorder. Arch Gen Psychiatry 48:1082–1088, 1991

Teichman Y, Teichman M: Interpersonal view of depression: review and integration. Journal of Family Psychology 3:349–367, 1990

Teichman Y, Bar-El Z, Shor H, et al: A comparison of two modalities of cognitive therapy (individual and marital) in treating depression. Psychiatry 58:136–148, 1995

Teri L, Lewinsohn PM: Individual and group treatment of unipolar depression: comparison of treatment outcome and identification of predictors of successful treatment outcome. Behavior Therapy 17:215–228, 1986

Thase M, Simons A, Cahalance J, et al: Severity of depression and response to cognitive therapy. Am J Psychiatry 148:784–789, 1991

Thase ME, Simons AD, McGeary J, et al: Relapse following cognitive behavior therapy of depression: potential implications for longer-term forms of treatment. Am J Psychiatry 149:1046–1052, 1992

Thase ME, Simons AD, Reynolds CF: Psychobiological correlates of poor response to cognitive behavior therapy: potential indications for antidepressant pharmacotherapy. Psychopharmocol Bull 29:293–301, 1993

Thase ME, Reynolds CF III, Frank E, et al: Response to cognitive-behavioral therapy in chronic depression. J Psychother Pract Res 3:204–214, 1994

Thompson LW, Gallagher DE: Efficacy of psychotherapy in the treatment of late-life depression. Psychological treatment of unipolar depression: special issue. Advances in Behavior Research and Therapy 6:127–139, 1984

Thompson LW, Gallagher DE, Breckenridge JS: Comparative effectiveness of psychotherapies for depressed elders. J Consult Clin Psychol 55:385–390, 1987

Turner RW, Wehl CK: Treatment of unipolar depression in problem drinkers. Advances in Behavior Research and Therapy 6:115–125, 1984

Usaf SO, Kavanagh DJ: Mechanisms of improvement in treatment for depression: test of a self-efficacy and performance model. Journal of Cognitive Psychotherapy: An International Quarterly 4:51–70, 1990

van den Hout JHC, Arntz A, Kunkels FHJ: Efficacy of a self-control therapy program in a psychiatric day-treatment center. Acta Psychiatr Scand 92:25–29, 1995

Van Gent EM, Zwart FM: Psychoeducation of partners of bipolar manic patients. J Affective Disord 21:15–18, 1991

Waring EM: Enhancing Marital Intimacy Through Cognitive Self-Disclosure. New York, Brunner/Mazel, 1988

Waring EM: The role of marital therapy in the treatment of depressed married women. Can J Psychiatry 39:568–571, 1994

Waring EM, Chamberlaine CH, Carver CM, et al: A pilot study of marital therapy as a treatment for depression. Journal of Family Therapy 23: 3–10, 1995

Weissman MM, Myers JK: Affective disorders in a US urban community: the use of research diagnostic criteria in an epidemiologic study. Arch Gen Psychiatry 35:1304–1311, 1978

Weissman MM, Klerman GL, Paykel ES, et al: Treatment effects on the social adjustment of depressed patients. Arch Gen Psychiatry 30:771–778, 1974

Wilkes TCR, Belsher G, Rush AJ, et al: Cognitive Therapy for Depressed Adolescents. New York, Guilford, 1994

Wilson JD, Enoch MD: Estimation of drug rejection by schizophrenic in-patients, with analysis of clinical factors. Br J Psychiatry 113:209–211, 1967

Wilson KCM, Scott M, Abou-Saleh M, et al: Long-term effects of cognitive-behavioural therapy and lithium therapy on depression in the elderly. Br J Psychiatry 167:653–658, 1995

Wollersheim JP, Wilson GL: Group treatment of unipolar depression: a comparison of coping, supportive, bibliotherapy, and delayed treatment groups. Professional Psychology—Research and Practice 22:496–502, 1991

Wollersheim JP, McFall ME, Hamilton SB, et al: Effects of treatment rationale and problem severity on perceptions of psychological problems and counseling approaches. Journal of Counseling Psychology 27: 225–231, 1980

Wright JH, Thase ME: Cognitive and biological therapies: a synthesis. Psychiatric Annals 22:451–458, 1992

Wulsin L, Bachop M, Hoffman D: Group therapy in manic-depressive illness. Am J Psychother 2:263–271, 1988

Yost E, Beutler LE, Corbishley MA, et al: Group Cognitive Therapy: A Treatment Approach for Depressed Older Adults. New York, Pergamon, 1986

Youssel FA: Compliance with therapeutic regimens: a follow-up study for patients with affective disorders. J Adv Nurs 8:513–517, 1983

Zettle RD, Haflich JL, Reynolds RA: Responsivity to cognitive therapy as a function of treatment format and client personality dimensions. J Clin Psychol 48:787–797, 1992

Efficacy, Indications, and Mechanisms of Action of Cognitive Therapy of Depression

Brian F. Shaw, Ph.D., C.Psych.

Zindel V. Segal, Ph.D., Psych.

Cognitive theorists and therapists are currently directing their attention to the significant clinical problem of relapse and recurrence in major depression and, to a lesser degree, the work of secondary prevention of emotional and behavioral disorders. For psychological therapies to "survive," both in human and economic terms, progress in cognitive, social, and behavioral models related to major depression is essential. Most readers accept that we are years away from the ideal treatment for the multidimensional depressions — indeed, psychopharmacology appears to be exploring the limits of applicability of newer agents (e.g., the use of SSRIs in a range of disorders and problems beyond major depression). Gene therapies, if applicable, are even more distant innovations, in part awaiting the discovery of specific genes for affective disorders (McGuffin et al. 1996).

This perspective on survivability is, of course, a simplistic one; the more pressing issue is the functional value of cognitive theories and therapies in restoring people to productive, quality lives in a cost-effective way (Sturm and Wells 1995). More appropriate care for the depressive disorders increases total *costs of care*, but also improves functioning outcomes, thereby offsetting the actual burden of illness costs to society.

This chapter surveys recent advances in theory, treatment efficacy and psychotherapy methodology (both outcome and processes) related to cognitive therapy of depression (Beck et al. 1979; Segal and Shaw 1996). Cognitive therapy (or cognitive-behavior therapy [CBT]) is one of the best studied psychological treatments for unipolar depression (Dobson 1989). We review the theoretical bases for relapse prevention and risk reduction in major depression from this perspective followed by a review of the efficacy, indications, and putative mechanisms of action of cognitive therapy.

Disrupting the Cognitive "Interlock" in Major Depression

In this section we briefly review the basic premises concerning cognitive risk factors for major depression. It is now well established that chronicity of depression, many previous episodes, and residual symptoms are important predictors of relapse or recurrence in major depression (Shaw 1989), but how are these clinical history variables understood from the cognitive perspective? Furthermore, how can this information be used to achieve the desirable goal of designing therapies that reduce this risk for relapse or recurrence? Several investigators, but mostly Teasdale et al. (1995), have employed a theory-driven conceptualization of the cognitive vulnerabilities in depression to devise a therapeutic intervention.

The recognition of important changes in a person's thinking and reasoning as the result of being depressed has been one of the main tenets of the cognitive behavioral approach to this disorder (Beck et al. 1979). Alternations from the manner in which these processes operate under conditions of normal mood have been extensively documented and researched (Blaney 1986). On the basis of these studies, a number of theoretical models of mood dependent processing have been developed. These have recently been applied to explain vulnerability to onset, relapse, and recurrence in depression (Segal et al. 1996; Teasdale and Barnard 1993).

These analyses converge on the conclusion that vulnerability to depressive recurrence is determined by the increased risk of particular negative patterns of information processing being activated in depressed states. The likelihood of such cognitive patterns being activated is dependent on their frequency of past usage, and greater experience of these patterns of processing makes it easier for their future activation to be achieved on the basis of increasingly minimal cues (Post 1992). Once depression-related cognitive patterns have been activated, a number of theories (Bower 1981; Collins and Loftus 1975) predict that positive information would be less accessible, and so would be less available to moderate the production of negative, depression-maintaining interpretations.

Through these processes it is hypothesized that the instantiation of depressive cognitive patterns increase the chances that mild dysphoric states are amplified through further ruminative processing, eventuating in a downward spiral of depression (Teasdale 1988). Repeated activation of negative patterns of thinking also mean that a wider range of stimuli are associated with these states of mind, and they become, therefore, easier to elicit in the presence of minimal cues. In fact, evidence suggests that even patients whose depression is in remission revert to a depressive information processing style when tested under conditions of mild and transient negative mood.

Seen from this model, patients who have experienced a greater number of depressive episodes are more likely to shift into a depressive response mode when they experience mild levels of depressed mood, because, within each episode, the links between dysphoric mood and depression-related constructs or patterns of processing are strengthened by their repeated co-occurrence. We would expect that the affective states required to selectively activate negative constructs would decrease in intensity over time (Post 1992; Segal et al. 1996).

This analysis suggests that the processes associated with recurrence of depression represent a retriggering of the patterns of information-processing activity that characterize the initial episode (Teasdale and Barnard 1993), and that it is important to distinguish between 1) the processes responsible for the escalation or "wind-up" of mild dysphoric states to more intense and persistent states of depressive relapse and recurrence, and 2) the processes responsible for the maintenance of these states once established. The implication for treatment is that interventions designed specifically to prevent the triggering and escalation of depression-related thinking patterns that seem central to relapse may be helpful. Such prophylactic treatments may differ in emphasis from those primarily designed to alleviate established depressions.

Other models of cognitive diathesis have also been emphasized. For example, the interaction between a biased attributional style (Abramson et al. 1986) and negative life events has been shown to predict depression. Working in the area of social cognition, Higgins (1989) has proposed a self-concept discrepancy as important to our understanding of the cognitive diatheses. Discrepancies essentially refer to accessible differences between a person's actual, ideal, and expected attributes. The discrepancies are relevant to both interpersonal and intrapersonal dimensions (see Strauman 1989).

Personality theorists such as Blatt (1995) and Beck (1983) have described comparable personality adaptations in dependent (sociotropic) and self-critical (autonomous) domains as vulnerability factors in depression. Zuroff and colleagues (Zuroff 1992, 1994; Zuroff and Fitzpatrick 1995) have conducted methodologically sophisticated evaluations of these potential diatheses in normal adults but have not as yet extended these analyses to patients with depression. Blatt (1995) observed that perfectionism was predictive of poor outcomes of depression treatment, whether medication (imipramine) or psychotherapy (cognitive therapy or interpersonal therapy) was used. Perfectionism may, in fact, be the most powerful predictor of suicidal behavior, being even more powerful than hopelessness.

The challenge may be to identify reliable vulnerability factors and then test whether CBT has specific effects on these factors. In this way, we reduce risk to future episodes, much like smoking cessation reduces the risk of cancer where the risk reduction is not absolute. There are many other cancer risk factors (family history, genetics, environment), but we know that smoking risk is independently significant. The task before us is to use multiple approaches to reduce the risk of major depression. Cognitive theory is part of the broader system of psychotherapy (theory, empirical foundation of central constructs, defined therapeutic interventions) and consistent with a multifaceted approach to treatment.

The organizing model of Shaw (1989) and colleagues (Katz et al. 1994; Segal and Shaw 1996) is to apply risk reduction strategies to health risk factors. Depression is accepted as a complex phenomenon with multiple causal variables. The ideal, single modality treatment may not be available for some time, if ever, and prevention of episodes is *always* preferable. We want to develop an approach to reducing the risk of major depressive episodes by engaging our patients in risk reduction strategies. In depression, these changes include building positive behaviors (exercise, diet, pursuing pleasurable activities) and decreasing risky attitudes (e.g., negative social comparisons, taking responsibility for the feelings and actions of other adults, ascribing self-worth to achievements or specific interpersonal relationships.

Risk Adaptation Model (RAM)

Risk expectancy variables provide the foundation for *risk reduction expectancies.* A risk must be experienced as sufficiently relevant, probable, and severe before risk reduction is contemplated or initiated. Cognitive-behavior change is affected by outcome expectations, decisional balance (the weights ascribed to the pros and cons of change), and the amount and quality of attention directed toward this change. Briefly put, to initiate and maintain change (adherence), one has to *want* to do it, feel it is the *right thing* to do, and feel relatively *confident in the ability to do it consistently.* The RAM predicts how psychological factors, in combination, influence maintenance of and adherence to behavior change (Katz et al. 1994; Ritvo 1994).

Risk Expectancies

Risk expectancy variables have been identified in each of the significant cognitive models of health-oriented change developed during the last two decades (Ajzen and Fishbein 1980; Janz and Becker 1984; Maddux and Rogers 1983; Weinstein 1988). In each of these models, there is emphasis on the perceived *probability* and *magnitude of* harm if no risk reduction measures are taken. In the context of adherence, risk expectancy variables refer specifically to beliefs about the consequences of nonadherence (i.e., interrupting therapy, skipping medication). Because risk expectancy measures have been important predictors of preventative health behavior in numerous studies (Aizen and Fishbein 1980), interventions designed to motivate adherence usually begin with raising awareness about the risks of nonadherence. The significant principle in this regard is that either too little *or* too much emphasis on risk produces either little effect or avoidance altogether. Despite our preferences for linear relationships, there appears to be a *curvilinear* relationship (actually an inverted U) between risk expectancy (and the experience of threat associated with it) and the motivation to reduce risk.

In understanding risk expectancy some people, particularly nonadherent individuals, see themselves as *less* vulnerable to the recurrence of depression than their peers, a phenomenon called *unrealistic optimism* (Meyerowitz et al. 1989; Weinstein 1983, 1988; Weinstein et al. 1988). To overcome such optimistic bias, risk communications interventions have typically been aimed at increasing fear and awareness of risk vulnerability. However, messages that are too threatening may increase fear beyond adaptive levels resulting in avoidance or denial (Job 1988; Leventhal et al. 1965; Leventhal and Watts 1966; Meyerowitz and Chaiken 1987; Sherbourne et al. 1992). On the other hand, findings suggest that people not intending to change health risk behavior retain an optimistic bias, whereas those preparing to change manifest less bias (McCoy et al. 1992). Thus, there should be a range of risk expectancies that produces a threat level to mobilize health behavior change but not avoidance. Information about risk expectancy should be combined with information about risk reduction expectancy. Simply put, people are more likely to attend to a risk they think they can reduce.

Risk Reduction Expectancy

Risk reduction expectancy variables combine judgments of *response* and *self-efficacy* (confidence in available risk reduction methods and in personally using them in specific situations) (Bandura 1986). These variables build on a substantial body of research supporting self-efficacy as a consistent predictor of behavior change (Bandura 1986). Both response and self-efficacy are affected by global outcome expectancies (pessimism–optimism) (Carver et al. 1993; Scheier et al. 1989; Taylor et al. 1992). Past failure or success influence such expectancies by setting the stage for learned helplessness or learned efficacy (Lin and Peterson 1990; Peterson et al. 1987; Vaillant 1978). Learned helplessness revolves around one's beliefs, derived from a series of unsuccessful change attempts, that actions do not lead to expected outcomes (Peterson et al. 1987) resulting in a pessimistic outcome expectancy (typical of patient dysthymia). Conversely, learned optimism, derived through a series of successful change attempts, reinforces the belief that actions do result in expected outcomes and results in a more optimistic outcome expectancy.

How do pessimism and optimism relate to adherence behavior? General optimism predisposes to positive outcome expectancies about specific risk reduction efforts, decreasing avoidance of risk-relevant information while increasing motivation for reduction efforts. Optimism thereby reinforces adherence if the consequences of these efforts are viewed positively.

Substantial evidence supports the association between optimism and better health outcomes. For example, pessimists are less likely to initiate health care practices such as going for a routine medical checkup (Lin and Peterson 1990) and are at higher risk, generally, for diseases and premature mortality (Peterson and Seligman 1987; Vaillant 1978). Optimists, on the other hand, are more likely to make use of active coping strategies in recovering from coronary artery bypass surgery (Scheier et al. 1989) and in adapting to breast cancer (Carver 1993). In men testing positive for HIV, optimism has been associated with better adherence to health protective practices (Taylor et al. 1992).

Findings suggest that pessimists experience risk information as distressing and react passively without adaptively changing cognition and behavior. Optimism, on the other hand, appears to promote more positive risk reduction expectancies and assists attention to health risks and their resolution through behavior change. Indeed, optimism may explain the observation that more adherent patients have better health outcomes even when the treatments to which they adhere are placebo tablets.

Attention Regulation

Attention regulation (the ability to deploy attention toward a specific activity amidst competing demands) also affects risk appraisal, risk reduction expectancies, and change efforts. Difficulties with attention regulation are linked to fluctuations in anxiety, depression, and stress (Horowitz et al. 1979). Following treatment for stress disorders, improvements are seen in attention regulation as measured by fewer intrusive thoughts and a reduced use of avoidance procedures (Horowitz et al. 1979). Without therapeutic intervention, however, attention regulation problems may be more fixed.

On the other side of the phenomenon from cognitive intrusions is the avoidance of anxiety-provoking cognition. Such avoidance is characteristic of individuals who deny elevated anxiety levels while exhibiting heightened physiological responses similar to individuals reporting high levels of anxiety (Weinberger et al. 1979). Such individuals have been observed to avoid situations and disturbing cognition across a variety of perceptual, projective, and learning tasks. In cognitive therapy, these individuals present a significant challenge, because they are "not thinking" about their feelings or problems.

Attention regulation can be facilitated by anxiety and arousal management. Optimal approaches take into account the reciprocal relationship between attention and *motivation*: attention is typically directed toward goals for which motivations are higher, whereas motivations are stronger for goals in the proximal ranges of attention. Thus attention-control techniques are an important fundament of anxiety management. Attention must first be directed away from intrusive cognition and toward rational, planned activities before anxiety-management approaches can be implemented. On the other hand, reductions in anxiety, once achieved, support rational responses to risk-related situations and strategies.

Motivation

Motivation (commitment to change) is affected by all of the risk adaptation variables already described. Motivation to engage in risk reduction behaviors is high when the risk is seen as probable and severe, the reduction methods are viewed as effective and practical, and the goal is in sight. Motivation that is too high, especially in the early active phase of risk reduction, however, may be counterproductive to adherence (Brownell et al. 1988). High motivation may result in unrealistic goals for change (e.g., I want to increase my self-esteem in 10 days). This can result in the unanticipated problems in changing behavior being viewed globally as failures. Commitment to change is best accomplished by a goal setting process that is realistic *and* optimistic. We call this process of goal setting *realistic optimism,* based on the view that optimism and realism exist on a continuum rather than as distinct categories. When engaged in adaptive change, people intentionally or unintentionally locate themselves on this continuum. Their position on the continuum can facilitate commitment to change when it represents the integration of reality testing skills on one hand and a positive vision reflecting effort-outcomes linkage on the other. The pursuit of this best-of-both-worlds combination may shift with circumstances but remains relatively consistent because people *need* to define a realistic-optimistic boundary.

These concepts must be understood in terms of motivation being a dynamic process fluctuating over time and situation (Miller and Rollnick 1991). Assessing the individual's eagerness for change at a specific time or in a specific situation helps determine the strength of his or her motivation. Assessing the individual's beliefs regarding the other factors (i.e., risk expectancy, risk reduction expectancy, attention regulation) serves to clarify which areas in the individual's risk adaptation process facilitate or undermine a commitment to adherence. Motivation may be most simply conceived of as the probability of a certain action being taken or adhered to. The probability of adherence may be expressed as *decisional balance* between the pros and cons of adherence.

Decisional balance summates the degree to which the pros of attempting risk reduction outweighs the cons or vice versa. Health behavior change is viewed as a cohesive process reliably divided into six stages: *precontemplation* (the individual is not thinking of making changes), *contemplation* (the individual is considering change within the next 6 months), *preparation* (the individual is considering change within the next month), *action* (taking steps), and finally, *maintenance* of the desired change. *Relapse*, a sixth stage, is considered a normative event as many depressed patients relapse, at any stage, often more than once, before reaching maintenance. It is assumed that several attempts to change a habitual behavior are required. Furthermore, people can get stuck in the early stages, where they become demoralized and discouraged about sustaining change.

The *decisional balance* determines whether an individual progresses, remains at that stage, or relapses. In precontemplation, the pros and cons of change are both low (i.e., not salient or personally relevant) with cons outweighing pros. The salience of pros and cons increases in contemplation and preparation with pros eventually outweighing cons. During action and maintenance their salience again decreases suggesting that to reinforce adherence to the change, it may be important to reinforce and support the salience or value of adherence.

The individual's decisional balance in relation to a specific behavior change, particularly during euthymic periods, is critical to the *adoption* and maintenance of cognitive behavior change. Ensuring the continued *valuing* of a particular change, particularly during euthymic periods, is critical to ensuring its maintenance or adherence. The value or pros of adherence is supported by perceptions of continued risk relevance (i.e., risk expectancy), treatment efficacy and self-efficacy (risk reduction expectancy), and reinforcement of change efforts. The effects of these factors, in turn, rests upon the individual's ability to regulate attention effectively for tasks related to making and maintaining change. Attention regulation supports the integration of risk expectancy and risk reduction in decisions regarding behavior change. Together they fuel motivation for adoption of and adherence to risk reducing practices (Prochaska et al. 1992).

Efficacy and Specific Indications

The efficacy of cognitive therapy has been extensively evaluated over the past decade. Despite many controversies, the evidence indicates that CBT is an effective treatment for unipolar, nonpsychotic, major depression of a mild to moderate severity. In many clinical trials, CBT has been compared with other treatments, particularly psychophar- macology. The focus here is not on the comparative efficacy of CBT but on clinical acceptance, outcomes, and prophylactic value. In all the scientific literature, 730 patients have participated in 30 systematic trials. (More than 730 patients have participated in CBT trials, but we have limited our review to CBT studies using the Beck et al. [1979] protocol.)

Overviews of Theory

We have detailed the theory and conceptualization of risk reduction in major depression to reveal the complexity of the areas and to reflect the advances in this work. As a group, we remain committed to an evidence-based model, and thus, the reader should view the previous discussion with appropriate caution. The main point is that major de- pression carries a significant risk for relapse and certain changes are required to reduce this risk. The model for risk reduction is compa- rable to other difficult cognitive and behavior changes. The significant problem is how to engage the patient with depression in the work of change when, during euthymic phases *and* during depressed phases, motivation for change is low. If we are able to overcome these serious problems we improve our patients' coping skills to reduce the escala- tion of depressive thinking and behavior. At the same time, if we place these changes in the context of other health risk behaviors, we may reduce stigma and enhance effort (Table 7–1). Seeing that only 22% of patients in these studies had a complete response and recovery, this table illustrates the need for intensive efforts with the estimated 568 (78%) other patients who will do less well.

TABLE 7–1

Estimated recovery rates based on controlled published literature on CBT for depression

Patients entering trial = 730
a) Dropouts across studies range from 8% to 30% Assuming 20% dropout (146), leaves: 584
b) Completers of protocol (more than 12 sessions out of 20) range from 60% to 90% Assuming 75% completer rate, leaves: 338
c) Of the completers, 39%–83% will obtain a full remission (BDI ≤ or HRSD ≤ 6) Assuming 60%, leaves: 203
d) Of the recovered sample, 15%–36% will suffer a relapse within two years Assuming 20%, leaves: 162 162/730 is a 22% rate of complete response and recovery.

The study of preventing future depressive episodes (or relapses) is in its early stages. In CBT as symptoms remit, the focus of therapy shifts to the acquisition of skills (primarily attitude change) to improve coping with a recurrence of symptoms. To observe the longer term effects of treatment, studies have followed patients who initially responded and examined their outcome over a subsequent 12- or 24-month period (Blackburn et al. 1986; Evans et al. 1992; Kovacs et al. 1981; Shea et al. 1992; Simons et al. 1986). As a relevant baseline, patients who respond to pharmacotherapy in these trials were generally discontinued after the acute treatment phase of the study and showed a high probability of relapse in the follow-up: 50% at 12 months (Shea et al. 1992); 50% at 24 months (Evans et al. 1992); 66% at 12 months (Simons et al. 1986); 78% at 24 months (Blackburn et al. 1986).

In comparison, patients who received CBT had significantly lower rates of relapse: 20% (Evans et al. 1992); 20% (Simons et al. 1986); 20% (Blackburn et al. 1986). Kovacs et al. (1981) report a trend in this direction with 44% of CBT patients reporting a recurrence at 12 months compared with 65% in the group treated with imipramine. Shea et al. (1992) found no differences in relapse rates among the CBT, interpersonal therapy, imipramine, and pill-placebo/clinical management groups over 18 months. She did report, however, that at

12 months CBT patients had the lowest rates of relapse if a more liberal criterion was used, which included either a diagnosis of major depressive disorder or return to treatment for depression (rates are 14%, 43%, 50%, and 31%, respectively. Finally, the 12-month relapse rate of 32% reported in Thase et al. (1991) for patients who only received CBT is in line with the figures cited earlier. The possible prophylactic effect of cognitive treatment may be due to its effects on the attentional system (Teasdale et al. 1995). Effective cognitive therapy may train patients to redeploy their attention away from the more automatic modes of processing associated with escalating ruminative elaborations of depressogenic meanings and toward more neutral sources of attention and alternative meanings. A clinical trial with patients recovered from depression comparing Attentional Control Training (a modification of cognitive therapy for depression based upon this formulation) against standard psychiatric care is currently being conducted (Segal et al. 1996). In addition, Jarrett and colleagues at Southwestern Medical School in Texas are conducting an extensive study of the maintenance of CBT effects over time.

With respect to other disorders, Clark et al. (1994) compared cognitive therapy, applied relaxation, and imipramine in the treatment of panic disorder. All three treatments were superior to a waiting list control condition. Cognitive therapy was superior to both the relaxation and imipramine groups, in most measures, at 3 months. Cognitive therapy and imipramine were equivalent in effect and superior to relaxation at 6 months. At 15 months cognitive therapy was superior to imipramine and relaxation, although on fewer measures than at 3 months. Data supporting a possible learning or prophylactic effect have been reported for cognitive treatment of generalized anxiety disorder (Butler et al. 1991), eating disorders (Fairburn et al. 1991), hypochondriasis (Warwick 1991), antisocial behavior in children (Kazdin et al. 1989), psychological sequelae of HIV infection (Kelly and Murphy 1992) and later life insomnia (Morin et al. 1993).

For major depression, qualitative reviews of the literature have been provided by several scientists (Shaw 1989). Dobson's (1989) meta-analysis of 27 studies reported a significant benefit of CBT compared with no treatment and a relative advantage over other psychotherapies.

Comparison of CBT with psychopharmacology has demonstrated few differences between the two and, interestingly, little evidence favoring combined treatment over either modality alone.

Cognitive therapy is generally well tolerated with relatively low dropout rates. Typically, 8%–30% of patients drop out of short-term therapy (approximately 20 sessions in 3–4 months). Most patients (60%–90%) complete the CBT protocol, and of these 25%–30% will recover fully, as defined by a Beck Depression Inventory (BDI) score (Beck et al. 1961) or a Hamilton Rating Scale for Depression (HRSD) 17-item score of <6 (Hamilton 1967). This relatively low "complete" recovery rate seems shocking, particularly when compared with general statements about the efficacy of antidepressant treatments but we are evaluating those who enter trials, drop out, or complete treatments, and who recover with few residual symptoms. Interestingly, these recovery data are comparable with the results obtained with addictions (e.g., smoking or alcohol abuse). Assessing the extant literature, 39%–83% of those who completed treatment experienced a full remission. Of these, 15%–36% relapse by two years.

The most significant controversy concerning CBT alone concerns selection criteria. It raises the question of whether depression severity (e.g., HRSD >20) can predict a poorer outcome in CBT. The other controversy aroused by the NIMH Treatment of Depression Collaborative Research Program (Elkin et al. 1995) is whether cognitive therapy is more effective than pill-placebo with clinical management. This latter question has only been examined in only one study, and although other studies have shown a better response, with severely depressed patients, the question lingers. We must remember how relatively few studies have included a CBT group; there are also many failures in the literature to differentiate active antidepressant drug from pill-placebo.

Returning to the severity issue, Elkin et al. (1995, 1996) observed that patients who initially had an HRSD score of >20 had a relatively poor response to CBT (i.e., worse than imipramine plus clinical management and interpersonal therapy). Other investigators (Hautzinger and deJong-Meyer 1995; McLean and Taylor 1992; Thase et al. 1991) have not observed this pattern. Only Hautzinger and deJong-Meyer

(1995) used a prospective design. Our initial conclusion is that the severity issue may be an artifact but clearly needs to be studied further.

In addition to depression severity, the other predictors of treatment response also need replication and include 1) higher level of dysfunctional attitudes (negative); 2) married (positive); 3) brief duration of current episode (positive); 4) several previous episodes (positive); 5) later age of onset (positive); 6) patient expectations (positive-optimistic); 7) no family history (positive).

We need more studies of outcome to determine the best predictors of response. Realistically, with the tiered approach to treatment (i.e., combining therapies or using one intervention and then another), it is difficult to complete this type of research.

Mechanisms of Action

How does psychotherapy, specifically CBT, work? There are many perspectives on this question, and it is fair to say that we do not know the answer. Some perspectives focus on such therapist factors as adhering to the treatment protocol, developing a strong therapeutic alliance (Bordin 1979), and providing skillful or competent interventions (Schaffer 1983; Shaw and Dobson 1988), on patient factors such as patient difficulty and the severity of the disorder (B. F. Shaw, I. E. Elkin, J. Yamaguchi, et al., unpublished data, January, 1998), and on process factors in the therapy itself (e.g., therapist-patient-therapy match, patient "externalizing" style and a "coping skills" therapy).

One salient observation from psychotherapy research is that theory-driven predictions of mechanisms are much stronger than the typical post hoc analyses, particularly given the relatively low power in studies (Beutler 1991). For example, one widely held view is that the connection between the therapist's and the patient's explanation for the patient's depression has a strong impact on the process and outcome of treatment (Fennell and Teasdale 1987). Perhaps the strongest empirical evidence for a factor including CBT outcome concerns homework. In CBT, therapists are expected to assign a specific self-help, homework assignment during the session. Typical assignments include monitoring activities, assessing pleasurable experiences, obtaining information from others and trying out new attitudes (e.g., assertion vs. approval seeking). The skillful assignment of homework as part of structuring the therapy session has been associated with positive outcomes (B. F. Shaw, I. E. Elkin, J. Yamaguchi, et al., unpublished data, January, 1998).

From a clinical research perspective, we speculate that a series of variables are worthy candidates. On meeting the patient with depression, the CBT therapist would want to assess the compatibility of the treatment rationale, patient optimism for treatment, and the level of hopelessness. (Lower hopelessness reduces the risk for suicidal behavior and potential for dropout.) During therapy one might evaluate the patient's compliance with early behavioral activation, willingness to follow through on homework or self-help and adoption of a coping skills or compensatory skills orientation. The latter variable concerns the acquisition of skills such as that proposed by Segal et al. (1996) and Ritvo et al (1994).

Limitations of Research

All research evolves and psychotherapy research is in its relative infancy. Cognitive therapists adopted an empirical approach to their field and as such, expect to develop improved methods and analyses within the tradition of critical appraisal. Four issues limit our understanding of the value of CBT for major depression.

The specification and assessment of the independent variable is a hallmark of CBT (Shaw 1984). Many studies have utilized carefully supervised CBT therapists who are carefully monitored for protocol adherence. Increasingly, therapist competence (skillfulness) has been measured using the Cognitive Therapy Scale (Shaw and Dobson 1988; J. E. Young and A. T. Beck, unpublished data, November, 1980). Whether the independent variable was delivered as expected is as important a question in psychotherapy research as is adequate dosing and clinical management to pharmacology. The current literature is limited by the uncertainty of the best (i.e., most valid) way to measure therapist competency. An even more important issue concerns when to exclude therapists (actually therapist-patient data as competency is a function of the therapeutic context and not the individual per se). For example, ignoring the competency, we reviewed data from 37 CBT completers in the NIMH Treatment of Depression Collaborative Research Program. In this trial, 27% of sessions were judged *a priori* to outcome assessment to be less than adequate (according to a standard set prior to the outcome trial). Depending on where one sets the criterion (e.g., a score <39 on the Cognitive Therapy Scale [J. E. Young and A. T. Beck, unpublished data, November, 1980]), future studies with an acceptable competency evaluation system will be of considerable interest.

Another controversy in psychotherapy research concerns the necessity to evaluate site differences before aggregating data. Few CBT trials have included multisite comparisons, and thus, the problem has only recently emerged. In contrast to the site difference debate, critics have pointed to *allegiance* effects (also known as the Mecca effect) whereby a therapy to which the researchers have the greatest allegiance does the best in an outcome trial (e.g., CBT would tend to fare better if conducted at the Philadelphia Center for Cognitive Therapy). We agree with Klein (1996) and Jacobson and Hollon (1996) that the multisite studies are desirable *but* allegiances must be controlled *within* sites by having comparable enthusiasts for each treatment approach at each site.

Several years ago Jacobson and Truax (1991) recommended analyses of clinical significance testing for all outcome trials. For the most part, these recommendations have, unfortunately, not been heeded. The advantage of clinical significance testing is to improve our understanding of the extent to which our treatment help return patients to functioning within normal limits. Earlier we reviewed data to the extent to which patients recover fully (defined by generally accepted standards), and further, the significant number who suffer a relapse or recurrence within a few years of their recovery.

Each of the aforementioned limitations (compromising the independent variable, allegiance or site differences, failing to test clinical significance) affect our ability to generalize findings from clinical trials to the field. The field of psychotherapy has a long (and *not* distinguished) history of spawning many different, untested forms of psychotherapy.

Cognitive therapy holds considerable promise as a treatment to reduce relapse or recurrence in major depression. To realize this advance, researchers would be wise to follow specific guidelines for clinical research and to redesign interventions in a way that is both theoretically sophisticated and evidence-based.

References

Abramson LY, Metalsky GI, Alloy LB: Hopelessness depression: a theory-based subtype of depression. Psychol Rev 96:358–372, 1986

Ajzen I, Fishbein M: Understanding Attitude and Predicting Behavior. Englewood Cliffs, NJ, Prentice-Hall, 1980

Bandura A: The explanatory and predictive scope of self-efficacy. Journal of Society and Clinical Psychology 4:359–373, 1986

Beck AT: Treatment of depression: old controversies and new approaches, in American Psychopathological Association. Edited by Clayton PJ, Barnett JE. New York, Lippincott-Raven, 1983

Beck AT, Ward CH, Mendelson M, et al: An inventory for measuring depression. Arch Gen Psychiatry 42:667–675, 1961

Beck AT, Rush AJ, Shaw BF, et al: Cognitive Therapy of Depression. New York, Guilford, 1979

Beutler LE: Have all won and must all have prizes? Revisiting Luborsky et al's verdict. J Consult Clin Psychol 59:226–232, 1991

Blackburn IM, Eunson KM, Bishop S: A two year naturalistic follow-up of depressed patients treated with cognitive therapy, pharmacotherapy, and a combination of both. J Affective Disord 10:67–75, 1986

Blaney PH: Affect and memory: a review. Psychol Bull 99:229–246, 1986

Blatt SJ: The destructiveness of perfectionism: implications for the treatment of depression. Am Psychol 50(12):1003–1020, 1995

Bordin ES: The generalization of the psychoanalytic concept of the working alliance. Psychotherapy: Theory, Research and Practice 16:252–260, 1979

Bower GH: Mood and memory. Am Psychol 36:129–148, 1981

Brownell KD, Lichtenstein E, Marlatt GA, et al: Understanding and preventing relapse, in Biological Barriers in Behavioral Medicine. Edited by Linden W. New York, Plenum, 1988, pp 281–313

Butler G, Fennell M, Robson P, et al: Comparison of behavior therapy and cognitive behavior therapy in the treatment of generalized anxiety disorder. J Consult Clin Psychol 59:167–175, 1991

Carver CS, Pozo C, Harris SD, et al: How coping medicates the effect of optimism on distress: a study of women with early stage breast cancer. J Consult Clin Psychol 65:375–390, 1993

Clark DM, Salkovskis PM, Hackman A, et al: A comparison of cognitive therapy, applied relaxation, and imipramine in the treatment of panic disorder. Br J Psychiatry 164:759–769, 1994

Collins AM, Loftus EF: A spreading-activation theory of semantic processing. Psychol Rev 82:407–428, 1975

Dobson KS: A meta-analysis of the efficacy of cognitive therapy for depression. J Consult Clin Psychol 57:414–419, 1989

Elkin, Gibbons RD, Shea MT, et al: Initial severity and differential treatment outcome in the NIMH Treatment of Depression Collaborative Research Program. J Consult Clin Psychol 63:841–847, 1995

Elkin I, Gibbons RD, Shea MT, et al: Science is not a trial (but it sometimes can be a tribulation). J Consult Clin Psychol 64:92–103, 1996

Evans MD, Hollon SD, DeRubeis RJ, et al: Differential relapse following cognitive therapy and pharmacotherapy for depression. Arch Gen Psychiatry 49:802–808, 1992

Fairburn CG, Jones R, Peveler R, et al: Three psychological treatments for bulimia nervosa. Arch Gen Psychiatry 48:463–469, 1991

Fennell M, Teasdale J: Cognitive therapy for depression: individual differences and the process of change. Cognitive Therapy and Research 11:253–271, 1987

Hamilton M: Development of a rating scale for primary depressive illness. British Journal of Social and Clinical Psychology 6:278–296, 1967

Hautzinger M, deJong-Meyer R: [Effectiveness of psychological treatment of depression.] Zeitschrift fur Klinische Psychologie 24(2), 1995

Higgins ET: Self-discrepancy theory: what patterns of self beliefs cause people to suffer? Advances in Experimental Social Psychology 22:93–136, 1989

Horowitz M, Wilner N, Alverez W: Impact of Event Scale: A measure of subjective stress. Psychosom Med 41:209–218, 1979

Jacobson NS, Hollon SD: Prospects for future comparisons between drugs and psychotherapy: lessons from the CBT versus pharmacotherapy exchange. J Consult Clin Psychol 64:104–108, 1996

Jacobson NS, Truax P: Clinical significance: a statistical approach to defining meaningful change in psychotherapy research. J Consult Clin Psychol 59:12–19, 1991

Janz NK, Becker MH: The health belief model: a decade later. Health Educ Q 11:1–47, 1984

Job RFS: Effective and ineffective use of fear in health promotion campaigns. Am J Public Health 78:163–167, 1988

Katz J, Ritvo PG, Irvine MJ, et al: Maximizing adherence with nonpharmacological treatment. Can J Cardiol (Pfizer Suppl.):6–8, 1994

Katz J, Ritvo PG, Irvine MJ, et al: Coping with chronic pain, in Handbook of Coping. Edited by Seidner M, Endler NS. New York, Wiley, 1996, pp 252–278

Kazdin AE, Bass D, Seigel T, et al: Cognitive behavioral therapy and relationship therapy in the treatment of children referred for antisocial behavior. J Consult Clin Psychol 55:522–535, 1989

Kelly JA, Murphy DA: Psychological interventions with AIDS and HIV: prevention and treatment. J Consult Clin Psychol 60:576–585, 1992

Klein DF: Preventing hung juries. J Consult Clin Psychol 64:81–87, 1996

Kovacs M, Rush AJ, Beck AT, et al: Depressed out-patients treated with cognitive therapy or pharmacotherapy: a one-year follow-up. Arch Gen Psychiatry 38:33–39, 1981

Leventhal H, Singer R, Jones S: Effects fear and specificity of recommendation upon attitudes and behaviour. J Pers Soc Psychol 2:20–29, 1965

Leventhal H, Watts JC: Sources of resistance to fear-arousing communications on smoking and lung cancer. J Personal Disord 34:155–175, 1966

Lin EH, Peterson C: Pessimistic explanatory style and response illness. Behav Res Ther 28:243–248, 1990

Maddux JE, Rogers RW: Protection motivation and self-efficacy: a revised theory of fear, appeals, and attitude change. J Exp Soc Psychol 19:469–479, 1983

McCoy SB, Gibbons FX, Reis TJ, et al: Perceptions of smoking risk as a function of smoking status. J Behav Med 15:469–488, 1992

McGuffin P, Katz R, Watkins S, et al: A hospital-based twin register of the heritability of DSM-IV unipolar depression. Arch Gen Psychiatry 53:129–136, 1996

McLean P, Taylor S: Severity of unipolar depression and choice of treatment. Behav Res Ther 30:443–451, 1992

Meyerowitz BE, Chaiken S: The effect of message framing on breast self-examination: attitudes, intentions, and behavior. J Pers Soc Psychol 52:500–510, 1987

Meyerowitz BE, Sullivan CD, Premeau CL: Reactions of asbestos-exposed workers to notifications and screening. Am J Ind Med 15:463–475, 1989

Miller WR, Rollnick S: Motivational Interviewing. Preparing People to Change Addictive Behaviour. New York, Guilford, 1991

Morin CM, Kowatch RA, Barry T, et al: Cognitive-behavior therapy for late-life insomnia. J Consult Clin Psychol 61: 137–146, 1993

Peterson C, Seligman ME: Explanatory style and illness. J Pers 55(2):237–265, 1987

Peterson C, Maier SF, Seligman MEP: Learned Helplessness. A Theory for the Age of Personal Control. New York, Oxford University Press, 1993

Post RM: Transduction of psychosocial stress into the neurobiology of recurrent affective disorder. Am J Psychiatry 149:999–1010, 1992

Prochaska JO, DiClemente CC, Norcross JC: In search of how people change. Applications to addictive behaviors. Am Psychol 47:1102–1114, 1992

Ritvo PG: Quality of life and prostrate cancer treatment: decision-making and rehabilitative support. Can J Oncol 4(Suppl 1):43–46, 1994

Schaffer ND: Methodological issues of measuring skillfulness and therapeutic techniques. Psychotherapy: Theory, Research and Practice 20:486–493, 1983

Scheier MF, Mathews KA, Owens JF: Dispositional optimism and recovery from coronary artery bypass surgery: the beneficial effects on physical and psychological well-being. J Pers Soc Psychol 57:1024–1040, 1989

Segal, ZV, Shaw BF: Cognitive therapy, in American Psychiatric Press Review of Psychiatry, Vol 15. Edited by Dickstein LJ, Oldham JM, Riba MB. Washington, DC, American Psychiatric Press, 1996

Segal ZV, Williams JM, Teasdale JD, et al: A cognitive science perspective on kindling and episode sensitization in recurrent affective disorder. Psychol Med 26:371–380, 1996

Shaw BF: Specification of the training evaluation of cognitive therapists for outcome studies, in Psychotherapy Research: Where Are We and Where Should We Go? Edited by Williams JBW, Spitzer RL. New York, Guilford, 1984, pp 173–189

Shaw BF: Cognitive-behavior therapies for major depression: current status with an emphasis on prophylaxis. Psychiatr J Univ Ott 14(2):403–408; discussion 409–412, 1989

Shaw BF, Dobson KS: Competency judgements in the training and evaluation of psychotherapists. J Consult Clin Psychol 56:666–672, 1988

Shea MG, Elkin I, Imber SD, et al: Course of depressive symptoms over follow-up: findings from the National Institute of Mental Health treatment of depression collaboration research program. Arch Gen Psychiatry 49:782–787, 1992

Sherbourne CD, Hays RD, Ordway L, et al: Antecedents of adherence to medical recommendations: results from the Medical Outcomes Study. J Behav Med 15(5):447–468, 1992

Simons AD, Murphy GE, Levine JL, et al: Cognitive therapy and pharmacotherapy for depression. Arch Gen Psychiatry 43:43–50, 1986

Strauman TJ: Self-descriptions in clinical depression and social phobia: cognitive structures that underlie affective disorders? J Abnorm Psychol 98:14–22, 1989

Sturm R, Wells KB: How can care for depression come more cost-effective? JAMA 273:51–58, 1995

Taylor SE, Kemeny ME, Aspinwall LG, et al: Optimism, coping psychological distress, and high-risk sexual behavior among men at risk for Acquired Immunodeficiency Syndrome (AIDS). J Pers Soc Psychol 63:460–473, 1992

Teasdale JD: Cognitive vulnerability to persistent depression. Cognition and Emotion 2:247–274, 1988

Teasdale JD, Barnard PJ: Affect, Cognition and Change: Re-modelling Depressive Thought. Hillsdale, NJ, Lawrence Erlbaum Associates, 1993

Teasdale JD, Segal ZV, Williams JMG: How does cognitive therapy prevent depressive relapse and why should attention control (mindfulness) training help? Behav Res Ther 33:25–39, 1995

Thase ME, Simons AD, McGeary J, et al: Relapse after cognitive therapy of depression: potential implications for longer courses of treatment. Am J Psychiatry 149:1046–1052, 1991

Vaillant GE: Natural history of male psychological health IV: what kinds of men do not get psychosomatic illness. Psychosom Med 40:420–431, 1978

Warwick HMC: A controlled trial of cognitive therapy for hypochondriasis. Paper presented at the 20th Annual Conference of the British Association of Behavioural Psychotherapy, Oxford, England, September 1991

Weinberger DA, Schwartz GE, Davidson RJ: Low-anxious, high-anxious, and repressive coping styles: psychometric patterns and behavioral and psychological responses to stress. J Abnorm Psychol 88:369–380, 1979

Weinstein ND: Reducing unrealistic optimism about illness susceptibility. Health Psychol 7:11–20, 1983

Weinstein ND: The precaution adoption process. Health Psychol 7:355–386, 1988

Weinstein ND, Klotz ML, Sandman PM: Optimistic biases in public perceptions of the risk of radon. Journal of Public Health 78:796–800, 1988

Zuroff DC: New directions for cognitive models of depression. Psychological inquiry 3:274–277, 1992

Zuroff DC: Depressive personality styles and the five factor model of personality. J Pers Assess 63:453–472, 1994

Zuroff DC, Fitzpatrick DA: Depressive personality styles: Implications for adult attachment. Personality and Individual Differences 18:253–265, 1995

CHAPTER 8

Cognitive-Behavioral Therapy for the Eating Disorders

W. Stewart Agras, M.D.

Research into the treatment of anorexia nervosa has the longest history of any of the eating disorders, despite being the rarest of these entities. In the early days, almost every imaginable approach to treatment was tried in uncontrolled studies. Once controlled research began, it became clear that behavior therapy aimed at weight gain was helpful in shortening hospitalization (Agras and Kraemer 1983) and that antidepressant treatment, although superior to placebo, was not clinically useful (Walsh and Devlin 1992). However, despite detailed descriptions of cognitive-behavioral therapy (CBT) for anorexia nervosa (e.g., Garner and Bemis 1985), only one study of CBT has been reported to date, and this study reported equivocal results (Channon et al. 1989). Hence, this chapter focuses on cognitive-behavioral treatments for bulimia nervosa and binge eating disorder.

Although both bulimia nervosa and binge eating disorder have been described in the psychiatric and medical literature for centuries, it was not until the influx of cases into outpatient clinics in the 1970s that controlled research began. Over the past 15 years rapid strides have been made in the treatment of bulimia nervosa, with CBT becoming the standard therapy, antidepressant treatment being useful but less effective that CBT, and interpersonal therapy (IPT) being a possible alternative treatment. Advantages of CBT include the relatively large number of controlled treatment trials attesting to its effectiveness, continuing research with larger patient populations in multicenter research, and the existence of therapy manuals allowing for dissemination and standardization of the therapeutic procedures (Agras and Apple 1997).

Curiously, binge eating disorder was neglected until very recently. Hence, treatment research is still in its infancy, although researchers were able to borrow from the findings noted in the treatment of bulimia nervosa. At the present time, even short-term follow-up data are rare. Because of the complication of obesity, treatment must focus on binge eating and weight, and the weight loss treatment literature does not inspire confidence in the effectiveness of standard weight loss treatment.

Theoretical Background of CBT

Clinical observation spurred by the remarkable increase in the number of cases of bulimia nervosa seen in the clinics of all industrialized societies in the late 1970s (Garner et al. 1985) led to a hypothetical model of bulimia nervosa upon which CBT is based. It is thought that society changed its ideal body shape for women toward a thin body habitus (Agras and Kirkley 1986), and that may have led to an increase in the proportion of dieting young women. It is also likely that those of low self-esteem, generated from any cause, may be more sensitive about their body weight and shape, predisposing them to severe dietary restriction. This, in turn, is thought to lead to disinhibition of eating by various stimuli, and to binge eating, experienced as being out of control, followed in bulimia nervosa by compensatory purging, usually self-induced vomiting. A further risk factor for the development of binge eating appears to be adolescent overweight, confirmed in a longitudinal study in the United Kingdom (Patton et al. 1990), a factor that would increase the weight and shape concerns of adolescents and leading to dieting.

CBT is aimed at the two principal components of the disorder: first, the behavior component (severe dietary restriction) and second, the cognitive component (unrealistic food rules and distorted thinking concerning weight and shape). It is hypothesized that self-esteem improves as patients master their eating disorder. The procedures used in the therapy were derived from those commonly used in CBT for other conditions (e.g., Beck 1976) and modified for use in the eating disorders. The usual treatment is about 18–20 sessions over the course of 6 months. Therapy is divided into three phases. The first phase, lasting between 8 and 10 sessions, is aimed at remediating the dietary restriction, using self-monitoring of the disturbed eating behavior, binge eating, and purging, as well as education and formal problem solving. If binge eating and purging have not been significantly reduced in this phase, little further progress is likely to be made, and alternative treatments should be considered. The second phase, often overlapping the first, spans the remaining sessions and focuses on treating cognitive issues along with maintaining and extending gains in regular eating habits. In the last two or three sessions of treatment, relapse prevention procedures are added (Marlatt and Gordon 1980). In this final phase of treatment the factors associated with any remaining binge eating episodes or urges to eat are examined in detail, and the patient develops specific methods of coping with such situations.

Evidence for Efficacy

Bulimia Nervosa

In the 10 to 15 years following the initial case series, both in individual and group modes (Fairburn 1981; Schneider and Agras 1985), that demonstrated the potential efficacy of CBT in bulimia nervosa, with recovery in about half the patients, nearly 30 controlled studies have appeared. In the case of individual treatment, a median of 55% of patients recovered, with 87% reduction in binge eating and purging. For group treatment, 44% recovered, with a 70% reduction in binge eating and purging. These overall figures suggest that group treatment may be slightly less effective than individual treatment, a not overly surprising finding, although in a controlled comparison of group and individual behavioral therapies, no differences were found (Freeman 1988). The range of outcomes in both individual (13%–92% recovered) and group (13%–70% recovered) therapies is large, attesting in part to differences in the therapeutic procedures used, to differences in defining *recovered*, and probably to differences in patient populations.

CBT has been demonstrated to be more effective that nondirective psychotherapy, a short-term focal psychotherapy (Fairburn 1981), behavior therapy (Fairburn et al. 1991), psychodynamically oriented psychotherapy (Garner et al. 1993), stress management (Laessle 1991), and antidepressant medication (Agras et al. 1991; Mitchell et al. 1990). This is an impressive array of different and plausible treatments, some of which are effective in their own right, suggesting that CBT should be regarded as the first choice for the treatment of bulimia nervosa.

These studies also throw light on the effective components of CBT. Agras et al. (1989) report that nondirective therapy, which included monitoring eating behavior but none of the cognitive-behavioral elements of CBT, was found less effective than CBT. This suggests that the cognitive-behavioral elements of treatment are an important addition to the therapeutic relationship when combined with self-monitoring of eating behavior. Following up on these findings, a study by Fairburn et al. (1991) found that adding the cognitive elements of treatment led to greater improvement over the behavioral elements (mainly overcoming dietary restriction) alone. There is evidence not only that CBT is effective, but that specific elements of therapy are crucial to a successful outcome.

What then are the longer term outcomes of treatment with CBT? Overall, the results appear satisfactory with good maintenance in studies with follow-up periods of 6 months or 1 year. However, these overall statistics may hide some interesting findings. For example, in a 1-year follow-up of CBT, 41% of patients were recovered posttreatment and 54% at the follow-up, suggesting continued improvement over the follow-up period (Agras et al. 1994). However, 22% of the recovered patients had relapsed, whereas 38% of those not recovered posttreatment now met criteria for recovery (in this case, abstinence from binge eating and purging). This suggests that both relapse and further improvement occur during follow-up, and a substantial proportion of individuals can expect to improve in the year following CBT without any further treatment. This makes some sense, because skills learned during therapy can be applied by the motivated patient in the months thereafter, leading to recovery.

The longest follow-up study of CBT reported to date spanned 5 years (Fairburn et al. 1995). Fifty percent of those receiving CBT were abstinent at the 5-year follow-up. Interestingly, only 18% of those receiving behavior therapy (with no cognitive component) were abstinent at follow-up, a further indication of the importance of the cognitive components of treatment. Again, a substantial proportion of those who improved had relapsed by the 5-year follow-up, whereas a similar proportion were now abstinent. Overall, only 19% of patients met criteria for bulimia nervosa at the 5-year follow-up, 3% met criteria for anorexia nervosa, and 24% met criteria for eating disorder not otherwise specified. These long-term results suggest that some form of follow-up treatment may be necessary to prevent relapse in patients who recover following initial treatment. They also suggest that bulimia nervosa can be successfully treated, and that treatment gains are maintained over long periods.

These data continue to confirm that CBT is the most effective form of treatment for bulimia nervosa. One study, however, stands in sharp contrast to the remainder of the research literature. In this study, IPT and behavior therapy were compared with CBT in a randomized controlled trial (Fairburn et al. 1991, 1993). The three therapies appeared equivalent in their effects on binge eating and purging. However, CBT was more effective than either of the treatments in reducing disturbed attitudes toward weight and shape, an important aspect of the psychopathology of bulimia nervosa. At 1-year follow-up, nearly half of those receiving behavior therapy had dropped out of the study or had been withdrawn, and few were abstinent from binge eating and purging (Fairburn et al. 1993). On the other hand, IPT was now as effective as CBT both in reducing binge eating and purging behaviors and psychopathology. Patients receiving IPT demonstrated improvement over the follow-up period, whereas those receiving CBT leveled off. This is an intriguing finding because IPT does not directly address eating disorder symptomatology except in the first four assessment sessions. However, because only slightly more than half of all patients with bulimia recover with these therapies, it raises the question as to what to do with treatment failures.

Unfortunately, little is known concerning additive or second line treatments for bulimia nervosa. Three studies have addressed the question of the additive effects of CBT and antidepressant medication (Agras et al. 1991; Mitchell et al. 1990; Walsh et al. 1997). In the first of these studies, medication was found to add nothing to the effectiveness of CBT in reducing binge eating and purging, although depression was reduced more effectively in the combined condition than in the CBT alone condition (Mitchell et al. 1990). The second study has similar findings, although the combined treatment more effectively reduced dietary preoccupation, an aspect of the core psychopathology of bulimia nervosa (Agras et al. 1991). In a 1-year follow-up, 78% of those in the combined condition had recovered compared with 54% in the CBT group alone (Agras et al. 1994). However, this finding was not statistically significant, raising doubt about whether combining CBT with antidepressant medication routinely is useful. In the third study a medication sequence (desipramine followed by fluoxetine) was used. This sequence appeared to be as effective as CBT and to enhance the efficacy of CBT when added to the latter treatment.

Binge Eating Disorder

Because this disorder has only recently been rediscovered and diagnostic criteria defined in DSM-IV (American Psychiatric Association 1994), treatment research is less developed than in bulimia nervosa. Nonetheless, an interesting start has been made, illuminating some complexities involved in treating this disorder. Because binge eating disorder shares many characteristics with bulimia nervosa, the first step in treatment research has been to test the utility of treatments useful in that condition. However, because binge eating disorder is frequently associated with obesity, and because the latter disorder is usually treated in group format, the published studies to date have all used group treatment. In the first of these studies, patients with binge eating disorder (at the time referred to as nonpurging bulimia) were allocated at random to either group CBT or to a waiting list control group (Telch et al. 1990). Nearly 80% of the patients treated with CBT became abstinent as a result of the 10-week program, whereas none of those in the control group recovered. When the latter group was treated, those patients did equally well. Abstinence, however, was assessed over a 1-week period, probably inflating the total recovered. In an uncontrolled study of group CBT in binge eating disorder, in which abstinence was assessed over a 4-week interval, 50% of patients recovered. The percentage would have been greater had a 1-week interval been used (Smith et al. 1992).

The next study was directed toward improving both binge eating and weight (Agras et al. 1995). The principal comparison was between CBT aimed at reducing binge eating and weight loss treatment. After 12 weeks of CBT, participants then engaged in weight loss therapy, with half the group also receiving desipramine. The results were somewhat surprising. In the first 12 weeks of treatment, CBT reduced binge eating more effectively than did weight loss therapy, whereas the reverse was true for weight loss therapy. However, after that time, no differences in either binge eating frequency or weight were detectable between the weight loss and CBT groups. Procedures used in the weight loss treatment may have affected dietary behavior (e.g., eating regularly), and therefore reduced binge eating. The group receiving desipramine lost significantly more weight than the group receiving CBT alone, suggesting that in this group of patients antidepressants may have useful weight loss inducing properties. Previous research has shown that desipramine reduces hunger in patients with binge eating disorder, and may, therefore, act as a weak appetite suppressant (McCann and Agras 1990). However, as in bulimia nervosa, the antidepressant did not add to the effectiveness of CBT in reducing binge eating. It also appeared that patients who stopped binge eating lost more weight than those who did not, suggesting that treating binge eating successfully is an important goal in the treatment of the obese binge eater.

As with bulimia nervosa, it seems that IPT is as effective as CBT in reducing binge eating in patients with binge eating disorder (Wilfley et al. 1993). In the one study designed to examine this issue, patients were allocated at random either to group CBT, group IPT, or to a waiting list condition. Patients receiving active treatment did equally well, and both treatment groups were superior to the waiting list control in reducing binge eating. At 1-year follow-up both treatment groups continued improvement, although some degree of relapse was demonstrated. Because these two treatments are procedurally distinct, they may achieve their therapeutic effects through different mechanisms and may be effective in different types of patients with binge eating disorder. Because only one-half of the patients with binge eating disorder become abstinent from binge eating, it seems likely that IPT would be useful as a treatment for those patients who do not respond to CBT.

This issue was examined in a study in which patients meeting criteria for binge eating disorder were treated with group CBT (Agras et al. 1995). Those who responded to treatment continued with weight loss therapy, whereas those who did not respond were treated with group IPT. Unfortunately, no patient treated with IPT became abstinent, no change in binge eating was noted, nor did these individuals lose weight in this phase of treatment. A high score on the binge eating scale and early onset of binge eating, both denoting a more severe clinical status, were shown to be predictors of failure to improve with CBT. On querying the patients who received IPT about what had been most helpful to them, they chose some ingredients of CBT as most efficacious. This led to the next study that was recently completed. In this study, the hypothesis was tested that extended CBT might prove helpful for those failing the 12-session group program. Hence, patients with binge eating disorder who failed to improve with CBT, 50% of the group, were treated with an additional 12 sessions of group CBT. Unlike IPT, this additional treatment resulted in significant improvement, with some 65% of patients becoming abstinent after the 24 weeks of treatment. Determining the optimal length of CBT was also possible because no patient became abstinent with treatment beyond the 18th session (Eldredge et al. 1997). This number is similar to the length of treatment for bulimia nervosa, suggesting that in most of the studies of binge disorder to date, the length of CBT has not been optimal. Because there is evidence that group treatment for bulimia nervosa may be less effective than individual treatment, perhaps individual treatment with CBT would further enhance outcome.

Current Issues in Research

It can be concluded that CBT is the treatment of choice in bulimia nervosa, that antidepressant medication is also effective, although not as effective as CBT, and that IPT may be as effective as CBT, the former treatment being the only treatment to demonstrate equivalent effectiveness. These successes lead to the next series of questions.

Models of Bulimia Nervosa

In the first place, these finding raise questions as to the adequacy of the cognitive-behavioral model of bulimia nervosa. Because IPT is effective in the treatment of binge eating, both in bulimia nervosa and binge eating disorder, and does not address eating behavior directly, it must work by another mechanism. As noted earlier, this mechanism is likely to be through a reduction of the emotional triggers of binge eating, triggers arising from faulty interpersonal interactions. The cognitive-behavioral model of bulimia nervosa might be modified to include negative emotions as an alternative pathway leading to binge eating.

Recent laboratory experiments suggest that this model is not complete (Telch and Agras 1996a). In the first of these experiments in which participants with bulimia nervosa and binge eating disorder spent the day in the laboratory and were either food deprived for 1 or 6 hours, it appeared that eating disordered participants regulated their caloric intake exactly over the laboratory day. Whereas those who were deprived of food for 6 hours ate more at a buffet in the afternoon than those deprived for 1 hour, the whole day intake totals and 24-hour caloric intakes were identical between groups. One might speculate that in a binge, individuals with bulimia nervosa simply compensate for previous dietary restriction (and calories lost through purging); i.e., binge eating is a normal phenomenon regarded as abnormal by the bulimic because the large amount of food consumed.

The second study addressed the effects of negative mood on caloric intake in a laboratory buffet (Telch and Agras 1996b). Patients with binge eating disorder were allocated at random to either a negative or neutral mood induction prior to a laboratory buffet. As in the previous experiment, caloric intake at breakfast and lunch had been standardized in the laboratory. Negative mood did not lead to increased caloric intake at the buffet. However, the greater the negative affect the more likely the participant was to label the eating episode as a binge. In addition, negative affect was related to feeling more out control during the buffet. The findings suggest that the notion of disinhibition leading to a binge may be erroneous. Instead, caloric compensation for dietary restriction may be labeled as a normal meal or overeating if the patient is not in a negative mood, and as a binge if the patient is in a negative mood. Therefore, IPT may work by altering the labeling of eating episodes toward a normal meal as negative affect is reduced.

Questions Regarding the Treatment of Eating Disorders

One of the most pressing questions in the treatment of the eating disorders is whether IPT is as effective as CBT, or whether the apparent equivalence of the treatments is an artifact of small sample sizes. The question is presently being pursued in a multicenter study that will have an ample sample size. In addition, the question as to the mechanism by which IPT works is being evaluated in the same study. If the two therapies prove equally effective, a further question arises as to the sequencing of the treatments. Should treatment begin with IPT or CBT, and is either of the treatments effective when the first fails to produce improvements? The answer to such questions requires a large sample, and may require a multisite study. Of current interest is the question about how to treat patients with bulimia nervosa who do not respond to an adequate trial of cognitive therapy. Two possibilities exist: first, to use IPT as a secondary treatment, and second, to use antidepressant medication as a secondary treatment. To date, medication treatment trials in bulimia nervosa have used only one antidepressant. From a clinical viewpoint this appears too restrictive; hence two medications (e.g., a tricyclic antidepressant and a serotonin reuptake inhibitor) might be used in future trials. These considerations have been taken into account in the design of another ongoing multicenter study, in which patients not responding adequately to individual CBT are randomized to either medication or individual IPT.

In these days of managed care, the cost-effectiveness of different treatment approaches to bulimia nervosa is important. A preliminary analysis of this issue was recently completed (Koran et al. 1995). Although cost-effectiveness studies are complex, in this study the cost-effectiveness of CBT and desipramine and their combinations were compared using data from a previously described outcome study (Agras et al. 1991, 1994). Six months after treatment had been discontinued, it was apparent that desipramine given for 24 weeks was the most cost-effective treatment, costing nearly $2,000 per recovered patient, followed by CBT costing just over $3,000 per recovered patient. This might suggest that antidepressant medication should be given a short trial (e.g., 6–8 weeks) in the treatment of bulimia nervosa followed by CBT for the nonresponder.

The search for the most cost-effective treatment of bulimia nervosa has led to initial testing of self-help manuals given in an initial therapy session, with 1 follow-up visit 8 weeks later (Treasure et al. 1994). The manual was less effective than CBT, but more effective than a waiting list control condition, with about one-quarter of the subjects with bulimia receiving the manual becoming free of binge eating and purging. These are encouraging results, and they suggest that a stepped-care treatment for bulimia nervosa might be considered and tested against standard treatment (e.g., CBT). A stepped-care treatment might, for example, begin with a self-help manual, followed by medication, and finally by CBT for nonresponders. At the very least this approach might lead to the same rates of improvement as CBT while using less costly treatment, thus providing an overall cost-benefit. It is also possible, however, that patients experiencing a failure with one treatment might drop out of the treatment sequence, leading to higher dropout rates than those usual with CBT.

Research questions regarding the treatment of binge eating disorder at this time are those regarding the interaction between binge eating and weight loss. It seems possible that weight control treatment may be as effective as CBT and that antidepressant medication may also increase weight loss. Further investigation of the relative effectiveness of weight loss treatment and CBT, and the role of medication alone or combined with these therapies would appear important, as well as investigations into the mechanisms by which these different treatments work. Information on the longer term outcome of these treatments is also a priority at this time, because the immediate and long-term results of treatment may differ from short-term results.

Considerable progress has been made in the treatment of bulimia nervosa and binge eating disorders in a relatively short period. The progress has resulted in a marked improvement in treatment for patients suffering from these disorders, especially in the treatment of bulimia nervosa, where CBT has become the standard treatment. Further refinement of the treatment procedures may result in improved outcomes for our patients.

References

Agras WB, Apple RF: Overcoming Eating Disorders: A Cognitive-Behavioral Treatment for Bulimia Nervosa and Binge Eating Disorder. San Antonio, TX, The Psychological Corporation, 1997

Agras WS, Kirkley B: Bulimia: theories of etiology, in Handbook of Eating Disorders: Physiology, Psychology, and Treatment of Obesity, Anorexia and Bulimia. Edited by Brownell K, Fortney J. New York, Basic Books, 1986

Agras WS, Kraemer HC: The treatment of anorexia nervosa: do different treatments have different outcomes? in Eating and its Disorders. Edited by Stunkard AJ, Stellor E. New York, Raven, 1983

Agras WS, Rossiter E, Arnow B, et al: Pharmacologic and cognitive-behavioral treatment for bulimia nervosa: a controlled comparison. Am J Psychiatry 159:325–333, 1991

Agras WS, Rossiter E, Arnow B, et al: One-year follow-up of psychosocial and pharmacologic treatments for bulimia nervosa. J Clin Psychiatry 55:179–183, 1994

Agras WS, Schneider JA, Arnow B, et al: Cognitive-behavioral and response-prevention treatments for bulimia nervosa. J Consult Clin Psychol 57:215–221, 1989

Agras WS, Telch C, Arnow B, et al: Does interpersonal therapy help patients with binge eating disorder who fail to respond to cognitive-behavioral therapy? J Consult Clin Psychol 63:356–360, 1995

American Psychiatric Association: Diagnostic and Statistical Manual: Mental Disorders, 4th Edition. Washington, DC, American Psychiatric Association, 1994

Beck A: Cognitive Therapy and the Emotional Disorders. New York, International University Press, 1976

Channon S, deSilva P, Helmsley D, et al: A controlled trial of cognitive-behavioral and behavioral treatment of anorexia nervosa. Behav Res Ther 27:529–535, 1989

Eldredge KL, Agras WS, Arnow B, et al: The effects of extending cognitive-behavioral therapy for binge eating disorder among initial treatment non-responders. Int J Eat Disord 21:347–352, 1997

Fairburn C: A cognitive-behavioral approach to the management of bulimia nervosa. Psychol Med 11:701–707, 1981

Fairburn C, Jones R, Peveler R, et al: Three psychological treatments for bulimia nervosa: a comparative trial. Arch Gen Psychiatry 48:463–469, 1991

Fairburn C, Jones R, Peveler R, et al: Psychotherapy and bulimia nervosa: The longer term effects of interpersonal psychotherapy, behavior therapy, and cognitive-behavior therapy. Arch Gen Psychiatry 50:419–428, 1993

Fairburn C. Norman S, Welch M, et al: A prospective study of outcome in bulimia nervosa and the long-term effects of three psychological treatments. Arch Gen Psychiatry 52:304–312, 1995

Freeman CP, Barry F, Dunkell-Turnbull J, et al: Controlled trial of psychotherapy for bulimia nervosa. Journal of Clinical Research 296(6621):521–525, 1988

Garner D, Bemis K: Cognitive therapy for anorexia nervosa, in Handbook of Psychotherapy for Anorexia Nervosa and Bulimia. Edited by Garner D, Garfinkel P. New York, Guilford, 1985

Garner D, Olmsted M, Garfinkel P: Similarities among bulimic groups selected by weight history. J Psychiatr Res 19:129–134, 1985

Garner D, Rockert W, Davis R: Comparison of cognitive-behavioral and supportive-expressive therapy for bulimia nervosa. Am J Psychiatry 150:37–46, 1993

Koran L, Agras WS, Rossiter E, et al: Comparing the cost-effectiveness of psychiatric treatments: bulimia nervosa. J Psychiatr Res 58:13–21, 1995

Laessle RG, Beaumont PJ, Butow P, et al: A comparison of nutritional management with stress management in the treatment of bulimia nervosa. Br J Psychiatry 159:250–261, 1991

Marlatt G, Gordon J: Determinants of relapse: implications for the maintenance of behavior change, in Behavioral Medicine: Changing Health Lifestyles. Edited by Davidson P, Davidson S. New York, Brunner/Mazel, 1980

McCann U, Agras WS: Successful treatment of nonpurging bulimia nervosa with desipramine: a double-blind, placebo-controlled study. Am J Psychiatry 147:1509–1513, 1990

Mitchell J, Pyle R, Eckert E, et al: A comparison study of antidepressants and structured intensive group psychotherapy in the treatment of bulimia nervosa. Arch Gen Psychiatry 47:149–160, 1990

Patton E, Johnson-Sabinem E, Wood A, et al: Abnormal eating attitudes in London schoolgirls — a prospective epidemiological study: outcome at twelve-month follow-up. Psychol Med 20:383–394, 1990

Schneider J, Agras WS: A cognitive behavioral group treatment of bulimia. Br J Psychiatry 146:66–69, 1985

Smith D, Marcus M, Kaye W: Cognitive-behavioral treatment of obese binge eaters. Int J Eat Disord 12:257–262, 1992

Telch C, Agras WS, Rossiter E, et al: Group cognitive-behavioral treatment for the nonpurging bulimic: an initial evaluation. J Consult Clin Psychol 58:629–635, 1990

Telch C, Agras WS: The effects of short-term food deprivation on caloric intake in eating disordered subjects. Appetite 26:221–234, 1996a

Telch C, Agras WS: Do emotional states influence binge eating in the obese? Int J Eat Disord 20:271–280, 1996b

Treasure J, Schmidt U, Troop N, et al: First step in managing bulimia nervosa: controlled trial of therapeutic manual source. BMJ 308(6930):686–689, 1994

Walsh BT, Devlin MJ: The pharmacologic treatment of eating disorders. Psychiatr Clin North Am 15(1):149–160, 1992

Walsh BT, Wilson GT, Loeb KL, et al: Medication and psychotherapy in the treatment of bulimia nervosa. Am J Psychiatry 154:523–531, 1997

Wilfley D, Agras WS, Telch C, et al: Group cognitive-behavioral therapy and group interpersonal psychotherapy for the nonpurging bulimic: a controlled comparison. J Consult Clin Psychol 61:296–305, 1993

PART IV

Interpersonal Therapy: Mechanisms and Efficacy

CHAPTER 9

Interpersonal Psychotherapy and the Health Care Scene

Myrna M. Weissman, Ph.D.

Interpersonal psychotherapy (IPT) is time-limited, specified psychotherapy developed by Gerald L. Klerman, M.D. and colleagues and tested for the treatment of adult patients with major depression (Klerman et al. 1984). Over time, IPT has been modified for the treatment of different groups of patients with depression (elderly, adolescents, pregnant women, patients with recurrent depression, breast cancer, or HIV-positive status); different types of mood disorders (dysthymia, bipolar disorder, adjustment disorders); different nondepressive disorders (bulimia, drug abuse, borderline personality, binge eating, a social phobia); and in different formats (in groups, by telephone) (Klerman and Weissman 1993). It is included in various treatment guidelines in the United States, New Zealand, and Holland (Depression Guideline

Presented in receipt of the Zubin Lecture Award to the author and her late husband, Gerald L. Klerman, M.D., from the American Psychopathological Association, March 1996.

Panel 1993a, 1993b, 1993c; Karasu et al. 1993). A patient book has been published (Weissman 1995), and training programs are developing. An IPT clinic has been opened in Canada and translations into languages other than English are underway. Furthermore, the PRITE exam last year included two questions on IPT.

The apparent success of IPT and other time-limited psychotherapies such as cognitive therapy is in part a reflection of the changing health care scene in the United States and elsewhere, and the diminishing financial coverage available for psychotherapy. This chapter describes IPT, how it got started, what it is, and the issues relevant to IPT raised in the current health care climate.

How IPT Got Started

Given Gerald L. Klerman's strong rooting in psychopharmacology in the 1960s (e.g., as a Clinical Associate at NIMH, he organized the first multicentered clinical trial to test the efficacy of the phenothiazines in schizophrenia), one may ask how he came to develop and test a form of psychotherapy.

The story of IPT began in the late 1960s at Yale University, when Dr. Klerman, with Eugene Paykel, M.D., then a young psychiatrist from London, initiated a collaborative study with Harvard University to test the relative efficacy of a tricyclic antidepressant alone and with psychotherapy as maintenance treatment for ambulatory nonbipolar depression. At that time, the evidence for the efficacy of tricyclic antidepressants for reducing the acute symptoms of depression was strong, yet the main treatment for depression was psychodynamic psychotherapy. The only well-done studies of psychotherapy were with behavioral treatments, and these were limited in scope and sample size. A manual for cognitive-behavioral treatment (CBT) was under development by Dr. A. Beck. Furthermore, it was clear that many patients with depression relapsed after termination of acute tricyclic antidepressant treatment. It was unclear how long psychopharmacologic treatment should continue, and whether psychotherapy had a role in the prevention of the relapse of depression. Many ideological debates erupted in the field. For example, it was debated whether psychotherapy interfered with drugs by undoing the symptomatic improvement caused by drugs. The possibility that drugs interfered with the doctor-patient transference, or undercut defenses, was also debated (see Rounsaville et al. (1981) for a review of empirical testing).

Gerry Klerman felt that a clinical trial of maintenance tricyclic antidepressants should, as much as possible, mimic clinical practice. Because many patients then received both psychotherapy and drugs, either together or in sequence, he felt that psychotherapy should be included in the maintenance treatment trial, if for nothing more than a milieu effect. Having read the work of Eysenck and others, he was not convinced that he would find a psychotherapy effect, but he was convinced that psychotherapy could be subjected to testing in a clinical trial. Our job was first to define the type of psychotherapy and specify the procedures to be used. Psychotherapists could then be trained, and the quality and stability of treatment could be insured. We felt that the psychotherapy should mimic what was called supportive treatment, and should be what made sense in a time-limited treatment of depression. Initially, IPT was called *high contact*.

Although Gerry's main interest was in psychopharmacologic treatment, this did not detract from the fact that he felt psychotherapy was important in the care of patients. He loved teaching and personally giving psychotherapy. Although he believed psychotherapy was a powerful tool, he did not think it was a universal solvent. Its effectiveness depended on the patient's diagnosis, the type of psychotherapy, knowledge of its usefulness, and required evidence, not opinions. Five guiding principles governed this early work:

1. Randomized control clinical trials were important for testing and establishing the efficacy of all the treatments studied.
2. A broad range of standardized assessments were needed for measuring outcomes, including quality of life and social functioning. (The Social Adjustment Scale [Weissman and Paykel 1974] was developed for the first trial.)
3. Treatment results needed to be replicated. (Gerry did not develop

training programs or make efforts for dissemination of IPT until findings were replicated outside the enthusiastic group of developers.)

4. The potential value of maintenance treatment for preventing recurrence needed to be understood.

5. It was necessary to integrate and prove the potential of new psychopharmacologic agents for reducing symptoms and preventing relapse. (Gerry was concerned about what he termed "pharmacologic Calvinism" in this country.)

Thinking about therapeutic pharmacology in the 1970s was influenced by the mushrooming use of illicit drugs. Because of a general distrust of drugs used for nontherapeutic purposes, there was concern that any drugs that made one feel good must be morally bad (Klerman 1972). This attitude still prevails in some circles and is partially reflected in the underprescribing of psychotropic drugs even today. In addition, concepts deriving from the 1970s included 1) the importance of interpersonal relationships in affecting the fluctuation in course and recurrence of illness; 2) the potential of psychotherapy for stabilizing interpersonal relations; 3) the need for a standing national group, whose function was more scientifically evaluative and less regulatory than the Food and Drug Administration, available to evaluate the safety and efficacy of psychotherapies; 4) the patient's right to be an educated consumer, one informed of treatment alternatives, their efficacy, and side effects (Klerman et al. 1984); and finally, 5) that the patient had the right to effective treatment and that this treatment should be grounded in empirical research and not ideology (Klerman 1983, 1990). These ideas, which evolved in the 1960s and 1970s, were a consistent theme in Gerry's research for over 25 years.

What Is IPT?

A full description of IPT can be found in the original manual (Klerman et al. 1984). An update of the manual will appear in 1999 (Weissman et al., in press). Adaptations are described in Klerman and Weissman

(1993), the modification for adolescents with depression in Mufson et al. (1993), and in the book for patients in Weissman (1995). The most recent review of efficacy studies is in Weissman and Markowitz (1994).

IPT was initially formulated as a time-limited, weekly outpatient treatment for depression. Based on the ideas of the interpersonal school, IPT conceptually makes no assumptions about the etiology of depression but uses the connection between an onset of depressive symptoms and current interpersonal problems as a treatment focus. IPT generally deals with current rather than past interpersonal relationships, focusing on the patient's immediate social context, and attempts to intervene in the symptom formation and social dysfunction associated with depression, rather than focusing on enduring aspects of personality.

When used as an acute treatment, IPT has three phases. The first phase, usually the first one to three sessions, includes obtaining a diagnostic evaluation and psychiatric history, and this phase sets the framework for the treatment. The therapist reviews symptoms, diagnoses depression by standard criteria, and gives the patient the *sick role*. This role may excuse the patient from overwhelming social obligations, but requires the patient to work in treatment to recover full function. During the initial session, the psychiatric history includes a review of the patient's current social functioning and close relationships, their patterns, and mutual expectations. Changes in relationships proximal to the onset of symptoms are elucidated (i.e., death of a loved one, children leaving home, worsening marital strife, or isolation from a confidant). This review provides a framework for understanding the social and interpersonal context of the onset of depressive symptoms and defines the focus of treatment.

The therapist assesses the need for medication based on symptom severity, history, response to treatment, and patient preference. The patient is then educated about depression through an explicit discussion of the diagnosis, including the constellation of symptoms that define the diagnosis and the treatment expectations. IPT sessions address present here-and-now problems rather than childhood or developmental issues. Sessions open with the question "How have things been since we last met?" This focuses the patient on recent interpersonal events and recent mood, which the therapist attempts to link. Therapists take an active, nonneutral, supportive, and hopeful stance. The therapist links the depressive syndrome to the patient's interpersonal situation within the framework of one of four interpersonal problem areas: 1) grief, 2) interpersonal role disputes, 3) role transitions, or 4) interpersonal deficits. In the middle phase, the therapist pursues strategies defined in the manual that are specific to the designated interpersonal problem area. These four problem areas, with examples of the concepts illustrated from literature, are described in the sections that follow.

Grief

Grief is defined as complicated bereavement following the death of a loved one. For this problem area, the therapist facilitates mourning and gradually helps the patient to find new activities and relationships to compensate for the loss. Tennyson gives an excellent description of unresolved grief, the lingering pain and suffering felt for a death that occurred long ago:

> Dead, long dead,
> Long dead!
> And my heart is a handful of dust,
> And the wheels go over my head,
> And my bones are shaken with pain,
> For into a shallow grave they are thrust,
> Only a yard beneath the street . . . [Tennyson 1991]

Likewise, K. Jamison describes facing the reality of the death of a loved one. This is the beginning of the healing process.

> . . . He talked to me a long time about David, about the many years he had known and worked with him, and what a wonderful doctor and person he had been. He also said he thought it might be "terribly difficult, but a good idea" if he read me portions of the autopsy report. Ostensibly, this was to reassure me that the massiveness of David's heart attack was such that no treatment or medical intervention would have helped. In actuality, it was clear he knew that cold-

blooded medical language would shock me into beginning to deal with the finality of it all. . . . It certainly helped, although it was not so much the gruesome medical details that lurched me toward reality, it was instead, the brigadier's statement that "a young officer had accompanied the body of Colonel Laurie on the royal Air Force plane. . . ." David no longer was Colonel Laurie; he no longer was Dr. Laurie; he was a body. *[Jamison 1995, p. 149]*

Interpersonal Role Disputes

Role disputes are conflicts with a significant other, such as a spouse or other family member, a co-worker, or close friend, in which the patient and at least one other person has different expectations about the relationship. In working on role disputes, the therapist helps the patient explore the relationship and the nature and stage of a dispute. Three stages of exploration of role disputes have been identified: 1) In renegotiation, the parties are aware of differences and are trying to bring about change. 2) In impasse, discussion has stopped. Resentment smolders, and there is no attempt to renegotiate. Options to resolve the problem are considered. Failing this, the parties may conclude that the relationship has reached an impasse and consider ways to end and replace it with better alternatives. 3) In dissolution, the dispute causes irretrievable disruption, and active efforts are underway to terminate the relationship.

Philip Roth's characters Sabbath and Drenka illustrate renegotiation:

Life was as unthinkable for Sabbath without the successful innkeeper's promiscuous wife, as it was for her without the remorseless puppeteer . . .

Since when? Drenka, I cannot take seriously what you are asking of me. How do you justify wishing to impose on me restrictions that you have never imposed on yourself? You are asking for fidelity of a kind that you've never bothered to bestow on your own husband and that, were I to do what you request, you would still be denying him because of me. You want monogamy outside marriage and adultery inside marriage. Maybe you're right and that's the only way to do it. [*Roth 1996*]

Henrik Ibsen illustrates a classic role dispute impasse:

HELMER: You loved me as a wife should love her husband. But do you imagine that you're any less dear to me for not knowing how to act on your own? No, no, you must simply rely on me — I shall advise you and guide you. I shouldn't be a proper man if your feminine helplessness didn't make you twice as attractive to me.

NORA: . . . Doesn't it strike you that there's something strange about the way we're sitting here? . . . For eight whole years — no, longer than that — ever since we first met, we've never exchanged a serious word on any serious subject.

HELMER: Was I to keep forever involving you in worries that you couldn't possibly help me with?

NORA: I'm not talking about worries; what I'm saying is that we've never sat down in earnest together to get to the bottom of a single thing.

HELMER: . . . but, Nora dearest what good would that have been to you? [*Ibsen 1998*]

Subsequently, Nora takes matters into her own hands and leaves the marriage, her children, and her home.

Finally, Anne Sexton presents a painful description of the dissolution of a relationship:

And I don't know
don't know,
if we belong together or apart,
except that my soul lingers over the skin of you
and I wonder if I'm ruining all we had,
and had not,
by making this break,
this torn wedding ring,
this wrenched life

this God who is only half a God,
having separated the resurrection
from the glory . . . *[Sexton 1981]*

Role Transitions

Role transition includes changes in life status (i.e., the beginning or the end of a relationship or career, a move, promotion, retirement, graduation, diagnosis of a medical illness). In working with role transitions, recognizing the positive and negative aspects of the new role helps the patient to deal with the change he or she is assuming, and the assets and liabilities of the old role this replaces.

Ishiguro illustrates a role transition as a man facing aging and retirement:

Don't keep looking back all the time, you're bound to get depressed. And all right, you can't do your job as well as you used to. But it's the same for all of us, see? We've all got to put our feet up at some point. Been happy as a lark since the day I retired. All right, so neither of us are exactly in our first flush of youth, but you've got to keep looking forward . . .

Perhaps, then, there is something to his advice that I should cease looking back so much, that I should adopt a more positive outlook and try to make the best of what remains of my day. *[Ishiguro 1995]*

Interpersonal Deficits

Interpersonal deficits, the residual fourth IPT problem area, define the patient as significantly lacking in social skills, including initiating or sustaining relationships. This is the most difficult type of problem to handle in brief treatment.

The Status of IPT

IPT adaptations are currently a growth industry. Table 9–1 describes the status of efficacy testing as of May 1997. Trials planned and/or

TABLE 9–1

Status of IPT (May 1997)

	Trials	
	Underway	Completed
MDD (acute Rx)		2
MDD (maintenance Rx)		2
Geriatric MDD	1	1
Adolescent MDD	2	1
Dysthymia	2	
Pregnant women	2	
Postpartum depression	1	
Primary care	1	1
Bipolar patients	1	
Marital disputes (conjoint)		1
Distress	1	2
Bulimia	1	1
Bulimia group	1	1
Drug abuse		2
Borderline personality	1	
Depressed HIV-positive		1
Depressed cancer patients	1	
Depressed patients over the telephone	1	
Depressed mothers	1	

Note. See Weissman and Markowitz (1994) for efficacy results and Klerman and Weissman (1993) for description of adaptations.

under way in the United States, New Zealand, Germany, Italy, and France have not been included because the details of their design are not available. IPT adaptations are under development for social phobias, panic, insomnia, depressed caregivers of traumatic brain-injured patients, newly abstinent alcoholics who are depressed, women with breast cancer, protracted bereavement, depression after cardiac surgery, IPT by telephone, and in a group format (see Klerman and Weissman [1993] for description of adaptations).

Efficacy of IPT

The efficacy of IPT for depression and other disorders has been reviewed (Weissman and Markowitz 1994). In that review, based on evidence from controlled clinical trials, we concluded that IPT is a reasonable alternative and/or adjunct to medication as an acute, continuation, and/or maintenance treatment for patients with major depression. It is a promising but still not fully tested treatment for adolescents and geriatric patients who are depressed, HIV-positive patients with depression, patients with dysthymia or bulimia, patients with mild depression seen in primary care, and patients diagnosed with depression and their spouses with marital disputes. More efficacy data are needed in these areas before any claims can be made clearly. Claims based on open trials alone cannot be considered evidence of efficacy. As an important negative finding, IPT is not effective, compared with standard drug treatment programs, for patients addicted to opiates and cocaine. Several IPT clinical trials are under way or in the planning stages, based on manual modifications, and several manuals are being developed. The manuals differ in the depth of their modifications, and some modifications for different disorders have not been formalized. There is little agreement on what a manual of an IPT adaptation should include.

We view the development of psychotherapy manuals as positive, as they will meet the growing request from third-party payers, managed care professionals, and patients for accountability and specification of treatment. Manuals are also a necessary first step for testing efficacy. However, basic guidelines and clarification should be developed for the content of manuals.

Teaching and Learning IPT

Until recently, the number of IPT practitioners has been quite small, and almost exclusively limited to participants in research studies. IPT is now being included at professional workshops and conferences. Training courses have been conducted at university centers in Canada, Switzerland, Germany, Italy, New Zealand, and Iceland, and the IPT manual has been translated into Italian, German, and Japanese. A training videotape has been produced and is available through Kingsley Communications in Houston, Texas. The tape contains an overall description of IPT and demonstrates the initial assessment phase of treatment.

Although the principles of IPT are straightforward, training beyond reading the manual is required. Candidates should have a graduate clinical degree (M.D, Ph.D., M.S.W, or R.N.) and several years of experience conducting psychotherapy. Training programs for IPT are designed to help experienced therapists refocus their treatment to learn a new technique, and are not designed to teach novices to be therapists. The training used in the NIMH Collaborative Study in the Treatment of Depression has become a model for subsequent research studies (Elkin et al. 1989). This training usually includes a brief didactic phase in which the manual is read and reviewed and a longer supervised practicum during which the therapist treats patients under supervision, monitored by observations of audio or videotapes of actual IPT sessions. Chevron and Rounsaville (1983) and Rounsaville et al. (1986) have demonstrated that experienced therapists committed to the IPT approach, who performed well on their first supervised case, did not require further intensive supervision.

Even for experienced therapists, training programs in IPT are still not widely available, but wider dissemination is planned. The established training criteria for conducting research have produced reliable therapists for clinical trials. However, the educational process for IPT in clinical practice requires further study. For example, what educational level and experience are required to learn IPT? Does an experienced therapist require supervision? Will reading the manual suffice?

Specific research on the components of IPT, often termed *dismantling studies*, may prove useful. For example, IPT scholars view the initial diagnostic and assessment phase of IPT as essential to the clinical treatment of all depression. The efficacy of using the initial IPT phase only versus the full treatment, in which the interpersonal context of the depression is managed, might be tested. Further research on how long to extend IPT before discarding it for another treatment in patients who do not respond initially is necessary. Data from the study by Frank et al. (1990) showed the value of monthly maintenance IPT for patients with recurrent depression. There needs to be a series of studies of IPT dosage (e.g., weekly, biweekly, or monthly). These studies would be comparable to phase one or two drug trials.

With respect to the training of psychiatrists and related professionals, psychiatric residency and other mental health care treatment training programs should include clinical instruction in the new time-limited psychotherapies described in manuals, in addition to providing exposure to long-term psychotherapy. To our knowledge, no accepted model psychotherapy curriculum is available.

Concerns

The recent success of IPT and other brief psychotherapies are, in part, a reflection of the restrictions on reimbursement for psychotherapy in the new health care scene. There are increasing limitations of coverage, training, efficacy studies, and erosion of patient confidentiality.

Limitations of Coverage

Although IPT is time limited, some patients may need treatment available over longer periods of time. Major depression, for which IPT was first developed, fits the model of a chronic illness in that it is often recurrent. Although a large number of patients with depression have only one episode, and a small minority are chronic, the great majority, about 60% have recurrences throughout their lifetime. Treatment, therefore, needs to be available when these episodes occur and possibly to prevent future episodes.

For many patients, IPT is available as needed during periods of stress, and the emergence of symptoms may be all that is required to begin or resume it. Even in conditions such as bipolar disorder, which is a lifelong condition, where psychotropic medications are clearly the major treatment and psychotherapy is adjunctive, psychotherapy may be important to deal with life events during the acute episodes, to help improve medication compliance, or to help the patient who for any number of reasons such as pregnancy, or a medical or surgical crisis wants to discontinue medication. Unfortunately, those who control the flow of dollars may not be sufficiently flexible to take into account the individual differences among patients.

The relationship of psychotherapy to biologic therapies, and the need to keep a flexible attitude in choosing treatment, is well illustrated by the case of those women of childbearing age who are at high risk for developing depression. Some recent studies are indicating no long-term effects on the offspring from the new psychotropic drugs taken during pregnancy. However, many pregnant women refrain from their use. Psychotherapy can be an alternative to medication should depression occur during pregnancy. Although a considerable body of evidence exists supporting the efficacy of psychotropic drugs in treating depression, in the few studies where psychotherapy has been included, both medication and time-limited psychotherapy have had equal efficacy in reducing depressive symptoms. Overall, drugs, as compared with psychotherapy for the treatment of depression, have a faster and more consistent onset of action. In the Frank et al. (1990) study, which included patients who had severe recurrent depression, IPT alone, delivered once a month, prevented recurrence in nearly 70% of patients over a 36-week period. If these results can be generalized to depression in pregnant women, psychotherapy could provide an effective alternative to antidepressant medication during gestation.

Even after pregnancy ends, reintroducing or continuing antidepressants in the postpartum period could pose a problem for nursing women. The long-term effect on the infant of antidepressants in breast milk has not been studied, and little information exists on the short-term effects. In the absence of this data, women who require antidepressants are usually advised to discontinue nursing. However, in some cases, this medical advice runs counter to strong social and maternal expectations that mothers nurse their babies. The availability of psychotherapy during this period may help a woman get through the lactation period.

Insurance policies and health care benefits that restrict access to psychotherapy may thus be detrimental to the health of some women who require treatment for depression during pregnancy and the postpartum period and who do not want to take medication.

The pressure is on for mental health professionals to make therapeutic interventions efficient. Demands for efficiency will focus most heavily on psychotherapy, with most managed care organizations tending to exclude it from the benefit package, or if included, to limit the benefit to only very few sessions. This exclusion is reflected in the recent Agency for Health Care Policy in Research (AHCPR) guidelines that recommend psychotherapy only when depression is mild to moderate, nonpsychotic, nonchronic, and not highly recurrent. These definitions seem to represent a great boost for brief time-limited treatments such as IPT. Unfortunately, most psychiatric illnesses do not fit into the category of being nonchronic and not recurrent.

Thus, we must ask, will psychotherapy only be reimbursed for acute episodes treated briefly? What about patients who have recurrent episodes or disorders that are lifelong, such as bipolar disorder, and may require interventions throughout life during periods of incipient symptoms? How will lifetime caps on coverage be handled? Who will make these decisions? Will the decisions be based on the clinical reality of the condition or on economic policies?

Training

Training a skilled therapist in the techniques of IPT is not the same as training a novice to do psychotherapy. Training experienced psychotherapists is relatively easy. If psychotherapy training is devalued or eliminated, we will be training IPT therapists who do not have a general background in psychotherapy. Inexperienced therapists often adhere closely to the manual and end up giving lectures. Perhaps psychotherapy should be a subspecialty in psychiatric residencies. Residents would get some exposure but only a few who are very interested would get more extended training.

Efficacy Studies

There is no question that there are far fewer efficacy studies of psychotherapy than of pharmacotherapy. There is no industry support of efficacy studies in psychotherapy. A typical drug before it gets to market goes through four phases and then undergoes postmarketing surveillance. During these studies, doses, feasibility, side effects, interaction, and efficacy are tested. Persons who are skilled to do a Phase 1 study (e.g., the chemists) are not the same people who are skilled to do a Phase 4 study (the clinicians). A similar model is applicable to psychotherapy. Most psychotherapy trials begin prematurely, because there has not been a series of open trials. Dose, specificity, or even what subgroups might benefit has not been tested. The absence of these data can be used as a rationale for eliminating the treatment. In the face of diminishing resources for this type of research, it is unlikely that this situation will change.

Cost Offset

With the spread of managed care, there is a strong financial incentive to limit treatment (Schowalter 1995). The assessment of a patient's clinical outcome tends to focus on short-term treatment costs. The data suggest that the assessment of outcomes should be expanded to include such issues as impact of a parent's depression on their offspring over time.

The focus in considering cost offset or treatment efficiency is in reducing symptoms, decreasing days lost from work, or eliminating days in a hospital. These are clearly not the major outcome for psychotherapy, nor are they outcomes that fully reflect the morbidity of illness. For example, for depression it has been well documented that the offspring of parents who are depressed are at high risk for developing depression as well as behavioral, school, and health problems. Cost offset studies need to have a long-term view, which includes assessment of the impact of the illness on the immediate family and other aspects of social functioning.

Confidentiality

Patients and therapists are quick to discover that, in the new health care scene, they have had to waive the confidentiality of their doctor-patient relationships to obtain treatment approval. Unlike traditional insurance plans, where a brief medical record summary may be sent for review, patients now find their problems explained in detail over the phone to a case coordinator who is often not trained in social work or psychology. The therapist is forced to bargain for more therapeutic time. The coordinator then determines if there is an emergency and gets the process rolling. A physician or other mental health professional, trying to get a continuation of patient care and to get further sessions approved, often has to go into very private details of the patient's illness to assure the screener or manager that the patient is sufficiently ill to warrant further psychotherapy. Disclosure about the patient's private life will be in far more detail than what has been done in the past in traditional insurance plans and inherently undercuts patient trust.

The Future

What do I see as the future of IPT or other brief psychotherapies? There will be increasing interest by managed care companies, increasing manualization, decreasing coverage, and the increasing treatment by persons of decreasing education and training. Treatment will be done by telephone or perhaps by computer and, under these circumstances, may show decreased efficacy.

My late husband, Gerald Klerman, M.D., the developer of IPT, was way ahead of his time. His vision would not have anticipated the great interest in IPT. He died in April 1992, exactly one year before the guidelines for the AHCPR *Clinical Practice for the Treatment of Depression in Primary Care* were published, and comparable guidelines were published by the American Psychiatric and the American Psychological Associations. However, his words about the patient's right to effective treatment in 1990 are still just as true today:

> In current psychiatric practice, where there are large areas of ignorance, it behooves individual practitioners and institutions to avoid relying on single treatment approaches or theoretical paradigms . . . Treatment programs based only on psychotherapy or only on drugs are subject to criticism. Professionalism required balancing available knowledge, clinical experience and promoting the advancement of

scientific knowledge. In the case of treatment practices such knowledge comes best from controlled trials. *[Klerman 1990]*

References

Chevron ES, Rounsaville BJ: Evaluating the clinical skills of psychotherapists: a comparison of techniques. Arch Gen Psychiatry 40:1129–1132, 1983

Depression Guideline Panel: Clinical Guideline: Depression in Primary Care: Detection and Diagnosis. Agency for Health Care Policy and Research Publication No. 93–0550. Rockville, MD, U.S. Department of Health and Human Services, 1993a

Depression Guideline Panel: Clinical Practice Guideline: Quick Reference Guide for Clinicians: Depression in Primary Care: Detection, Diagnosis, and Treatment. Agency for Health Care Policy and Research Publication No. 93–0552. Rockville, MD, U.S. Department of Health and Human Services, 1993b

Depression Guideline Panel: Clinical Practice Guideline: Depression is a Treatable Illness: A Patient's Guide. Agency for Health Care Policy and Research Publication No. 93–0553. Rockville, MD, U.S. Department of Health and Human Services, 1993c

Elkin I, Shea MT, Watkins JT, et al: National Institute of Mental Health Treatment of Depression Collaborative Research Program: general effectiveness of treatments. Arch Gen Psychiatry 46:971–982, 1989

Frank E, Kupfer DJ, Perel JM, et al: Three-year outcomes for maintenance therapies in recurrent depression. Arch Gen Psychiatry 47:1093–1099, 1990

Ibsen H: A Doll's House, in Four Major Plays. Oxford, England, Oxford University Press, 1998

Ishiguro K: The Remains of the Day. New York, Random House, 1995

Jamison KR: An Unquiet Mind. New York, Knopf, 1995

Karasu TB, Coherty JP, Gelenberg A, et al: Practice guideline for major depressive disorder in adults. Am J Psychiatry 150(Suppl):1–26, 1993

Klerman GL: Psychotropic hedonism versus pharmacological Calvinism. Hastings Center Report 2(4):1–3, 1972

Klerman GL: The efficacy of psychotherapy as the basis for public policy. Am Psychol 38(8):929–934, 1983

Klerman GL: The psychiatric patient's right to effective treatment: implications of Osheroff versus Chestnut Lodge. Am J Psychiatry 147(4):409–418, 1990

Klerman GL, Weissman MM: New Applications of Interpersonal Psychotherapy. Washington, DC, American Psychiatric Press, 1993

Klerman GL, Weissman MM, Rounsaville BJ, et al: Interpersonal Psychotherapy of Depression. New York, Basic Books, 1984

Mufson L, Moreau D, Weissman MM, Klerman GL (eds): Interpersonal Psychotherapy for Depressed Adolescents. New York, Guilford, 1993

Roth P: Sabbath's Theater. New York, David McKay, 1996

Rounsaville BJ, Chevron ES, Weissman MM, et al: Training therapists to perform interpersonal psychotherapy in clinical trials. Compr Psychiatry 27:364–371, 1986

Rounsaville BJ, Weissman MM, Klerman GL: Do psychotherapy and pharmacotherapy for depression conflict? Arch Gen Psychiatry 38:24–29, 1981

Schowalter JE: Managed care: income to outcome. J Am Acad Child Adolesc Psychiatry 34(9):1123, 1995

Sexton A: The Complete Poems. Boston, Houghton Mifflin, 1981

Tennyson: In Memoriam, Maud and Other Poems. Everyman's Classic Library. Boston, Charles E. Tuttle, 1991

Weissman MM: Mastering Depression: A Patient's Guide to Interpersonal Psychotherapy. Albany, NY, Graywind Publications, 1995

Weissman MM, Markowitz JC: Interpersonal psychotherapy: current status. Arch Gen Psychiatry 51(8):509–606, 1994

Weissman MM, Markowitz JC, Klerman GL: Comprehensive Guide to Interpersonal Psychotherapy. New York, Basic Books, in press

Weissman MM, Paykel ES: The Depressed Woman: A Study of Social Relationships. Chicago, IL, University of Chicago Press, 1974

CHAPTER 10

Interpersonal Psychotherapy

Alone and Combined With Medication

John C. Markowitz, M.D.

Other chapters in this volume have described interpersonal psychotherapy (IPT) and aspects of its efficacy in a long-term maintenance trial. This chapter addresses IPT outcome trials that inform our still limited knowledge of the uses of IPT, both as monotherapy and in combination with medication.

Psychiatry is gaining sophistication in differential therapeutics, the science of treatment selection for particular disorders (Frances et al. 1984). Differential therapeutics can increasingly rely on empirical evidence from controlled clinical research trials, rather than having to depend on clinical experience and on sometimes ideologically biased wisdom (Klerman 1991). Differential therapeutics has been more extensively developed for pharmacotherapy than for psychotherapy, but evidence for the latter is starting to emerge as well.

From its inception, IPT (Klerman et al. 1984) has been empirically validated in controlled comparisons with pharmacotherapeutic and

Supported in part by grant MN-46250 from the National Institute of Mental Health, and from a fund established in The New York Community Trust by DeWitt-Wallace.

psychotherapeutic treatment alternatives. The IPT therapist helps depressed patients understand the interpersonal context within which depression occurs, recognizing interpersonal problem areas that can be linked to the onset of the depressive episode. Therapist and patient agree on an interpersonal formulation (Markowitz and Swartz 1997) linking the onset of the mood disorder to one of four interpersonal problem areas: grief (complicated bereavement), role dispute, role transition, or interpersonal deficits. Using strategies to help the patient alter these affectively linked interpersonal problems, the therapist helps the patient ameliorate both their interpersonal problems and their mood.

IPT as a Monotherapy for Mood Disorders

Therapists can offer patients IPT with a confidence based not only on ideology but also on empirical efficacy data from outcome studies. Outcome research has focused on monotherapy (i.e., IPT alone) for theoretical and practical reasons. Theoretically, it is important to show that each ingredient works alone before combining them in a treatment cocktail. Practically, monotherapy is often sufficient to treat depression, leaving little room at the top to show advantages for combined therapy. Combined treatment studies also raise research design difficulties. One is differential attrition: subjects who have strong feelings about receiving pharmacotherapy or psychotherapy may drop out if randomized to the opposing condition, but remain in a combined treatment cell where they receive, at least in part, their desired treatment. Another problem is that large sample sizes are needed to show the potential differences between two active treatment conditions, yet the number of subjects per cell in most combination studies to date have been relatively small (Manning et al. 1992).

Studies have demonstrated acute, continuation, and maintenance efficacy of IPT alone in comparison with behavioral controls and reference medication conditions. The multisite NIMH Treatment of Depression Collaborative Research Program (TDCRP) (Elkin et al. 1989) is the most ambitious and elaborate acute outcome study of the psychotherapy of major depression. It compared IPT with cognitive-behavioral therapy (CBT) (Beck et al. 1979), imipramine plus clinical management (IMI/CM), and a placebo plus clinical management (PLA/CM). Unlike earlier tests of the efficacy of IPT (Klerman et al. 1974; DiMascio et al. 1979; Weissman et al. 1979), the TDCRP took place away from the centers where IPT and CBT had been developed. Therapists carefully trained and monitored for adherence to their treatment protocols treated 250 subjects.

Because the PLA/CM cell performed well, no statistical difference between treatments was noted overall. When post hoc analyses examined subjects who presented with more severe initial depression, defined as a Hamilton Rating Scale for Depression (HRSD; Hamilton 1960) score of at least 20, however, differences did emerge. Both IMI/CM and IPT produced improvements significantly better than that of the PLA/CM condition. CBT ran a distant third, not statistically different from any of the other treatments. Subjects with depression who had difficulties in concentrating, impairment in functioning, low social dysfunction, or greater initial symptom severity did better in IPT compared with CBT, whereas patients with severe interpersonal deficits performed better in CBT (Sotsky et al. 1991). Thus, building on patients' strengths, rather than confronting their deficits, seemed to determine the success of IPT and CBT. Subjects who were less depressed (initial HRSD ≤20) improved equally regardless of intervention.

We are currently analyzing data from an NIMH-funded study in New York for the treatment of depression in subjects who are HIV-positive, begun by the late Samuel Perry, M.D., that largely replicates the TDCRP. Subjects (N = 101) were randomly assigned to receive IPT, CBT, supportive therapy, or supportive therapy plus imipramine (Markowitz et al. 1995). Preliminary results suggest the superiority of IPT to supportive therapy—a psychotherapy control rather than the placebo control used in the TDCRP. Like the post hoc TDCRP findings, early analyses from this study show that the IPT and pharmacotherapy cells produced the best results, with CBT and supportive therapy faring less well.

In the special case of depression in HIV infection, IPT may have particular advantages over CBT. Whereas CBT minimizes the patient's distorted cognitions, implying that the patient is overreacting because he or she is depressed, IPT acknowledges the importance of life traumas as contributors to the patient's psychopathology before helping to solve them. IPT thus may provide a better fit than CBT for patients who have had recent severe traumata (e.g., HIV infection) occur. In contrast, CBT may have advantages for patients who have not had recent life events or interpersonal disturbances, whose depression is more internalized. The latter patients would fall into the IPT category of interpersonal deficits.

Research demonstrating the efficacy of IPT alone as a continuation treatment (i.e., roughly 6 months of treatment) and a maintenance treatment (greater than 6 months) are described later in this chapter (Frank et al. 1991b). This discussion does not pretend to exhaustively recount monotherapy trials for IPT, but should suffice to indicate its efficacy as a single modality in treating depression.

IPT in Combination With Pharmacotherapy

The concept of combining modalities is not new. In the first half of the seventeenth century, Robert Burton wrote in his *Treatise on Melancholia*: "First begin with prayer and then use physick; not one without the other but both together" (Burton 1651/1955). More feels better to many clinicians. Yet, it is not clear that more treatment is necessarily better, or that it is always necessary.

Combined psychotherapy and pharmacotherapy studies of depression sometimes show modest advantage for the combined therapies; combined treatment often proves no better but never does worse than its component monotherapies (Manning et al. 1992; Persons et al. 1996). There are no negative clinical indications, then, aside from patient disinclination. Economically, however, combined therapy may not be necessary or cost effective. A 1987 NIMH consensus conference concluded that discriminating between psychotherapy and pharmacotherapy effect was difficult, because both treatments were so effective and because sample sizes in most extant studies were small. Patients with severe and/or chronic depression (i.e., more difficult-to-treat patients) were deemed optimal for differentiating combined and mode-specific treatment benefits of antidepressant therapies (Prien and Hirschfeld 1987).

Three studies have assessed the benefits of IPT in combination and competition with tricyclic antidepressants. These three studies — one acute, one continuation, and one maintenance trial — provide mixed findings on the benefits of combined therapy of patients with major depression. Unlike some other psychotherapies, IPT espouses a medical illness model of depression, which makes its combination with depression straightforward. IPT therapists can present the mixture of psychotherapy and pharmacotherapy as a compatible two-pronged attack on the illness, much as physicians prescribe both behavioral and medical interventions for diabetes mellitus, hypertension, cardiovascular disease, and other syndromes.

Acute Study

A 1979 study by Weissman, Klerman, and colleagues found mono-therapy with IPT or amitriptyline (AMI) superior to a low contact condition, but each inferior to combined IPT and AMI (DiMascio et al. 1979; Weissman et al. 1979). Eighty-one patients with major depression diagnosed by the Schedule for Affective Disorders and Schizophrenia (SADS; Endicott and Spitzer 1978) were entered, 40% of whom were experiencing their first episode. Most were women, and about half were married. Subjects were randomized to 16 weeks of treatment with IPT, AMI, their combination, or a low contact condition. The dosage of amitriptyline ranged from 100 to 200 mg daily, somewhat lower than we would aim for today. IPT sessions were scheduled at least weekly, and contrasted with a low contact, nonscheduled treatment. Patients in the latter condition received telephone contact and 50-minute supportive sessions "on demand," as needed; those who required more than one session a month were dropped from the study and treated openly.

End point analysis of the 17-item HRSD scale found that both IPT and AMI alone were statistically superior to the low contact condition. Moreover, there was an additive effect for the combination of IPT and AMI. Combined treatment subjects ($n = 23$) were most likely to complete the 16-week trial (67% vs. 48% for IPT alone, 33% for AMI alone, 30% for nonscheduled subjects). Combined treatment subjects were also least likely to be dropped from the study for "symptomatic failure": 4% versus 12% for IPT, 21% for AMI, and 48% for nonscheduled controls. AMI produced an early beneficial effect on insomnia, whereas IPT improved anxious and depressed mood and apathy earlier in treatment. Furthermore, IPT was associated with the development of new social skills at 1-year follow-up (Weissman et al. 1981). Thus in this acute study, each active treatment appeared to have specific symptomatic targets, and their effects were additive.

Continuation Study

In contrast, a continuation study by Klerman et al. (1974) found no advantage for 8 months of combined IPT plus AMI over either component alone. In this inaugural IPT trial, 150 women with depression were randomized in a sequential, 6-cell design. The depressed women were typically in their late 30s, and the majority had no prior mood episode, although 5% reported a history of manic episodes. All subjects received an open trial of AMI 100–200 mg/day for 6 weeks, after which those patients who showed significant improvement were randomized to 8 months of AMI versus a placebo versus no pill, and high or low interpersonal contact (i.e., weekly IPT versus low contact [15 minutes per month] conditions). Note that randomization to the placebo condition meant withdrawal from active amitriptyline.

Both AMI and IPT proved superior to the low contact control condition, but this early version of IPT did not add to the antidepressant effect of AMI alone as a maintenance treatment. IPT was again associated with gains in interpersonal relations and social adjustment, however.

Maintenance Study

The 1990 Pittsburgh maintenance study (Frank et al. 1990) found monthly maintenance IPT (IPT-M) more effective than a PLA/CM condition in prophylaxis of patients who were at extremely high risk for recurrence of major depression. Patients who had multiple (a mean of 7) episodes of major depression were treated with combined high dose imipramine and weekly IPT. Responders continued in treatment for a total of about 5 months before random assignment ($n = 128$) to one of five conditions: 1) imipramine (IMI), maintained at the acute dose (mean >200 mg/day) plus clinical management; 2) IPT-M, a monthly maintenance form of IPT; 3) IPT-M plus placebo; 4) combined IMI and IPT-M; or 5) PLA/CM. This was the first study to use high maintenance doses of imipramine, and the first to use any maintenance psychotherapy, but also, at once monthly, the lowest dosage of IPT ever.

High dose imipramine was the key prophylaxis in this elegant 5-cell study, with no added benefit from the addition monthly (i.e., low dose) IPT over 3 years (Frank et al. 1990). However, there were intriguing hints that higher dose maintenance IPT might make a difference, particularly in the first maintenance year, when 18% of IMI-alone patients relapsed, versus 8% of combined IMI/IPT patients. Although Dr. Ellen Frank (personal and public communication, February 1996) assures me that this difference does not approach statistical significance, this early discrepancy raises the question of whether more intensive IPT (e.g., biweekly rather than monthly) might have augmented the benefits of the pharmacotherapy condition. One must also remember that patients in the "imipramine only" maintenance condition had already had months of inoculation with weekly IPT in the acute and continuation treatment prior to randomization: thus the study did not compare pure effects of medication alone versus medication combined with psychotherapy.

In summary, the three IPT-pharmacotherapy combinations studied to date show differing results. The overall box score shows one with no difference, one with additive difference, and one with an intriguing hint of a difference. Acutely, adding IPT and medication yielded a synergy. In the earliest IPT study, which we would now consider of continuation length (Frank et al. 1991a), the combination of IPT and antidepressant medication was no more efficacious than monotherapy. In the Pittsburgh maintenance study, monthly (low dose) IPT-M did not add to the effect of high dose medication alone in patients with prior IPT exposure.

The combined therapy data involving IPT are both rich and limited. On the one hand, IPT is the *only* antidepressant psychotherapy to have been tested as both an acute and longer term treatment. Only one cognitive therapy study, involving a few postacute booster sessions, approaches consideration as a continuation study (Blackburn et al. 1981); all other non-IPT psychotherapy studies of mood disorder have been acute. The Pittsburgh maintenance study is not only unique in testing psychotherapy maintenance, but stands as a paragon of outcome research, employing comprehensive psychological and physiological assessments, audiotaped adherence monitoring (Frank et al. 1991b), and suffering almost no dropouts despite its extended duration (Frank et al. 1990). Other long-term combined treatment studies of patients in the geriatric population (Reynolds et al. 1992) and patients with bipolar disorder are currently underway in Pittsburgh. In many respects we should feel fortunate that, in a field where outcome studies are relatively few, so much evidence exists to document the efficacy of IPT, both as monotherapy and combined treatment.

On the other hand, there is only one combined IPT-pharmacotherapy treatment study to date for each category of treatment duration (i.e., acute, continuation, and maintenance). Only tertiary amine tricyclic antidepressants (amitriptyline and imipramine) have been used in these research projects. We have no research data on the combination of IPT with selective serotonin reuptake inhibitors; albeit there is little reason to expect them to fare less well with IPT than the tricyclics.

IPT as Monotherapy for Non-Mood Disorders

Like many treatments, IPT's success in one area has bred attempts to apply it elsewhere. In this respect it may be compared with pharmacotherapies such as beta blockers, originally used to treat hypertension but later found to help social phobia and other conditions. IPT has demonstrated efficacy in the acute treatment of bulimia, both as an individual treatment (Fairburn et al. 1991, 1993) and a group therapy

(Wilfley et al. 1993). Yet, IPT is not a panacea. Although interpersonal issues are ubiquitous and the principles of IPT can thus be generalized, the treatment does not work universally, as treatments of substance dependence have shown (Carroll et al. 1991; Rounsaville et al. 1983). Psychiatric illnesses do occur in a social context, not in a vacuum, but whether that insight can be turned to therapeutic advantage appears to vary from syndrome to syndrome.

Discussion

When should IPT be used as monotherapy? When should it be used in a combined treatment? Despite a relatively rich array of studies, we know relatively little about its differential therapeutics. Here follow my speculations, based, insofar as possible, on the research just reviewed.

For mild or moderate depression, monotherapy is likely to suffice.

This has been the conclusion of several reviews of combined antidepressant literature (Frank et al. 1991b; Sotsky et al. 1991). The results of the TDCRP indicated that all its monotherapies, including the PLA/CM intervention, tended to yield good outcomes for patients whose initial 17-item HRSD score was less than 20 (Elkin et al. 1989). Given today's economic pressures, reserving the combination of psychotherapy and pharmacotherapy for more difficult patients seems sensible. Either psychotherapy or pharmacotherapy may be appropriate for patients with mild depression. (An inexpensive, quasi "combined" alternative approach might add an IPT patient book [Weissman 1995] to pharmacotherapy.) Treatment selection should depend largely on the patient's preference, which should rest upon an accurate knowledge of the full array of available treatments, their likely benefits, and side effects.

IPT helps people who have had something happen to them.

In my experience, most people accept the basic IPT premise as credible: it makes sense that what is happening in your interpersonal environment can affect your mood, and vice versa. Patients who have developed a depressive episode while undergoing life crises — losses, interpersonal disputes, transitions — are still more likely to believe this formulation (Markowitz and Swartz 1997). This is probably why IPT works so well for patients with depression resulting from knowledge of an HIV-positive status, many of whom have faced a surfeit of life stressors: multiple AIDS-related bereavements, interpersonal disputes deriving from their HIV-serostatus, and the inherent life transition of learning one has HIV infection. In contrast, patients who are socially isolated and depressed and who have major interpersonal deficits and little environmental perturbation may be better CBT than IPT candidates (Sotsky et al. 1991).

This is not to say that IPT works only for "reactive" depressions, nor that the IPT interpersonal deficit category is unworkable. It does, however, comprise a group of particularly difficult-to-treat patients who lack the interpersonal skills IPT builds upon. Interpersonal deficits are the least developed of the IPT interpersonal problem areas. Thus, for several reasons these patients may work better with a different antidepressant paradigm.

Combined treatment may benefit patients with more severe depression.

The 1979 Weissman et al. study (DiMascio et al. 1979) showed acute benefit for combined treatment in comparison with monotherapy. Overall, symptom severity has been considered a negative prognostic factor, requiring greater gains to attain a HRSD remission threshold. The IPT maintenance study did not show an augmentation of pharmacotherapy affect by monthly IPT-M, yet it is possible that combined therapy may have benefited all patients through the continuation phase of that study, with a hint of this benefit showing through even at a reduced, monthly dosage in the combined treatment group during the first post randomization year. Thase et al. (1994) have also reported that combined IPT and pharmacotherapy surpassed psychotherapy alone for outpatients with more severe depression, but not for outpatients who were less depressed.

Whereas vigorous pharmacotherapy may produce a faster remission of neurovegetative symptoms and provide surer prophylaxis against relapses, psychotherapy may help patients to reorient their lives as they recover from a depressive episode, and may help them to address ongoing life stressors that could precipitate a future episode. Indeed, IPT focuses on such interpersonal stressors and has been shown to improve social functioning (Klerman et al. 1974; Weissman et al. 1979).

My clinical impression is that many patients whose recurrent or chronic depression clears with pharmacotherapy benefit greatly from postdepressive or postdysthymic psychotherapy that helps them recover confidence, take social risks, and develop social skills (Markowitz 1993). For patients too severely depressed to respond to psychotherapy initially, the structure of the 1974 continuation study provides a treatment model: treatment with pharmacotherapy first, followed by the addition of psychotherapy as the medication takes effect (Manning et al. 1992).

Approach psychotherapy with a treatment algorithm.

Pharmacotherapists generally approach depression with the idea of treatment resistance in mind. If an adequate trial of one medication should not work, many augmentation and alternative strategies are available (Roose and Glassman 1990). The same approach should apply to antidepressant psychotherapy. Psychotherapy has traditionally been delivered as an open-ended treatment, with no such consideration of acute outcomes or alternatives. Changing gears from one psychotherapy to another is probably more complicated than switching antidepressant medications: the medication paradigm remains the same, whereas to switch from interpersonal to cognitive therapy, or vice versa, the patient must cast aside one perspective and adopt another. Yet if the psychotherapy is not making a difference after a reasonable time — say, 12 weeks — then such a change is worth discussing with the patient and may be warranted. The therapist's allegiance should be to the patient's improvement rather than to a particular psychotherapeutic approach.

Combined treatment is indicated for treatment-resistant patients.

This recommendation is based not on research evidence — the proposition has never been tested — but on common sense. Depression usually responds to treatment. If monotherapy fails, or fails repeatedly, combined psychotherapy and pharmacotherapy may be both clinically and economically efficient, attacking an illness from different aspects and by different mechanisms. Again, IPT melds nicely with pharmacotherapy in using a medical model of depressive illness and giving the patient the sick role (Parsons 1951).

Conclusion

Research to date provides reasons to be encouraged about this optimistic, pragmatic therapy. IPT can be easily combined with pharmacotherapy for depression. At least acutely, combined treatment may be beneficial, at least for more severe depression. Yet the differential therapeutics of antidepressant psychotherapy is still a nascent enterprise, inviting the academic axiom: more research is needed.

References

Beck AT, Rush AJ, Shaw BF, et al: Cognitive Therapy of Depression. New York, Guilford, 1979

Blackburn IM, Bishop S, Glen AIM, et al: The efficacy of cognitive therapy in depression: a treatment trial using cognitive therapy and pharmacotherapy, each alone and in combination. Br J Psychiatry 139:181–189, 1981

Burton R: The Anatomy of Melancholy (1651). New York, Tudor Publishing, 1955

Carroll KM, Rounsaville BJ, Gawin FH: A comparative trial of psychotherapies for ambulatory cocaine abusers: relapse prevention and interpersonal psychotherapy. Am J Drug Alcohol Abuse 17(3):229–247, 1991

DiMascio A, Weissman MM, Prusoff BA, et al: Differential symptom reduction by drugs and psychotherapy in acute depression. Arch Gen Psychiatry 36:1450–1456, 1979

Elkin I, Shea MT, Watkins JT, et al: National Institute of Mental Health Treatment Of Depression Collaborative Research Program: general effectiveness of treatments. Arch Gen Psychiatry 46:971–982, 1989

Endicott J, Spitzer RL: A diagnostic interview: the Schedule for Affective Disorders and Schizophrenia. Arch Gen Psychiatry 35:837–844, 1978

Fairburn CG, Jones R, Peveler RC, et al: Three psychological treatments for bulimia nervosa: a comparative trial. Arch Gen Psychiatry 48:463–469, 1991

Fairburn CG, Jones R, Peveler RC, et al: Psychotherapy and bulimia nervosa. Arch Gen Psychiatry 50:419–428, 1993

Frances A, Clarkin JF, Perry S: Differential Therapeutics in Psychiatry: The Art and Science of Treatment Selection. New York, Brunner/Mazel, 1984

Frank E, Kupfer DJ, Perel JM, et al: Three-year outcomes for maintenance therapies in recurrent depression. Arch Gen Psychiatry 47:1093–1099, 1990

Frank E, Prien RF, Jarrett RB, et al: Conceptualization and rationale for consensus definitions of terms in major depressive disorder. Arch Gen Psychiatry 48:851–855, 1991a

Frank E, Kupfer DJ, Wagner EF, et al: Efficacy of interpersonal psychotherapy as a maintenance treatment of recurrent depression. Arch Gen Psychiatry 48:1053–1059, 1991b

Hamilton M: A rating scale for depression. J Neurol Neurosurg Psychiatry 25:56–62, 1960

Klerman GL: Ideological conflicts in integrating pharmacotherapy and psychotherapy, in Integrating Pharmacotherapy and Psychotherapy. Edited by Beitman BD, Klerman GL. Washington, DC, American Psychiatric Press, 1991, pp 3–19

Klerman GL, DiMascio A, Weissman MM, et al: Treatment of depression by drugs and psychotherapy. Am J Psychiatry 131:186–191, 1974

Klerman GL, Weissman MM, Rounsaville BJ: Interpersonal Psychotherapy of Depression. New York, Basic Books, 1984

Manning DW, Markowitz JC, Frances AJ: A review of combined psychotherapy and pharmacotherapy in the treatment of depression. J Psychother Pract Res 1:103–116, 1992

Markowitz JC: Psychotherapy of the post-dysthymic patient. J Psychother Pract Res 2:157–163, 1993

Markowitz JC, Swartz HA: Case formulation in interpersonal psychotherapy of depression, in Handbook of Psychotherapy Case Formulation. Edited by Fels TD. New York, Guilford, 1997, pp 192–222

Markowitz JC, Klerman GL, Clougherty KF, et al: Individual psychotherapies for depressed HIV-positive patients. Am J Psychiatry 152:1504–1509, 1995

Parsons T: Illness and the role of the physician: a sociological perspective. Am J Orthopsychiatry 21:452–460, 1951

Persons JB, Thase ME, Crits-Christoph P: The role of psychotherapy in the treatment of depression: review of two practice guidelines. Arch Gen Psychiatry 53:283–290, 1996

Prien R, Hirschfeld RMA: Combined medication and psychotherapy in depression. NIMH workshop, Washington, DC, September 1997

Reynolds CF, Frank E, Perel JM, et al: Combined pharmacotherapy and psychotherapy in the acute and continuation treatment of elderly patients with recurrent major depression: a preliminary report. Am J Psychiatry 149:1687–1692, 1992

Roose SP, Glassman AH (eds): Treatment Strategies for Refractory Depression. Washington, DC, American Psychiatric Press, 1990

Rounsaville BJ, Glazer W, Wilber CH, et al: Short-term interpersonal psychotherapy in methadone-maintained opiate addicts. Arch Gen Psychiatry 40:629–636, 1983

Sotsky SM, Glass DR, Shea MT, et al: Patient predictors of response to psychotherapy and pharmacotherapy: findings in the NIMH Treatment Of Depression Collaborative Research Program. Am J Psychiatry 148:997–1008, 1991

Thase ME, Greenhouse J, Frank E, et al: Correlates of remission of major depression during standardized trials of psychotherapy, pharmacotherapy, or their combination: results from the Pittsburgh 600 (abstract). Psychopharm Bull 30:642, 1994

Weissman MM: Mastering Depression: A Patient's Guide to Interpersonal Psychotherapy. Albany, NY, Graywind Publications, 1995

Weissman MM, Prusoff BA, DiMascio A, et al: The efficacy of drugs and psychotherapy in the treatment of acute depressive episodes. Am J Psychiatry 136:555–558, 1979

Weissman MM, Klerman GL, Prusoff BA, et al: Depressed outpatients: results one year after treatment with drugs and/or interpersonal psychotherapy. Arch Gen Psychiatry 38:52–55, 1981

Wilfley DE, Agras WS, Telch CF, et al: Group cognitive-behavioral therapy and group interpersonal psychotherapy for the nonpurging bulimic individual: a controlled comparison. J Consult Clin Psychol 61:296–305, 1993

CHAPTER 11

Maintenance Interpersonal Psychotherapy for Recurrent Depression

Biological and Clinical Correlates and Future Directions

Cynthia A. Spanier, Ph.D.

Ellen Frank, Ph.D.

Ann B. McEachran, M.A.

Victoria J. Grochocinski, Ph.D.

David J. Kupfer, M.D.

Mood disorders treatment research in the last decade has experienced a paradigm shift, from a focus on recovery from an acute episode to a focus on prevention or maintenance of the well state. This broadening of focus has been stimulated by a convergence of epidemiological and clinical evidence indicating that major depression follows a chronic or recurrent course for most individuals (Kessler et al. 1994), and thus, the critical problem in the treatment of depression is the prevention of relapse and recurrence. This view of depression and its treatment is not new (Klerman et al. 1974), although it is only in the last decade that the importance of prevention has gained widespread acceptance. The aim of preventive treatment for depression, be it psychotherapeutic, pharmacological, or both, is to alter the short- and long-term course of the disorder by either preventing or delaying a recurrence of a sub-

This work was supported in part by National Institute of Mental Health Grants MH 29618 (Dr. Frank) and MH30915 (Dr. Kupfer).

sequent depressive episode and thus increasing the length of the well state following recovery from an acute episode.

Much recent research has focused on the development and evaluation of improved maintenance treatment strategies for patients with a history of recurrent depressive episodes. Although strong evidence exists to support the efficacy of long-term antidepressant medications in the prevention of recurrence (Frank et al. 1990, 1993b; Glen et al. 1984; Kupfer et al. 1992; Prien et al. 1984), even on maintenance pharmacotherapy, the long-term course of patients with recurrent unipolar illness can be variable. In addition, a sizeable group of patients either chooses not to continue long-term pharmacotherapy in the absence of any depressive symptoms, cannot take medication due to a medical condition that precludes the use of antidepressants, or suffer from side effects that are intolerable to them. Furthermore, in a review of pharmacotherapy of mood disorders, Thase and Kupfer (1996) note that the risk of recurrence is significantly higher in patient samples following withdrawal of antidepressants in comparison to the risk of recurrence in naturalistic samples of patients. Clearly, if long-term preventive treatment of patients in remission with recurrent unipolar illness is to advance or improve significantly, considering the effects of biological *and* psychological factors is imperative as they affect vulnerability to depression, rather than focusing exclusively on protection of vulnerable patients by pharmacotherapy.

Taken together, these findings indicate the critical importance of developing and improving nonpharmacological alternatives that reduce the risk of recurrence. In spite of the American Psychiatric Association (1993) practice guidelines (Persons et al. 1996; Rush 1996), psychosocial treatments, such as interpersonal psychotherapy (IPT), have an important and empirically validated role in the treatment of major depressive disorder (see Frank and Spanier 1995, for a review). As one of the promising forms of psychosocial treatment for depression, IPT has shown consistent efficacy in a series of well-designed acute (DiMascio et al. 1979; Elkin et al. 1989), continuation (Klerman et al. 1974), and maintenance (Frank et al. 1990) treatment trials.

The focus in this chapter is not to debate the relative merits, efficacy, or effectiveness of somatic therapy in comparison to psychotherapy or their combination in the long-term treatment of depression. We still do not have enough empirical evidence to suggest one strategy over another in the long-term preventive treatment of major depression. Rather, using an integrative approach, the goal in this chapter is to examine more closely what variables moderate the effect of long-term preventive treatment of depression, in this case, IPT, after patients discontinue pharmacotherapy. Although much research has examined treatment response to pharmacotherapy, the purpose of this work is to identify and integrate psychological and biological processes that work to optimize response to psychotherapy. Such efforts advance our knowledge regarding ways to maximize the preventive capacity of IPT and increase our understanding of ways to match patients to treatment, be it psychotherapeutic, pharmacological, or both.

IPT as an Acute and Preventive Treatment for Depression

Since its inception as a research intervention over 25 years ago, IPT (Klerman et al. 1984) has emerged as a viable and well-researched psychotherapeutic intervention for the acute and preventative treatment of major depression (see Frank and Spanier 1995; Frank et al. 1993a; Klerman and Weissman 1991, 1993; Prochaska and Norcross 1994; Weissman and Markowitz 1994 for reviews). IPT focuses on the association between the onset and/or persistence of depression and current interpersonal stressors. In addition to being an efficacious short-term treatment, the maintenance form of IPT (IPT-M) (Frank 1991), has been particularly useful in reducing the risk of recurrence.

Maintenance IPT (IPT-M)

The adaptation of IPT to a maintenance treatment was based extensively on IPT as developed by Klerman et al. (1984). Both are manual-based treatments focusing on the analysis of social relations and on the alleviation of interpersonal problems. In addition, IPT-M preserves the four distinctive problem areas of IPT: role transitions, role disputes, interpersonal deficits, and grief. It also implements the strategies (e.g., exploration of feelings associated with loss of a role) and techniques of IPT (e.g., elicitation of feelings, nonjudgmental exploration of the affective quality of relationships, encouraging the development of satisfying and adaptive interpersonal behaviors). It differs from IPT, however, in terms of its goals and timing. The primary goal of IPT-M is to *prevent recurrence*, that is, sustain wellness in patients who are fully remitted; in contrast, the goal of IPT is to *bring about remission* from an acute episode of depression. Moreover, IPT-M is designed to treat patients in a maintenance format for several years. Patients were treated for up to three years with IPT-M in the Maintenance Therapies in Recurrent Depression (MTRD) study for which it was originally developed (Frank et al. 1990). Accordingly, the *number* of problem areas that are typically the focus of IPT-M is greater than in IPT for the acute treatment of depression. In addition, whereas the techniques used in IPT-M are similar to IPT, the time frame of IPT-M places a greater emphasis on the future.

The timing of IPT-M also differs from weekly IPT for short-term acute treatment. All patients participating in IPT-M in the MTRD protocol were fully remitted and IPT-M was scheduled once per month (Frank et al. 1990). Although monthly IPT sessions showed a significant effect in extending the interval between depressive episodes, it may be that more frequent contact, weekly or biweekly, could have produced an even better outcome, especially in patients who preferred more frequent contacts or who experienced loss or increased anxiety by moving from weekly IPT to monthly IPT-M. Currently underway is a clinical trial testing the efficacy of weekly, biweekly, and monthly maintenance IPT (IPT-M). The goal of this investigation (MH-49115, E. Frank, PI) is to maximize the preventive capacity of IPT-M by establishing the ideal contact frequency. Clearly, at least for a subset of patients in the MTRD protocol, moving from weekly to monthly contact was the optimal preventive strategy: "These individuals seemed able to benefit from the longer distance between therapy sessions as a direct consequence of having had more time between sessions to think about and observe the interpersonal context of their lives and to experiment with new interpersonal behaviors" (Frank 1991, p. 264).

Review of Results Concerning the Efficacy of IPT-M

The work reported in this chapter is based on data drawn from the Pittsburgh study of MTRD (Frank et al. 1990), a 3-year randomized clinical trial designed to determine the efficacy of five maintenance treatments that involved IPT (i.e., IPT-M) and/or antidepressant medication in preventing a recurrence of illness in a group of patients with recurrent unipolar illness. The five treatments included 1) IPT-M alone, 2) IPT-M with placebo tablet, 3) IPT-M with imipramine, 4) medication clinic visits with imipramine, 5) medication clinic visits with placebo tablet. Individuals participating in this clinical trial were initially seen during an acute episode of depression and received both IPT and antidepressant medication (i.e., imipramine hydrochloride, 150–300 mg). Initial treatment was provided weekly for 12 weeks, every other week for the next 8 weeks, and then monthly until patients' symptoms diminished to a remission range defined as an HRSD score <7 and a Raskin score <5. Once stabilized, patients continued to received both IPT and imipramine until they had maintained a symptom-free state (i.e., HRSD <7; Raskin <5) for 20 weeks.

Following this period of short-term and continuation treatment, the experimental maintenance phase began. The 128 patients who achieved a sustained remission of their acute depressive episode were randomly assigned to one of the five maintenance treatment conditions. Maintenance treatment sessions occurred monthly for 3 years or until the patient experienced a recurrence of illness. In addition, patients underwent sleep electroencephalographic (EEG) monitoring at baseline and periodically throughout the course of treatment, and thus biological variables, such as delta sleep ratio (DSR), REM latency, and slow wave sleep percentage, were incorporated as part of this treatment research.

Results of survival analyses showed that active imipramine, maintained at an average dose of 200 mg, provided a prophylactic effect to a larger proportion of patients over a longer period than in any previous study of maintenance therapy of recurrent depression (Frank et al. 1990). Of most relevance here, we also demonstrated that when patients received a combination of pharmacotherapy and IPT for the treatment of their acute episode, those who continued to receive IPT on a monthly basis following drug discontinuation remained well significantly longer than those who did not.

Variables Moderating the Effectiveness of Maintenance IPT in the Absence of Medication

In addition to examining the efficacy of preventive treatments, another overarching aim of this clinical trial was to identify and better understand potential risk and protective factors influencing the efficacy (i.e., response or nonresponse) to preventive treatments. Consistent with the integrative approach used in this long-term treatment trial, both biological and psychosocial *correlates* have been examined.

Before reviewing the findings, it is important to clarify our use of the term *correlate* as opposed to *risk factor* and how these terms pertain to treatment outcome in the MTRD protocol. Kraemer et al. (1997) have elaborated a model suggesting that the term *risk* should be used *only* when referring to the probability of some binary outcome (e.g., recurrence, no recurrence). Typically, the outcome is negative (i.e., death or disorder) but the model holds for positive outcomes (sustained wellness, no recurrence) usually noted by the term *protective factor*. In addition, when a factor has been shown to be associated with an outcome, we can infer from these findings only that the two are *correlated*. Until other conditions are met, for example, if the factor is associated with outcome and precedes the outcome, as might be determined in a longitudinal study, then we can begin to consider it a *true* risk factor. An important caveat is that a risk factor cannot be considered causal unless it can be demonstrated (e.g., through an experimental intervention study) that manipulation of the factor modifies the outcome.

How can this conceptual framework be applied to the work presented here? At this point in our study of treatment moderators, it is most accurate to consider these variables *correlates* of maintenance treatment outcome. Because the population in the MTRD study includes individuals in their third or greater episode of depression, the moderators examined in the current report (e.g., DSR, patient attitudes, and personality) cannot be shown to have preceded the outcome of interest (e.g., recurrence, no recurrence). Moreover, these variables have not been experimentally manipulated and thus would not be considered causal (i.e., causal risk factor).

Biological Correlates of Outcome

In this project of long-term preventive treatment, we examined whether specific biological factors, in this case, EEG sleep parameters, associated with sustained recovery could be identified. DSR, which represents the proportional distribution of delta (i.e., slow wave) sleep in the first and second non-REM (NREM) sleep periods, was highly predictive of the length of survival following the discontinuation of drug treatment (Kupfer et al. 1990). Specifically, individuals with a high DSR had a five times greater likelihood of remaining in remission than those with a low DSR.

Because a significant influence of monthly psychotherapy on length of survival had been noted, response to maintenance psychotherapy in relation to DSR was also examined, seeking to integrate biological measures with psychotherapeutic treatment. Patients who received IPT-M *and* had normal delta sleep in the first NREM period (i.e., high DSR) survived significantly longer. In contrast, patients with decreased delta sleep in the first NREM period were not significantly protected by monthly IPT-M. Thus, normal delta sleep was identified as a biological correlate associated with enhanced response to psychotherapy, in this case IPT-M, whereas decreased delta sleep was associated with a higher risk of recurrence.

Psychological Correlates of Outcome

We also ascertained whether higher quality IPT was associated with longer survival (Frank et al. 1991) in the group of patients assigned to IPT-M without active medication. Treatment quality was defined as the extent to which therapists conformed to specific principles, goals, and techniques of IPT, thus labeled *treatment specificity*. Analysis of treatment specificity ratings across sessions indicated that psychotherapy that was more specifically interpersonal was associated with significantly increased survival time ($P < .0001$) without a new episode of depression. We concluded that when the patient and therapist are able to maintain a consistent focus on interpersonal issues as opposed to somatic or depressive symptoms, monthly sessions of IPT have substantial protective benefits.

Interestingly, these results are consistent with data drawn from an earlier efficacy study of [continuation] IPT (Klerman et al. 1974) in which "discussion of mental symptoms" and "overt expression of anxiety" were significantly associated with relapse (Jacobson et al. 1977). Also relevant to our understanding of the robust effects of treatment specificity on survival, Jacobson et al. (1977) concluded that the group of patients who relapsed, in focusing primarily on "the self-oriented and static topic of mental symptoms" (p. 145), were able to avoid more adaptive work on current interpersonal issues or, in limiting discussion to symptomatic concerns, on what could be done to ameliorate them.

In several previous MTRD analyses (Bearden et al. 1996; Frank et al. 1987), personality functioning was associated with response to acute treatment. Specifically, we have shown that personality functioned as a moderator of response to combined pharmacotherapy and psychotherapy among patients in an acute episode of depression. Patients who responded more slowly and erratically during their acute phase treatment evidenced more personality pathology when fully recovered (Frank et al. 1987). In addition, these analyses corroborate extant literature suggesting that the personalities of patients recovered from unipolar illness can be characterized by two prototypes: the dependent, anxiously attached patient and the obsessive-compulsive character (i.e., excessive dependency and excessive autonomy), although the most prevalent among our group of recovered patients were the fearful, anxious personality dimensions.

Integrating Biological and Psychological Correlates of Treatment Outcome

Given these findings, and, in an effort to integrate biological and psychological correlates of treatment outcome following discontinuation of somatic therapy, in *this* work, we examined the *simultaneous* contribution of DSR, a presumably traitlike sleep EEG measure, and treatment specificity of IPT-M, a psychotherapy process measure, to survival time, in a group of patients with a history of recurrent depressive episodes. We also examined the contribution of several other patient characteristics, including patient attitudes/expectancies and personality to treatment specificity and time to recurrence to explore further the issue of the contribution of patients to preventive treatment outcome. The question of interest was whether patient attitude and personality parameters would moderate response to *maintenance* psychotherapy and thus influence the risk of recurrence in the absence of medication in patients in remission.

Methods

Participants in this study were drawn from the larger study of MTRD. The subjects, design, treatments, and measures have been described in detail elsewhere (Frank 1991; Frank et al. 1987, 1989, 1990, 1993a; Kupfer et al. 1990) and are described only briefly here. For entry into the study, subjects between the ages of 21 and 65 years were required to be seen initially in their third or greater episode of unipolar major depression meeting Research Diagnostic Criteria (RDC; Spitzer et al. 1978) with a minimum HRSD score of 15 and a minimum Raskin score of 7. Subjects were drawn from the group of patients randomly assigned to maintenance IPT who had discontinued somatic treatment following recovery from the acute episode ($n = 52$). Thus the potential confounding effects of maintenance medication was avoided. Altogether, 41 patient-therapist dyads were included in the analysis. We excluded patients whose therapist changed during the course of the 3-year maintenance phase ($n = 8$) and patients who had inadequate EEG sleep period data ($n = 3$). Table 11–1 shows the demographic and clinical characteristics of the 41 subjects. The four subgroups (LS/LD, LS/HD, HS/LD, HS/HD) refer to high and low treatment specificity and high and low DSR and are described in more detail later in this chapter.

Seven therapists with a range of 2 to 10 years of therapy experience but without prior training in IPT were selected (5 females, 2 males). Therapists were trained to predetermined competence levels in both IPT and medication clinic before being assigned protocol patients. Given the logistical restrictions of the clinic, patients were not randomly assigned to therapists, but instead were assigned to the next

TABLE 11–1

Demographic and clinical characteristics of the total sample and the four groups

	Total sample (N = 41) Mean (SD) Median	LS/LD (n = 7) Mean (SD) Median	LS/HD (n = 13) Mean (SD) Median	HS/LD (n = 8) Mean (SD) Median	HS/HD (n = 13) Mean (SD) Median	P[d]
Gender Male	27%	14%	15%	50%	31%	
Female	73%	86%	85%	50%	69%	.36
Age at entry[a]	39(10) 39	39(8) 39	40(9) 41	47(11) 46	35(11) 34	.18
Duration[b]	24(20) 16	34(28) 16	22(16) 16	22(20) 14	24(19) 16	.74
Age at onset[c]	27(11) 24	24(5) 22	27(11) 25	34(13) 34	25(10) 21	.21
HRSD at index episode	22(4) 21	25(4) 24	21(4) 20	23(5) 24	21(4) 20	.25
Number of previous episodes	8(7) 5	10(8) 8	9(9) 6	5(2) 5	6(3) 5	.41

[a] *Age at entry to study (in years).*

[b] *Duration of illness (in weeks).*

[c] *Age at onset of first episode (in years).*

[d] *The P value associated with gender is the exact P for Fisher's exact test. All other P values are those associated with the Kruskal-Wallis test statistic (df = 3).*

available therapist. Although little information had been collected specifically on therapist variables, we examined whether therapists from dyads in the high versus low treatment specificity groups differed in the average number of years of total therapy experience or years of IPT experience. We also examined the gender and age match between therapists and patients in the two groups. We found no statistically significant differences (Frank et al. 1991).

Measures

Treatment Specificity Ratings

Treatment specificity ratings were completed for all patients receiving monthly IPT-M who had reached the maintenance phase. Each maintenance therapy session was tape recorded and a 7-minute segment was later rated by trained raters using a 27-item Therapy Rating Scale (TRS; Wagner et al. 1992), a treatment fidelity scale developed for the study. The TRS was designed to distinguish between IPT-M and medication clinic sessions and to assess the degree to which therapists adhered to intended treatments. Raters were blind to the number of months patients had been in the maintenance phase and to patients' assigned treatment conditions.

Therapists provided both types of treatments and thus followed their patients through all phases of the study regardless of the treatment condition to which their patients were assigned in the maintenance phase. The TRS assessed the extent to which therapy sessions were characterized by interpersonal interventions, somatic interventions reflecting the medication clinic approach, and contamination interventions reflecting cognitive-behavioral or psychoanalytic approaches. As in our previous report (Frank et al. 1991), the primary analyses used only the average interpersonal score as the measure of treatment specificity of IPT-M.

The interpersonal items on the TRS assessed the extent to which an interpersonal focus was either achieved or maintained by the therapist-patient dyad. For example, when a patient assigned to IPT-M focused on various symptoms of the illness, appropriate in the medi-cation clinic approach, the therapist might *achieve* an interpersonal focus by translating the patient's concerns into an interpersonal con-text. If the patient assigned to IPT-M focused on interpersonal con-cerns, then the therapist could *maintain* an interpersonal focus by, for example, encouraging the patient to *elaborate* on a description of a relationship, by *exploring* ways in which the patient could develop or resume interpersonal relationships and social or occupational activi-ties, or by *eliciting* feelings associated with the content under dis-cussion. Psychometric evaluation of the TRS indicated that the scale possessed adequate psychometric properties, and that student raters achieved and maintained adequate interrater reliability.

Delta Sleep Ratio (DSR)

As described previously (Kupfer et al. 1990), DSR represents the av-erage delta wave counts per minute during the first NREM sleep pe-riod divided by the average delta counts during the second NREM period. DSR was computed from all-night sleep EEG studies that were completed at baseline during a 2-week drug-free period. Delta wave sleep was measured at two baseline nights, and the average of the two comparable nights was used in all analyses. It is important to note that normal healthy people have about twice as much delta (i.e., slow wave) sleep in the first NREM period as in the second NREM period. In age-matched normal control subjects, the average DSR is about 2. In contrast, the median DSR in this group of patients with recurrent unipolar illness was 1.1. For purposes of creating high and low DSR groups in data analyses, the subjects were divided at this score.

Patient Attitudes

We measured patient attitudes using a 20-item Patient Attitudes and Beliefs Scale (PAB) developed for the NIMH Treatment of Depression Collaborative Research Program (TDCRP; Elkin et al. 1989). This scale was designed to assess patients' beliefs regarding the cause(s) of their depression along three factors: biological, cognitive, and social. *Biological* items assess the extent to which patients believe the cause of their illness is related primarily to neurotransmitter dysfunction or genetic factors, for example: "An imbalance of certain substances in my brain is a cause of my problems." *Cognitive* items assess the extent to which patients believe the cause of their depression is due to the way they think about themselves and the world, for example: "Pessimistic attitudes about many things are a cause of my problems." *Social* items assess the extent to which patients believe the cause of their depression is due to factors in their social environment, for example: "Marital or family problems are a cause of my problems."

We measured patient attitudes at three time periods: baseline, continuation, and premaintenance. The results reported here come from only the premaintenance evaluations, when all patients were asymptomatic and had been so for an extended period, ≥ 20 weeks.

Patient Personality

To increase the validity of the data, personality data used in these (and earlier) analyses were gathered at premaintenance when all patients were fully recovered and in the well state. We measured patient personality using a self-report measure of personality traits, the Hirschfeld-Klerman Personality Battery (Hirschfeld et al. 1983), as well as a clinician-rated measure of personality disorder dimensions, the Personality Assessment Form (Jacob and Turner 1983, cited in Frank et al. 1987), developed for the NIMH TDCRP (Elkin et al.1989). Factors from each inventory were calculated for each patient by adding the appropriate scores together.

Outcome-Recurrence

Because patients began the experiment in remission, the outcome measure of primary interest is time to recurrence (in weeks). A recurrence (i.e., the onset of a new episode of depression) could be declared at any time during the maintenance phase of treatment. The procedures for the assessment of recurrence involved several stages. When a patient presented in a state of clinical worsening, the patient was observed and examined twice within a 7-day period. A new episode was confirmed only when an independent clinical evaluator rated the patient as having a minimum HRSD score of 15 and a minimum Raskin score of 7 on both occasions *and* when the clinical evaluation of an independent senior psychiatrist who was blind to the patient's maintenance treatment assignment indicated the presence of an episode of major depression according to the RDC.

Results of Survival Analyses

Survival methods were used for the analyses. We first tested four co-variates by examining their individual association with survival time: clinician, HRSD score at index episode, gender, and age. When examining the relationship of the variable clinician to survival time, we found a significant association with outcome ($P = .016$). Further, when we categorized the clinicians as having patients with shorter (3 clinicians, 17 patients), average (2 clinicians, 14 patients), or longer (2 clinicians, 8 patients) times to recurrence, and allowing us to include the therapist whose only two subjects survived the full 3 years in the survival analysis, we found a significant association with outcome ($P = .0003$, df = 2). Thus, we covaried for the three clinician types throughout subsequent proportional hazards analyses. Higher mean HRSD scores were also found to be significantly and negatively associated with time to recurrence ($P = .02$, df = 1) and thus we covaried for the HRSD scores in subsequent analyses. It is important to note that there was *no* evidence of differences in the HRSD score among the patients of the three different clinician types ($F = .07$, $P = .93$, df = 2, 38). The other demographic variables, gender ($P = .64$) and age ($P = .63$), were not associated with time to recurrence after covarying for index HRSD and clinician type.

    Using the Cox proportional hazards model, next we examined the relationships among treatment specificity, DSR, and time to recurrence with the covariates clinician type and index HRSD score in the model. Treatment specificity was significantly associated with time to recurrence ($P = .013$, df $= 1$) after covarying for clinician type, HRSD score at the index episode, and DSR. DSR was also significantly associated with outcome ($P = .0003$, df $= 1$) after covarying for the other three variables. There was no evidence, however, of an interaction effect between treatment specificity and DSR ($P = .80$, df $= 1$) and no evidence of association between treatment specificity and DSR ($r = -.09$, $P = .56$, df $= 39$).

Following these analyses, Kaplan-Meier analyses were run to elucidate the results from the Cox proportional hazards model and to confirm that trends within the groups were as expected. We divided the sample into four groups: 1) high treatment specificity and high DSR (HS/HD; $n = 13$), 2) high treatment specificity and low DSR (HS/LD; $n = 8$), 3) low treatment specificity and high DSR (LS/HD; $n = 13$), and 4) low treatment specificity and low DSR (LS/LD; $n = 7$). The first Kaplan-Meier analysis involved examining all four groups. The Mantel-Cox statistic was highly significant ($P < .0001$, df $= 3$). Post hoc tests were run using a Bonferroni correction. The results (Figure 11–1) indicated several significant differences among groups. First, time to recurrence was significantly longer for the HS/HD group as

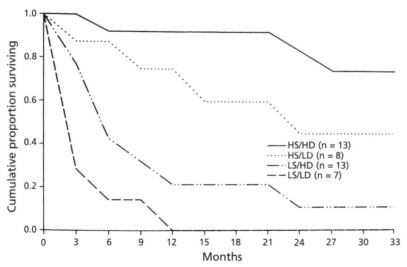

FIGURE 11–1. *Relationship of treatment specificity and DSR to time to recurrence.*

compared with the low specificity groups with either high or low DSRs (LS/HD and LS/LD). Second, time to recurrence was significantly longer for the HS/LD group as compared with the LS/LD group. In contrast, DSR did not have a significant effect within groups with comparable treatment specificity. That is, time to recurrence was not significantly different between the two groups with high specificity (the HS/HD group vs. the HS/LD group) or between the two groups with low specificity (the LS/HD group vs. the LS/LD group). In addition, time to recurrence for the two middle groups, each with one vulnerability factor, either decreased delta sleep or low specificity (i.e., HS/LD versus LS/HD), was not significantly different.

When examining the cumulative proportion of patients surviving within each group, the HS/HD group demonstrated the greatest proportion of patients surviving at every time point over the 3 years. In fact, 73% of the patients in this group survived the entire 3-year maintenance trial, whereas only 44% survived in the HS/LD group. In the low specificity groups, 11% of the patients with high DSR survived the 3-year trial compared with none with low DSR. Even though time to recurrence was not significantly different between the two groups with high specificity or between the two groups with low specificity in this particular demonstration, Figure 11–1 shows a positive effect for high DSR, suggesting that having *both* high specificity and high DSR is of significant clinical benefit.

Earlier we found that specific clinicians could be ranked by their patients' times to recurrence (i.e., shorter, average, and longer times to recurrence). To display this effect, we used life table methods to produce the cumulative proportion of patients surviving at various times, while the data were stratified according to clinician type and grouped by treatment specificity within each clinician group. The results (Table 11–2) show two main points. First, even when we divide clinicians into groups based on their patients' survival times, we *still* see the robust and prophylactic effect of treatment specificity; that is, within each clinician group, proportionately more patients in the higher specificity dyads survived relative to patients in lower specificity dyads. Second, we confirmed that trends within the groups were as expected. For example, it would be anticipated that the proportion of patient-therapist dyads with low treatment specificity would decrease

TABLE 11–2

Cumulative proportion of patients surviving grouped by time to recurrence and treatment specificity

Time to recurrence	HS or LS	3 months (SE)	6 months (SE)	1 year (SE)	2 years (SE)	3 years (SE)
Shorter	LS ($n = 13$)	0.54 (.14)	0.21 (.12)	0.00 (.00)	0.00 (.00)	0.00 (.00)
	HS ($n = 4$)	1.0 (0.0)	0.75 (.22)	0.38 (.29)	0.38 (.29)	0.38 (.29)
Average	LS ($n = 7$)	0.71 (.17)	0.56 (.19)	0.37 (.20)	0.19 (.16)	0.19 (.16)
	HS ($n = 7$)	0.85 (.13)	0.85 (.13)	0.71 (.17)	0.71 (.17)	0.54 (.20)
Longer	LS ($n = 0$)	—	—	—	—	—
	HS ($n = 10$)	1.0 (0.0)	1.0 (0.0)	1.0 (0.0)	0.79 (.13)	0.79 (.13)

as the clinician group time to recurrence increases. This expected result was demonstrated in Table 11–2. At the same time, this association between clinician and treatment specificity did not change the significant independent effect of specificity on time to recurrence because we covaried for the three clinician types throughout all Cox proportional hazards analyses.

When examining how patient attitude and personality parameters might influence the risk of recurrence, we first examined the relationship between the three PAB factors and time to recurrence using the Cox proportional model. The three factor scores were not found to have any association with outcome ($P = .36$ biological, .33 cognitive, and .41 external). However, when the *difference* between the biological and cognitive plus external scores was examined (Table 11–3), we found a highly significant association with outcome.[1]

Patients with a larger positive difference, that is, patients who reported that their biological beliefs were greater relative to their cognitive plus external beliefs, demonstrated a shorter time to recurrence. This association remained highly significant when the covariates of DSR and clinician were included in the model. When including treatment specificity scores in the model, patient attitude difference scores were no longer significant whereas treatment specificity remained sig-

---

1. We computed PAB difference scores for each patient by summing standardized cognitive plus external scores and then subtracting them from biological scores.

TABLE 11–3

Survival analyses of patient attitudes, treatment specificity, and time to recurrence using the Cox proportional model

PAB difference scores and time to recurrence	P
Difference between biological and cognitive plus external scores	< .0006
Including the covariates DSR and clinician in the model	< .0001
Including the covariates DSR, clinician, and treatment specificity	< .14
Treatment specificity and time to recurrence with DSR and clinician in the model	< .024

Note. *PAB difference and treatment specificity scores* (r = .31; P < .05; n = 41).

nificantly associated with time to recurrence. Of particular interest is the finding of a significant association between treatment specificity and the PAB difference scores. In contrast, we did not find any of the personality factors to be significantly associated with outcome.

Finally, using the Cox proportional hazards model, we also explicitly compared survival times among high specificity IPT-M, low specificity IPT-M, and no IPT-M groups, while covarying for DSR (Figure 11–2). Subjects ($n = 21$) who were randomly assigned to the medication clinic plus placebo group (and thus did not participate in IPT treatment and were unmedicated), and had DSR measurements, were compared with the 41 subjects examined here. Figure 11–2 shows the expected differences among the groups. Significant differences in survival time were observed between the high specificity IPT-M group and the no IPT-M group ($P < .0002$). In contrast, no significant differences were observed between the low specificity IPT-M group and the no-IPT-M group ($P = .23$).

Conclusions

The present findings must be considered in light of our design, which precludes conclusions about the effect of either high quality IPT-M or

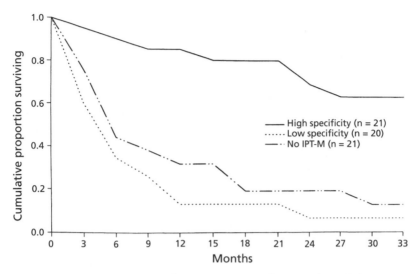

FIGURE 11-2. *Relationship of treatment specificity and no IPT-M to time to recurrence.*

DSR on time to recurrence in patients treated acutely with IPT alone rather than a combination of medication and IPT. Despite this limitation, our results provide compelling evidence that good-quality IPT-M is effective in preventing or delaying a recurrence of illness in patients with unipolar illness who have discontinued their medication, even when their baseline EEG sleep is markedly abnormal.

In the group of 52 patients who were randomly assigned to the two (out of five) maintenance treatments involving IPT-M alone without active medication, the outcome survival analysis showed that 35% of these patients survived the full 3 years (Frank et al. 1990). In contrast, this subsequent analysis shows that in the absence of biological (decreased delta sleep in the first NREM period) or psychotherapeutic (lower quality therapy) vulnerability factors, 73% of the patients treated with IPT-M alone without active medication survived the 3-year trial. With both vulnerability factors present, none (0%) of the patients survived; in fact all patients participating in lower quality IPT-M with reduced delta sleep had recurred within the first year of the 3-year trial. When one compares these rates, it becomes clear that both the quality of the psychotherapy and pretreatment sleep parameters, such as normal delta sleep, have highly significant effects for maximizing the preventive capacity of maintenance psychotherapy. In fact, the 73% survival rate does not appear to be significantly different from antidepressant therapy in this study of maintenance treatments for recurrent depression. For at least a subgroup of patients with recurrent depressive episodes and healthy delta sleep, good quality monthly IPT-M is a powerful preventive treatment. It may be that, for this subset of patients, moving from weekly to monthly sessions of IPT-M was the ideal contact frequency.

It is also important to note the 44% 3-year survival rate for patients characterized by decreased delta sleep, but whose therapy sessions were rated above average. This suggests that good-quality psychotherapy provides significant protection even for patients with a biological vulnerability factor for recurrence. Perhaps above average therapy serves as a buffer, mitigating the negative effects of biological vulnerabilities, in this case, EEG sleep disturbance. At the same time, patients with abnormal sleep profiles were less responsive to good-quality preventive IPT (44% survival vs. 73% survival). What remained uncertain was how to identify which patients with reduced delta sleep would be protected by above average therapy; as discussed shortly, our findings with respect to patient attitudes shed light on this important issue.

The finding of a 0% survival rate suggests that IPT-M was an ineffective preventive treatment for patients characterized by decreased delta sleep who participated in lower quality therapy. This fact is even more pronounced when one compares survival rates between patients assigned to the medication clinic-pill placebo treatment in the MTRD study (13%) to survival rates in patients participating in low specificity psychotherapy in the absence of medication, 7% (see Figure 11–2). The finding that these survival rates are not significantly different suggests that participation in below average therapy is no more effective (in fact, it is less effective clinically) than being assigned to the control condition, in this case, no *active* psychotherapy or medication. Thus, it is the quality and not simply the occurrence of IPT-M that contributes to its protective capacity.

Our findings also suggest that both patient and therapist factors are important moderators of response to preventive psychotherapy. The finding of a significant association among therapist, treatment specificity, and outcome, and the absence of any differences among the three clinician types on patients' HRSD scores at the index assessment suggests that therapists differ in effectiveness and that this has an impact on treatment specificity of IPT-M and survival time. At the same time, we found an effect of treatment specificity beyond the significant effects of therapists on outcome, suggesting a patient contribution to specificity (i.e., some patients make it easier than others for therapists to achieve or maintain the interpersonal focus). Thus, it is important to note our finding of the significant association between patient attitudes, treatment specificity, and outcome. It appears that in addition to the influence of therapists, patients' attitudes about their illness are related to at least a part of the process of therapy. It may be that patients in the well state who believe (correctly or not) the cause of their illness is primarily biological, with psychological or social factors (e.g., distorted cognitions, conflictual relationships) of lesser causal importance, make it more difficult for therapists to achieve a consistent focus on interpersonal concerns in IPT-M, and this lowered treatment specificity is, in turn, reflected in these patients' shorter times to recurrence.

That patient attitudes are related to treatment specificity, which is, in turn, related to survival time suggests that these perceptions are causally related to treatment specificity of IPT-M. These findings are consistent with extensive empirical data indicating that patient expectancies and attitudes are significant correlates of successful outcome in psychotherapy (see Stiles et al. 1986 for a review), and may in fact reflect the degree of patient capacity to become actively engaged in the therapeutic interaction. Patient attitudes in the effectiveness of long-term preventive IPT appears to be an extremely important influence on a patient's engagement in therapy.

These findings are also consistent with a treatment matching approach to therapy; that is, one option for maximizing the effectiveness of psychotherapy would be to select only those patients who evidence a mind set to actively participate in the therapeutic process. As Klein (1996) suggests, mismatching patients and treatments might "promote demoralization" (p. 82). In addition, being prudent about who to consider for which treatments is no longer a luxury but a necessity in the face of shrinking health care dollars. Alternative interventions need to be considered for patients who do not appear willing to commit to long-term preventive psychotherapy or who do not appear able to assume responsibility for change.

Future Directions

The results of this study have illustrated that both patient and therapist factors are related to the quality and efficacy of psychotherapy, in this case, monthly IPT. They provide support for the importance of matching patients with treatments and they additionally provide support for our earlier conclusion (Frank et al. 1991) of the bidirectional nature of the patient-therapist relationship. However, additional questions concerning the role of the patient and therapist in determining the course of long-term preventive psychotherapy have been raised. Even though attitudes had a significant influence on a patient's capacity to engage in IPT-M, our finding of a significant association between individual therapists and outcome suggests that certain kinds of therapists behaviors appear to influence the development of positive (or conversely negative or defensive) attitudes toward therapy. Studies examining factors associated with competent therapists and committed patients need to be conducted so that we might further our understanding of how IPT-M serves to protect patients from a recurrence of illness and so that our procedures for selecting, training, and monitoring therapists might more effectively enhance their ability to consistently provide high-quality treatment across a range of patients.

Given the importance of developing strategies to match optimal patient-therapist dyads, our next set of questions explore factors associated with competent therapists and committed patients. IPT provides a unique opportunity to study what we call "universal interpersonal changes processes" or how work on improving interpersonal relationships can lead to longer wellness intervals. We need to more clearly articulate these taken for granted interpersonal changes processes; for example, what kinds of therapist interventions and patient responses inspire a patient to take responsibility for his or her relationships and for taking an active stance to interpersonal problem solving. Some data (Weissman and Giacomo 1994) suggest that with successful psychotherapy, patients begin to take responsibility for the quality of their relationships, are provided with options and thus come to see that they have choices and are competent, and develop a more flexible stance toward life's dilemmas. Perhaps some of the answers to questions about process and successful therapeutic interventions in IPT will be found in social psychology, especially in research on social cognition and processes in relationship formation, maintenance, and dissolution.

Finally, in our study of long-term preventive treatments in recurrent depression, it has become clear that more complex longitudinal models of vulnerability to affective illness need to be developed, consistent with treatment models for chronic (rather than acute typically single episode) illnesses. Using an integrative approach, a next step is to integrate interpersonal and biological vulnerability factors with cognitive vulnerability or risk factors in the study of recurrence in depression as well as in the development of expanded or enhanced psychotherapeutic treatments for depression. The goal of this work would be to increase understanding and enhance response to effective preventive treatments and thus reduce vulnerability to recurrence in depression.

References

American Psychiatric Association: Practice guidelines for major depressive disorder in adults. Am J Psychiatry 150(No 4, Suppl):1–26, 1993

Bearden C, Lavelle N, Buysse D, et al: Personality pathology and time to remission in depressed outpatients treated with interpersonal psychotherapy. J Personal Disord 10:164–173, 1996

DiMascio A, Weissman MM, Prusoff BA, et al: Differential symptom reduction by drugs and psychotherapy in acute depression. Arch Gen Psychiatry 36:1450–1456, 1979

Elkin I, Shea MT, Watkins JT, et al: NIMH Treatment of Depression Collaborative Research Program: 1. General effectiveness of treatments. Arch Gen Psychiatry 46:971–982, 1989

Frank E: Interpersonal psychotherapy as a maintenance treatment for patients with recurrent depression. Psychotherapy 28:259–266, 1991

Frank E, Spanier CA: Interpersonal psychotherapy for depression: overview, clinical efficacy, and future directions. Clinical Psychology: Science and Practice 2:349–369, 1995

Frank E, Kupfer DJ, Jacob M, et al: Personality features and response to acute treatment in recurrent depression. J Personal Disord 1:14–26, 1987

Frank E, Kupfer DJ, Perel JM: Early recurrence in unipolar depression. Arch Gen Psychiatry 45:397–400, 1989

Frank E, Kupfer DJ, Perel JM, et al: Three-year outcomes for maintenance therapies in recurrent depression. Arch Gen Psychiatry 47:1093–1099, 1990

Frank E, Kupfer DJ, Wagner EF, et al: Efficacy of interpersonal psychotherapy as a maintenance treatment of recurrent depression: contributing factors. Arch Gen Psychiatry 48:1053–1059, 1991

Frank E, Kupfer DJ, Cornes C, et al: Maintenance interpersonal psychotherapy for recurrent depression, in New Applications of Interpersonal Psychotherapy. Edited by Klerman GL, Weissman MM. Washington, DC, American Psychiatric Press, 1993a, pp 75–102

Frank E, Kupfer DJ, Perel JM, et al: Comparison of full-dose versus half-dose pharmacotherapy in the maintenance treatment of recurrent depression. J Affective Disord 27:139–145, 1993b

Glen AIM, Johnson AL, Shepherd M: Continuation therapy with lithium and amitriptyline in unipolar depressive illness: a randomized, double-blind, controlled trial. Psychol Med 14:37–50, 1984

Hamilton M: A rating scale for depression. J Neurol Neurosurg Psychiatry 23:56–62, 1960

Hirschfeld RMA, Klerman GL, Clayton PJ, et al: Personality and depression: empirical findings. Arch Gen Psychiatry 40:993–998, 1983

Jacobson S, Deykin E, Prusoff B: Process and outcome of therapy with depressed women. Am J Orthopsychiatry 47:140–148, 1977

Kessler RC, McGonagle KA, Zhao S: Lifetime and 12-month prevalence of DSM-III-R psychiatric disorders in the United States: results from the National Comorbidity Survey, I. Arch Gen Psychiatry 51:8–19, 1994

Klein DF: Preventing hung juries about therapy studies. J Consult Clin Psychol 64:81–87, 1996

Klerman E: Treatment of depression by drugs and psychotherapy. Am J Psychiatry 131:186–191, 1974

Klerman GL, Weissman MM: Interpersonal psychotherapy: research program and future prospects, in Psychotherapy Research: An International Review of Programmatic Studies. Edited by Beutler LE, Crago M. Washington, DC, American Psychological Association, 1991, pp 33–40

Klerman GL, Weissman MM: Interpersonal psychotherapy for depression: background and concepts, in New Applications of Interpersonal Psychotherapy. Edited by Klerman GL, Weissman MM. Washington, DC, American Psychiatric Press, 1993, pp 3–50

Klerman GL, DiMascio A, Weissman M, et al: Treatment of depression by drugs and psychotherapy. Am J Psychiatry 131:186–191, 1974

Klerman GL, Weissman MM, Rounsaville BJ, et al: Interpersonal Psychotherapy of Depression. New York, Basic Books, 1984

Kraemer HC, Kazdin AE, Offord DR, et al: Coming to terms with the terms of risk. Arch Gen Psychiatry 54(4):337–343, 1997

Kupfer DJ, Grochocinski VJ: Five-year outcome for maintenance therapies in recurrent depression. Arch Gen Psychiatry 49:769–773, 1992

Kupfer DJ, Frank E, McEachran AB, et al: Delta sleep ration: a biological correlate of early recurrence in unipolar affective disorder. Arch Gen Psychiatry 47:1100–1105, 1990

Kupfer DJ, Frank E, Perel JM, et al: Five-year outcome for maintenance therapies in recurrent depression. Arch Gen Psychiatry 49:769–773, 1992

Persons JB, Thase ME, Crits-Christoph P: The role of psychotherapy in the treatment of depression: review of two practice guidelines. Arch Gen Psychiatry 53:283–290, 1996

Prien RF, Kupfer DJ, Mansky PA, et al: Drug therapy in the prevention of recurrences in unipolar and bipolar affective disorders: a report of the NIMH Collaborative Study Group comparing lithium carbonate, imipramine, and a lithium carbonate-imipramine combination. Arch Gen Psychiatry 41:1096–1104, 1984

Prochaska JO, Norcross JC: Interpersonal therapies, in Systems of Psychotherapy: A Transtheoretical Analysis, 3rd Edition. Pacific Grove, CA, Brooks/Cole, 1994, pp 191–225

Raskin A, Schulterbrandt J, Reatig N, et al: Replication of factors of psychopathology in interview, ward behavior, and self-report ratings of hospitalized depressives. J Nerv Ment Dis 148:87–98, 1969

Rush AJ: The role of psychotherapy in the treatment of depression: review of two practice guidelines. Arch Gen Psychiatry 53:301–302, 1996

Spitzer RL, Endicott J, Robins E: Research diagnostic criteria: rationale and reliability. Arch Gen Psychiatry 35:773–782, 1978

Stiles WB, Shapiro DA, Elliott R: "Are all psychotherapies equivalent?" Am Psychol 7:165–180, 1986

Thase ME, Kupfer DJ: Recent developments in the pharmacotherapy of mood disorders. J Consult Clin Psychol 64:646–659, 1996

Wagner EF, Frank E, Steiner SC: Discriminating maintenance treatments for recurrent depression: development and implementation of a rating scale. J Psychother Pract Res 22:281–290, 1992

Weissman MM, Markowitz JC: Interpersonal psychotherapy: current status. Arch Gen Psychiatry 51:599–606, 1994

Weissmark MS, Giacomo DA: A therapeutic index: measuring actions in psychotherapy. J Consult Clin Psychol 62:315–323, 1994

PART V

Psychotherapy With the Medically Ill

CHAPTER 12

Psychotherapeutic Intervention With the Medically Ill

David Spiegel, M.D.

In an era when the utility of psychotherapy is increasingly questioned, expanding its application toward the problem of coping with life-threatening medical illness might seem strange. Yet there is growing evidence of the efficacy of such techniques in helping patients with cancer and other serious illnesses reduce anxiety and depression, develop more active and effective coping skills, and reduce pain and other disease-related symptoms. New work in this area are reviewed in this chapter, with an emphasis on group psychotherapeutic intervention with cancer patients.

As oncological treatment has become more effective, cancer is now better thought of as a chronic rather than a terminal illness. However, given the progressive nature of the disease, and the fact that approximately half of all people diagnosed with cancer eventually die of it, assistance in coping with a life threat is needed. Currently, medical treatment focuses almost exclusively on the model of providing a cure, no matter whether it is possible. We pay far less attention to the process of helping ill people live with cancer as well, and as long, as possible.

Several recent studies of psychotherapeutic treatments for cancer patients have provided evidence of increases in survival time and improved adjustment. This is currently an active arena of research.

Theoretical Basis for Psychosocial Intervention

Anxiety Among Cancer Patients

The diagnosis of cancer is a universally stressful life event, and it is clearly associated with some increase in distress at a population level. As many as 80% of patients with breast cancer report significant distress during initial treatment (Hughes 1982), most often anxiety about recurrence (Koocher and O'Malley 1981; Quigley 1989; Rieker et al. 1985), difficulties with sexual functioning (Maguire et al. 1978; Morris et al. 1977), death anxiety, and vocational difficulties (Fobair et al. 1986). The treatment itself also stimulates recurrent anxiety that may promote conditioned anticipatory nausea (Cella et al. 1986) and reduce compliance (Itano et al. 1983). Although several early studies showed good long-term adjustment of patients with breast cancer (Craig et al. 1974; Schottenfeld and Robbins 1970), others demonstrated that 20%–30% of patients suffer severe distress for 2 years or more postsurgery (Ganz et al. 1992; Irvine et al. 1991; Itano et al. 1983). In one study cited for its methodological rigor (Morris et al. 1977) and in Irvine et al. (1991), a careful review of the literature, patients with breast cancer suffered 12% more sexual problems than those with benign breast disease, and 46% experienced significant psychological distress. The proportion declined only to 30% by the end of a year after diagnosis. Omne-Ponten et al. (1992) found significant anxiety and depression among 45% of a sample of 99 women 1 year after diagnosis. At 6-year follow-up, 10% continued to have severe maladjustment, and breast-sparing surgery did not reduce the rate of emotional disturbance (Omne-Ponten et al. 1994). Thus, a substantial minority of women with breast cancer experience persistent emotional disturbance, which is intertwined with their understandable anxiety about recurrence and disease progression.

Indeed, significant medical variables contributing to distress include recency of diagnosis and more advanced disease (Vinokur et al. 1989). In contrast, demographic variables are not associated with psychological distress. Ganz et al. (1992) did not find race, marital status, educational level, or income to be influential on adjustment. Conflicting results have been found in looking at age as a factor in distress (Northouse and Swain 1987; Vinokur et al. 1990). Thus, more advanced disease stage, through its relationship with mood disturbance, should predict greater sensitivity to variables influencing treatment.

A large collaborative study compared patients with breast cancer at 1-year follow-up with women who had undergone cholecystectomy, had a breast biopsy with benign outcome, or were healthy control subjects ("Psychological response to mastectomy," 1987). They found statistically higher somatic distress, self-denigration, psychosocial impairment, and physical complaints, although the rate of psychiatric illness was not higher in women who had good prior mental health. In a carefully conducted study of 274 patients with breast cancer drawn from a community sample, and therefore with more generalized findings than those from convenience samples, Vinokur et al. (1990) found, similar to the previous study, persistent mental health problems throughout the year after diagnosis, including anxiety, depression, and somatic preoccupation. Interestingly, one of the strongest predictors of poor mental health at 1-year follow-up was an appraisal of the threat, more than initial stages of disease. This provides evidence that threat appraisal (whether accurate or inaccurate) is a more powerful determinant of adjustment to breast cancer than initial prognostic indicators, such as staging. The authors suggest that better education of patients may reduce long-term distress.

Depression and Cancer

Several studies have documented a substantial prevalence of depression and anxiety among patients with cancer, independent of pain status. In random samples of hospitalized patients with cancer, reported rates of depressive states vary roughly from 16% to 50% (Craig and Abeloff 1974; Derogatis et al. 1983; Dworkin et al. 1990; Greer

1991; Helliwell et al. 1992; Lansky et al. 1985; Levine et al. 1978; Maguire 1985; Massie and Holland 1987, 1990; ; Plumb and Holland 1977). Overall, the more narrowly the term *depression* is defined, the lower the prevalence of depression reported. Factors (in addition to the presence of pain) associated with greater prevalence of depression are a higher level of physical disability and more severe illness.

Derogatis et al. (1983) examined the prevalence of psychiatric disorders in 215 oncology inpatients randomly selected from three cancer centers (excluding those gravely physically disabled) and found that 47% had clinically apparent psychiatric disorders (6% major affective disorders, 12% adjustment disorders with depressed mood, and 13% adjustment disorders with mixed emotional features). Nearly 90% of the psychiatric disorders observed were judged to be reactions to, or manifestations of, disease or treatment.

Lansky et al. (1985) argue that the highest depression rates derive mainly from studies of patients with cancer who were either referred for psychiatric consultation, hospitalized, or had advanced disease. In their study of 500 "everyday" patients with cancer (i.e., ambulatory outpatients), they found that only 5.3% had major depression, still a greater rate than the 3% 6-month prevalence found in the general population (Bukberg et al. 1984). However, depression in patients with cancer has been underdiagnosed and undertreated. This is due, in part, to the belief that depression is a normal and universal reaction to serious disease (Rodin and Voshart 1986), and because the neurovegetative signs (weight loss, sleep disturbance) or emotional/cognitive signs are often attributed to the medical illness itself (Craig et al. 1974).

Mermelstein et al. (1992) report that the rate of depressive disorders in their population of oncology patients may be as high as four times that of the general population. Elevated rates of mood disturbance have been observed throughout the course of the disease, from undiagnosed breast lumps (Hughes et al. 1986; Morris and Greer 1982) to biopsy (Greer and Morris 1975) and recurrence (Holland 1989; Hughes et al. 1986). Others (Maraste et al. 1992) found a 14% incidence of anxiety disorders in a sample of patients with breast cancer, but only 1.5% of this sample met criteria for a depressive disorder.

Initial levels of mood disturbance are strong predictors of subsequent distress (Ell et al. 1989). Other predictors are a history of depression (Maunsell et al. 1992), low self-esteem (Felton et al. 1984; Timko and Janoff-Bulman 1985), an external locus of control (Northouse and Swain 1987), and neuroticism (Morris et al. 1977), as reviewed in Irvine et al. (1991).

Rates of depressive states reported for cancer inpatients are roughly comparable to those reported for comparably ill patients with other medical diagnoses. Studies of medical inpatients show that about one-third report mild or moderate symptoms of depression, and up to one-fourth may suffer from a depressive syndrome (Maguire et al. 1974; Myers et al. 1984; Steckel 1982; Stewart et al. 1965). These studies suggest that the severity of the medical illness, irrespective of its underlying cause, is the factor most closely associated with the frequency of both depressive symptoms and syndromes. Efficacious treatments that reduce the severity of illness also reduce, based on this research, the prevalence and severity of depression, anxiety, and other psychiatric disorders.

Coping Style

Coping patterns, including attitudes toward the illness, have been relatively stable predictors of adjustment. Carver and Scheier (1994) studied 70 Stage I–Stage II patients with breast cancer and found that a general attitude of optimism at the time of diagnosis presurgery was predictive of better 3-, 6-, and 12-month subjective well-being as measured by scores on the Profile of Mood States (McNair et al. 1971) and measures of life satisfaction, sexual fulfillment, thought intrusion, and pain. Optimism accounted for between one-quarter and one-third of the variance in outcomes. Thus, information that would make a patient unduly pessimistic would be likely to increase thought intrusion and reduce life satisfaction. Similarly, the meaning associated with a symptom such as pain is associated with more pain intensity, independent of the site or number of metastases (Spiegel and Bloom 1983b). The difference in coping style is well summarized by Carver and Scheier (1994): "In particular, optimistic women appear to accept more readily the reality of the challenge they face, whereas pessimistic women try to push this reality away. Acceptance was tied to positive mood changes, and denial was tied to adverse changes. In considering this pattern, we suggest that acceptance is important, in part, because it keeps the patients engaged in the active pursuit of the goals that define their lives." (p. 1219). Consistent with this observation, fatalism, a coping construct similar to pessimism as measured by the Mental Adjustment to Cancer Scale (Watson et al. 1988), has been positively correlated with a tendency to suppress anger, anxiety, and depression on the Courtauld Emotional Control Scale (Watson et al. 1991).

There is evidence that patients' patterns of coping with a cancer diagnosis (Dunkel-Schetter et al. 1992) and the types of psychosocial needs expressed (Liang et al. 1990) do not change significantly after the initial diagnosis (Heim et al. 1993; Nelson et al. 1994). Concerns expressed by patients with cancer in one survey included family members, emotional stress, and acquiring further information as the top three priorities of 96% of patients (Liang et al. 1990; Mahon et al. 1990). Patients at higher risk for poor coping include those who are socially isolated, have a history of recent losses, have multiple obligations, or employ inflexible or fewer coping strategies (Cooper and Faragher 1992). On the other hand, patients with breast cancer who learn to use more direct and confrontational coping strategies are less distressed than those who use avoidance and denial (Holland and Holland 1990). Thus, emotional distress is common among patients newly diagnosed with breast cancer. Some are at higher risk for mood disturbance than others, and certain coping strategies improve adjustment, suggesting that psychosocial support should be potentially effective in improving the outcome.

Social Support and Cancer

Recent research provides growing evidence for a moderating effect of social relationships on health. Social isolation elevates the risk of mortality from all causes as much as high serum cholesterol levels or smoking (House et al. 1988). Decreased survival has been associated with low quantity or quality of social relationships in several prospective studies (Berkman and Syme 1979; Funch and Marshall 1983; Ganster and Victor 1988; Goodwin et al. 1987; House et al. 1982; Joffres et al. 1985; Kennedy et al. 1988; Rodin and Voshart 1986). Reynolds and Kaplan (1990) examined data on 6,928 adults and found that women who were socially isolated were at elevated risk for dying of cancer. Those who had few social contacts and felt isolated had an almost twofold increase in incidences and a fivefold increase in relative risk for mortality from hormone-related cancers. Another clear example of the effect of social support on cancer progression is the finding that married patients with cancer survive longer than unmarried persons (Goodwin et al. 1987). Emotional support is associated with longer survival following a diagnosis of breast, colorectal, or lung cancer (Ell et al. 1992). In particular, expressive-social activities and social support, not merely extroversion, have been related to longer survival time (Hislop et al. 1987; Waxler-Morrison et al. 1991). These data confirm observations that emotional expression is associated with a better medical outcome (Derogatis et al. 1979; Greer and Morris 1975; Greer et al. 1979; Stavraky et al. 1988; Temoshok 1985). Maunsell and colleagues (1993) found that among 224 women with newly diagnosed breast cancer, married women had a relative death rate of 0.86 compared with unmarried women over a 7-year follow-up. In contrast to women who had no confidants in the few months after surgery, those who had support show a relative death rate of 0.55. Thus, the availability of social support is a robust predictor of subsequent mortality.

Besides the diagnosis of cancer itself, these patients must contend with other stressful life events. Maunsell et al. (1993) also demonstrated that levels of distress following initial treatment for breast cancer were predicted by, among other things, a history of multiple stressful life events. If social support can moderate the effects of such difficult life stressors and decrease the incidence of mood disorders, then patients with cancer have a clear need for such support mechanisms. Maunsell and colleagues (1993) studied 224 women with newly diagnosed breast cancer and examined the relationship between social support and mortality. Married women had a relative death rate of 0.86 compared with unmarried women over a seven-year follow-up. The death rate of women who had confidants in the few months after surgery was about half that of women who had no confidants at all. The death rate was even lower among those who used more than one. Thus, the availability of social support through marriage and confidants was a robust predictor of survival.

Ell and colleagues (1992) examined relationships between social support and survival following a diagnosis of breast, colorectal, or lung cancer. Of 294 patients, 74 had died. Most of the sample had been diagnosed with breast cancer (57%), although the bulk of the mortality occurred among those who had been diagnosed with lung or colorectal cancer. Emotional support protectively affected survival for patients with earlier stages of disease, but only one out of three measures of social support did. Specifically, perceived adequacy of emotional support was positively related to survival but marital status and social integration were not. No effect was found with more advanced disease. The analyses in this study should be accepted with caution because it was unclear what tests were performed, especially in the multivariate analyses. Furthermore, no mention was made of effects of interactions between site and stage. The cancer sites included in this study have differing means and ranges of survival times so that when sites or stages are combined, true effects may be masked, if they exist at all. Finally, of the 24 separate estimates of relative risk for four measures of social and emotional support, only 6 were significant and supported the hypothesis that social or emotional support was related to survival in this population.

Hislop et al. (1987) and Waxler-Morrison et al. (1991) studied 133 patients diagnosed with primary intraductal breast cancer. At 4-year follow-up, 26 had died and 38 had recurred. Using the Cox Proportional Hazards Model, they found that 6 of 11 measures of social relationships were significantly associated with longer survival: marital status; support from friends; contact with friends; total support from friends, relatives, and neighbors; employment status; and social network size. In particular, expressive-social activities and social support, not merely extroversion, were related to longer survival time. Thus, certain forms of social support are related to survival.

Other studies have not found a relationship between social support and cancer progression. Neale (1994) carried out a well-designed analysis of the 10-year survival of 10,778 women diagnosed with invasive breast cancer. Neale found that marital status as a proxy variable for social support was not related to cancer survival. Using marital status as a proxy variable for social support, however, may have been problematic in Neale's study because of the different ways in which men and women benefit from marriage as social support. Recent work on long-term marriages has shown that men and women differ in their health outcomes depending on marital satisfaction (Levenson et al. 1994). Namely, women are healthy in happy marriages and unhealthy in unhappy marriages. Men receive health benefits from marriage regardless of whether the marriage is a happy or unhappy one. Thus, marriage may function as social support differently for men and for women. This may explain Neale's null finding, although further studies should specifically examine marital satisfaction, social support, and health outcomes in patients with cancer. Finally, Levy and colleagues (1991) assessed 90 women with stage I or stage II breast cancer about 5 days after surgery on immunological and psychosocial parameters. Among the psychosocial parameters evaluated was the patient's perception of interpersonal support in her environment, especially from family members. The patients were followed for about 5 years. Twenty-nine women reported disease recurrence during the follow-up period. The best predictor of disease recurrence was natural killer cell activity. Social support was not predictive of disease recurrence, however, the investigators admit that the measure used was refined and so may not have adequately reflected the social support of the women in this study.

Much evidence points to a positive relationship between social support and cancer survival, although the relationship is still unclear and deserves further study. Most studies provide evidence that the presence of social networks, via frequent daily contact with others or the presence of confidants, reduces mortality risk from cancer, as well as other diseases.

Effects of Psychotherapeutic Intervention

Psychosocial intervention for patients with cancer in our clinical research program, conducted in conjunction with appropriate psychopharmacologic, medical, and surgical treatment, typically involves meetings of 6–10 patients with similar illness and prognosis, meeting for weekly 90-minute sessions. Groups are time-limited for those with early stage disease, usually 3 months, but continue indefinitely with rolling recruitment to replace losses for those with advanced and life-threatening disease. Groups are led by trained co-therapists, often one with considerable group psychotherapy experience (psychiatrist, psychologist, or social worker) and another with disease-related experience (nurse or social worker). The groups are semistructured, meaning that there is no set agenda for a given meeting. However, therapists structure the discussion according to general group psychotherapy principles (Yalom 1995) and toward exploration of the following seven basic components:

1. Social Support

Psychotherapy, especially in groups, can provide a new social network with the common bond of facing similar problems (Spiegel 1993). Just at a time when the illness makes a person feel removed from the flow of life, when many others withdraw out of awkwardness or fear, psychotherapeutic support provides a new and important social connection. Indeed, the very thing that damages other social relationships is the ticket of admission to such groups, providing a surprising intensity of caring among members right from the beginning.

2. Emotional Expression

The expression of emotion is important in reducing social isolation and improving coping. Yet it is often an aspect of adjustment in patients with cancer that is overlooked or suppressed. Emotional suppression and avoidance are associated with poorer coping (Greer 1991; Greer et al. 1979). At the same time, much can be done in both group and individual psychotherapy to facilitate the expression of emotion appropriate to the disease. Doing so seems to moderate the repressive coping style that reduces expression of positive and negative emotion. Emotional suppression also reduces intimacy in families, limiting opportunities for direct expression of affection and concern. Indeed, evidence indicates that those who can ventilate strong feelings directly cope better with cancer (Derogatis et al. 1979; Greer 1991; Greer et al. 1979; Pettingale 1984; Spiegel 1993; Temoshok 1985).

The use of the psychotherapeutic setting to deal with painful affect also provides an organizing context for handling its intrusion. When unbidden thoughts involving fear of dying and death intrude, they can be better managed by patients who know that there is a time and a place during which such feelings will be expressed and dealt with. Furthermore, a disease-related dysphoria is more intense when amplified by isolation, leaving the patient to feel that she is deservedly alone with the sense of anxiety, loss, and fear that she experiences. Being in a group where many others express similar distress normalizes their reactions, making them less alien and overwhelming.

3. Detoxifying Dying

Death anxiety in particular is intensified by isolation, in part because we often conceptualize death as separation from loved ones. Feeling alone, especially at a time of strong emotion, makes one feel already a little bit dead, setting off a cycle of further anxiety. This can be powerfully addressed by psychotherapeutic techniques that directly address such concerns.

This component of the therapy involves looking the threat of death right in the eye rather than avoiding it. The goal is to help those facing death see it from a new point of view. When worked through, life-threatening problems can come to seem real but not overwhelming (Spiegel 1993). Following a diagnosis of cancer, a variety of coping strategies come into play, including positive reappraisal and cognitive avoidance (Jarrett et al. 1992). However, denial and avoidance have their costs, including an increase in anxiety and isolation. Facing even life-threatening issues directly can help patients shift from emotion-focused to problem-focused coping (Moos and Schaefer 1984; Spiegel 1990). The process of dying is often more threatening than death itself. Direct discussion of death anxiety can help to divide the fear of death into a series of problems: loss of control over treatment decisions, fear of separation from loved ones, anxiety about pain. Discussion of these concerns can lead to a means of addressing, if not completely resolving, each of these issues. Thus, even facing death can result in positive life changes.

One woman with metastatic breast cancer described her experience of group psychotherapy in this way:

> What I found is that talking about death is like looking down into the Grand Canyon (I don't like heights). You know that if you fell down, it would be a disaster, but you feel better about yourself because you're able to look. I can't say I feel serene, but I can look at it now. [*Spiegel 1993*]

Even the process of grieving can be reassuring at the same time that it is threatening. The experience of grieving others who have died of the same condition constitutes a deeply personal experience of the depth of loss that will be experienced by others after one's own death.

4. Reordering Life Priorities

The acceptance of the possibility of illness shortening life carries with it an opportunity for reevaluating life priorities. When cure is not possible, a realistic evaluation of the future can help those with life-threatening illness make the best use of remaining time. One cost of unrealistic optimism is the loss of time for accomplishing life projects, communicating openly with family and friends, and setting affairs in order. Facing the threat of death can aid in making the most of life (Spiegel et al. 1981). This can help patients take control of those aspects of their lives they can influence, while grieving and relinquishing those they cannot. Having a domain of control can be quite reassuring.

5. Family Support

Psychotherapeutic interventions can also be quite helpful in improving communication, identifying needs, increasing role flexibility, and adjusting to new medical, social, vocational, and financial realities. Spiegel et al. (1983) show that an atmosphere of open and shared problem solving in families results in reduced anxiety and depression among patients with cancer. Thus, facilitating the development of such open addressing of common problems is a useful therapeutic goal. The group format is especially helpful for such a task, in that problems expressing needs and wishes can be examined among group members as a model for clarifying communication in the family.

In addition to enhancing communication, group participants are encouraged to develop role flexibility, a capacity to exchange roles or develop new ones as the pressures of the illness demand. One woman, for example, who became unable to carry out her usual household chores, wrote an "owners' manual" for the care of the house so that her husband could better help her and carry on after her death. Others wrote letters to friends asking them to cook an extra bit of dinner on one evening a month to share with them and relieve them of the pressure of cooking.

We have also conducted monthly support groups for family members of patients with cancer, to give them the opportunity to ventilate their emotions and concerns in a supportive atmosphere where their problems, rather than those of the medically ill family member, take precedence. One husband of a patient with metastatic breast cancer said: "This is a place where I come to feel better about feeling bad."

6. Communication With Physicians

Support groups can be quite useful in facilitating better communication with physicians and other health care providers. Groups provide mutual encouragement to get questions answered, to participate actively in treatment decisions, and to consider alternatives carefully. Research has shown that patients diagnosed with cancer are more satisfied with the results of intervention, such as lumpectomy versus a modified radical mastectomy, to the extent that they have been involved in making the decision about which type of treatment to have (Fallowfield et al. 1990). Such groups must be careful not to interfere with medical treatment and decisions, but to encourage clarification and the development of a cooperative relationship between doctor and patient.

7. Symptom Control

Many treatment approaches involve teaching cognitive techniques to manage anxiety. These include learning to identify emotions as they develop, analyze sources of emotional response, and move from emotion-focused to problem-focused coping. These approaches help the patient take a more active stance toward the illness. Rather than feeling overwhelmed by an insoluble problem, they learn to divide problems into smaller and more manageable ones. If I don't have much time left, how do I want to spend it? What effect will further chemotherapy have on my quality of life?

Many group and individual psychotherapy programs teach specific coping skills designed to help patients reduce cancer-related symptoms such as anxiety, anticipatory nausea and vomiting, and pain. Techniques used include specific self-regulation skills such as self-hypnosis, meditation, biofeedback, and progressive muscle relaxation (Burish and Lyles 1981; Hilgard and Hilgard 1975; Morrow and Morrell 1982; Spiegel 1990; Spiegel and Bloom 1983a; Zeltzer and LeBaron 1982).

Outcome

Psychosocial

There is now clear evidence that various psychotherapies for cancer patients are effective in reducing anxiety and depression (Ferlic et al. 1979; Gustafson and Whitman 1978; Mulder et al. 1992; Spiegel and Bloom 1983a; Spiegel et al. 1981; Wood et al. 1978), improving coping skills (Fawzy et al. 1990; Turns 1988), and reducing symptoms such as pain and nausea and vomiting (Cain et al. 1986; Forester et al. 1985; Morrow and Morrell 1982). Supportive-expressive group therapy for patients with metastatic breast cancer has been shown to result in better mood, fewer maladaptive coping responses, fewer phobic symptoms (Spiegel et al. 1981), and reduced pain (Spiegel and Bloom 1983a). In a randomized prospective trial, this treatment model (Spiegel and Bloom 1983a; Spiegel et al. 1989) has been compared with cognitive-behavioral treatment in a sample of HIV-infected patients (Kelly et al. 1993) and found more effective in reducing mood disturbance.

Medical

Recent evidence indicates that the provision of social support via group and other forms of psychotherapy may affect the quantity as well as the quality of life. One such study involved a randomized trial of supportive-expressive group therapy for women with metastatic breast cancer (Spiegel et al. 1981). Fifty of 86 women were randomly assigned to weekly support groups, which emphasized building strong supportive bonds, encouraging emotional expression, dealing directly with fears of dying and death, reordering life priorities, improving relationships with family and friends, enhancing communication and shared problem solving with physicians, and learning self-hypnosis for pain control. Clear psychological benefits were evident after 1 year, including reduced mood disturbance (Spiegel et al. 1981) and pain (Spiegel and Bloom 1983a). At 10-year follow-up, an average of 18 months or longer statistically significant survival advantage for women in the group therapy condition was shown, although there was no difference in median survival. By 48 months after the study had begun, all of the control patients had died, and a third of the treatment patients were still alive (Spiegel et al. 1989).

This positive effect of psychotherapy on disease progression has been observed in two other randomized prospective trials. Richardson et al. (1990) found that lymphoma and leukemia patients who were offered a combination of counseling and home visiting lived significantly longer than control patients, even when observed differences in adherence to medical treatment were controlled. Fawzy and colleagues (1990) found that patients with malignant melanoma who were randomly assigned to a series of six structured support group meetings were less anxious and depressed than control patients 6 months later.

At 6-year follow-up, Fawzy and colleagues (1993) reported significantly lower rates of recurrence (7/40 vs. 13/40) and mortality (3/40 vs. 10/40). However, one study that used matching rather than random design indicated no survival advantage for patients with cancer who were trained in the Exceptional Cancer Patient Program (Gellert et al. 1993). One other randomized trial of a vaguely defined group psychotherapy that had no measurable positive emotional results also found no effect on survival time (Ilniyki et al. 1994).

Many psychotherapies that have shown promise in improving emotional adjustment and influencing survival time involve encouraging open expression of emotion and assertiveness in assuming control over the course of treatment, life decisions, and relationships (Spiegel et al. 1989; Spiegel et al. 1981; Watson et al. 1990). Adequate assessment of quality of life requires attention to multiple variables. Research has shown that beliefs that one has control over the *cause* of the disease leads to a poor outcome, while belief in control over the *course* of the disease leads to better outcomes (Watson et al. 1990).

Thus, there is provocative evidence that psychotherapy may affect not only adjustment to medical illness, but survival time with it. The mechanisms underlying such an effect may involve influence on daily activities such as diet, exercise, and sleep, on adherence to medical treatment, or may involve changes in endocrine and immune function (Spiegel 1991). Various psychotherapeutic stress management techniques have effects on the endocrine (Levine et al. 1989; Rose 1984) and immune (Ader et al. 1990; Irwin and Strausbaugh 1991; Kennedy et al. 1988) systems.

Preliminary results of stress management intervention for patients with malignant melanoma (Fawzy et al. 1990) that included relaxation, social support, cognitive restructuring, and education suggest that immune function may be positively affected. Fawzy found that patients in support groups had greater activity of natural killer cells, a measure of the functioning of cells in the immune system involved in combating cancer (Levy et al. 1987). Indeed, baseline levels of natural killer cell cytotoxicity (though not changes over time in these levels) predicted later recurrence and mortality (Fawzy et al. 1993). Thus, there is growing evidence that the nature of social relationships in coping with breast cancer has marked psychological and possible physical effects.

Conclusion

Evidence suggests that levels of distress, depression, and anxiety are substantially elevated among patients with breast cancer. These problems persist in a sizeable minority of patients even years after diagnosis. Coping styles are related to adjustment, and, in some studies, survival time. Social support in the form of integration, availability of confidants, and structured psychotherapy has been shown to affect both adjustment and survival time positively. Taken together, these studies indicate that the social, psychological, and medical environment of patients with breast cancer is crucial to their adjustment and can influence the course of the disease.

There is growing evidence that psychotherapy for the medically ill is a powerful and important treatment, with marked psychological and possible physical effects. The medicine of the future would do well to consider these psychosocial effects. When we rediscover the role of care as well as cure in medicine, we will help patients and their families better cope with disease, and may also better mobilize the mind and body's resources to fight illness.

References

Ader R, Felten D, Cohen N, et al: Interactions between the brain and the immune system. Annu Rev Pharmacol Toxicol 30:561–602, 1990

Berkman LF, Syme SL: Social networks, host resistance, and mortality: a nine-year follow-up study of Alameda County residents. Am J Epidemiol 109(2):186–204, 1979

Bukberg J, Penman D, et al: Depression in hospitalized cancer patients. Psychosom Med 46:199–212, 1984

Burish TG, Lyles JN: Effectiveness of relaxation training in reducing adverse reactions to cancer chemotherapy. J Behav Med 4(1):65–78, 1981

Cain EN, Kohorn EI, Quinlan DM, et al: Psychosocial benefits of a cancer support group. Cancer 57(1):183–189, 1986

Carver CS, Scheier MF: Situational coping and coping dispositions in a stressful transaction. J Pers Soc Psychol 66(1):184–195, 1994

Cella DF, Pratt A, Holland JC, et al: Persistent anticipatory nausea, vomiting, and anxiety in cured Hodgkin's disease patients after completion of chemotherapy. Am J Psychiatry 143(5):641–643, 1986

Cooper CL, Faragher EB: Coping strategies and breast disorders/cancer. Psychol Med 22(2):447–455, 1992

Craig TJ, Abeloff MD: Psychiatric symptomatology among hospitalized cancer patients. Am J Psychiatry 131(12):1323–1327, 1974

Craig TJ, Comstock GW, et al: Epidemiologic comparison of breast cancer patients with early and late onset of malignancy and general population controls. J Natl Cancer Inst 53(6):1577–1581, 1974

Derogatis LR, Abeloff MD, et al: Psychological coping mechanisms and survival time in metastatic breast cancer. JAMA 242(14):1504–1508, 1979

Derogatis LR, Morrow GR, et al: The prevalence of psychiatric disorders among cancer patients. JAMA 249(6):751–757, 1983

Dunkel-Schetter C, Feinstein LG, Taylor SE, et al: Patterns of coping with cancer. Health Psychol 11(2):79–87, 1992

Dworkin SF, VonKorff M, LeResche L, et al: Multiple pains and psychiatric disturbance: an epidemiologic investigation. Arch Gen Psychiatry 47(3):239–244, 1990

Ell K, Nishimoto R, Morvany T, et al: A longitudinal analysis of psychological adaptation among survivors of cancer. Cancer 63(2):406–413, 1989

Ell K, Nishimoto R, Mediansky L, et al: Social relations, social support and survival among patients with cancer. J Psychosom Res 36(6):531–541, 1992

Fallowfield L, Hall A, Maguire GP, et al: Psychological outcomes in women with early breast cancer (letter). BMJ 301(6765):1394, 1990

Fawzy FI, Kemery ME, Fawzy NW, et al: A structured psychiatric intervention for cancer patients, I: Changes over time in methods of coping and affective disturbance. Arch Gen Psychiatry 47(8):720–725, 1990

Fawzy FI, Fawzy NW, Hyun CS, et al: Malignant melanoma: effects of an early structured psychiatric intervention, coping, and affective state on recurrence and survival 6 years later. Arch Gen Psychiatry 50(9):681–689, 1993

Felton BJ, Revenson TA, Hinrichsen GA: Stress and coping in the explanation of psychological adjustment among chronically ill adults. Soc Sci Med 18(10):889–898, 1984

Ferlic M, Goldman A, Kennedy BJ: Group counseling in adult patients with advanced cancer. Cancer 43(2):760–766, 1979

Fobair P, Hoppe RT, Bloom J, et al: Psychosocial problems among survivors of Hodgkin's disease. J Clin Oncol 4(5):805–814, 1986

Forester B, Kornfeld DS, Fleiss JL: Psychotherapy during radiotherapy: effects on emotional and physical distress. Am J Psychiatry 142(1):22–27, 1985

Funch DP, Marshall J: The role of stress, social support and age in survival from breast cancer. J Psychosom Res 27(1):77–83, 1983

Ganster DC, Victor B: The impact of social support on mental and physical health. Br J Med Psychol 61(pt 1):17–36, 1988

Ganz PA, Schag AC, Lee JJ, et al: Breast conservation versus mastectomy. Is there a difference in psychological adjustment or quality of life in the year after surgery? Cancer 69(7):1729–1738, 1992

Gellert GA, Maxwell RM, Siegel BS, et al: Survival of breast cancer patients receiving adjunctive psychosocial support therapy: a 10-year follow-up study. J Clin Oncol 11(1):66–69, 1993

Goodwin JS, Hunt WC, Key CR, et al: The effect of marital status on stage, treatment, and survival of cancer patients. JAMA 258(21):3125–3130, 1987

Greer S: Psychological response to cancer and survival. Psychol Med 21(1):43–49, 1991

Greer S, Morris T: Psychological attributes of women who develop breast cancer: a controlled study. J Psychosom Res 19(2):147–153, 1975

Greer S, Morris T, Pettingale KW: Psychological response to breast cancer: effect on outcome. Lancet 2(8146):785–787, 1979

Gustafson J, Whitman H: Towards a balanced social environment on the oncology service. Soc Psychiatry 13:147–152, 1978

Heim E, Augustiny KF, Schaffner L, et al: Coping with breast cancer over time and situation. J Psychosom Res 37(5):523–542, 1993

Helliwell PS, Mumford DB, Smeathers JE, et al: Work related upper limb disorder: the relationship between pain, cumulative load, disability, and psychological factors. Ann Rheum Dis 51(12):1325–1329, 1992

Hilgard ER, Hilgard JR: Hypnosis in the Relief of Pain. Los Altos, CA, William Kauffman, 1975

Hislop TG, Waxler NE, Coldman AJ, et al: The prognostic significance of psychosocial factors in women with breast cancer. J Chronic Dis 40(7):729–735, 1987

Holland JC: Fears and abnormal reactions to cancer in physically healthy individuals, in Handbook of Psychooncology. Edited by Holland JC, Rowland JH. New York, Oxford University Press, 1989, pp 13–21

Holland J, Holland RJ (eds): Handbook of Psychooncology: Psychologic Care of the Patient With Cancer. Newark, NJ, Oxford University Press, 1990

House JS, Robbins C, Metzner HL: The association of social relationships and activities with mortality: prospective evidence from the Tecumseh Community Health Study. Am J Epidemiol 116(1):123–140, 1982

House JS, Landis KR, Umberson D: Social relationships and health. Science 241(4865):540–545, 1988

Hughes J: Emotional reactions to the diagnosis and treatment of early breast cancer. J Psychosom Res 26(2):277–283, 1982

Hughes JE, Royle GT, Buchanan R, et al: Depression and social stress among patients with benign breast disease. Br J Surg 73(12):997–999, 1986

Ilniyki A, Farber J, Cheong M et al: A randomized controlled trial of psychotherapeutic intervention in cancer patients. Annals of the Royal College of Physicians and Surgeons of Canada 27(2):93–96, 1994

Irvine D, Brown B, Crooks D, et al: Psychosocial adjustment in women with breast cancer. Cancer 67(4):1097–1117, 1991

Irwin MR, Strausbaugh H: Stress and immune changes in humans: biopsychosocial model, in Psychoimmunology Update. Edited by Gorman JM, Kertzner RM. Washington, DC, American Psychiatric Press, 1991, pp 55–79

Itano J, Tanabe P, Lum J et al: Compliance and Noncompliance in Cancer Patients: Advances in Cancer Control. New York, Allan R Liss, 1983

Jarrett SR, Ramierz AJ, Richards MA, et al: Measuring coping in breast cancer. J Psychosom Res 36(6):593–602, 1992

Joffres M, Reed DM, Nomura AM: Psychosocial processes and cancer incidence among Japanese men in Hawaii. Am J Epidemiol 121(4):488–500, 1985

Kelly JA, Murphy DA, Bahr GR, et al: Outcome of cognitive-behavioral and support group brief therapies for depressed, HIV-infected persons. Am J Psychiatry 150(11):1679–1686, 1993

Kennedy S, Kiecolt-Glaser JK, Glaser R, et al: Immunological consequences of acute and chronic stressors: mediating role of interpersonal relationship. Br J Med Psychol 61(pt 1):77–85, 1988

Koocher G, O'Malley J: The Damocles Syndrome: Psychosocial Consequences of Surviving Childhood Cancer. New York, McGraw Hill, 1981

Lansky SB, List MA, Herrmann CA, et al: Absence of major depressive disorder in female cancer patients. J Clin Oncol 3(11):1553–1560, 1985

Levenson RW, Carstensen LL, Gottman JM, et al: The influence of age and gender on affect, physiology, and their interrelations: a study of long-term marriages. J Pers Soc Psychol 67(1):56–58, 1994

Levine PM, Silberfarb PM, Lipowski ZJ: Mental disorders in cancer patients: a study of 100 psychiatric referrals. Cancer 42(3):1385–1391, 1978

Levine S, Coe C, Weiner SG, et al: Psychoneuroendocrinology of stress: a psychobiological perspective, in Psychoendocrinology. Edited by Brush FR, Levine S. New York, Academic Press, 1989, pp 341–377

Levy S, Herberman R, Lippman M, et al: Correlation of stress factors with sustained depression of natural killer cell activity and predicted prognosis in patients with breast cancer. J Clin Oncol 5(3):348–353, 1987

Levy SM, Herberman RB, Lippman M, et al: Immunological and psychosocial predictors of disease recurrence in patients with early-stage breast cancer. Behav Med 17(2):67–75, 1991

Liang LP, Dunn SM, Gorman A, et al: Identifying priorities of psychosocial need in cancer patients. Br J Cancer 62(6):1000–1003, 1990

Maguire P: Improving the detection of psychiatric problems in cancer patients. Soc Sci Med 20(8):819–823, 1985

Maguire GP, Julier DL, Hawton KE, et al: Psychiatric morbidity and referral on two general medical wards. BMJ 1:268–270, 1974

Maguire GP, Lee EG, Bevington DJ, et al: Psychiatric problems in the first year after mastectomy. Br Med J 1(6118):963–965, 1978

Mahon SM, Cella DF, Donovan MI, et al: Psychosocial adjustment to recurrent cancer. Oncol Nurs Forum 17(suppl 3):47–52; discussion 53–54, 1990

Maraste R, Brandt L, Olson H, et al: Anxiety and depression in breast cancer patients at start of adjuvant radiotherapy. Relations to age and type of surgery. Acta Oncol 31(6):641–643, 1992

Massie MJ, Holland JC: The cancer patient with pain: psychiatric complications and their management. Med Clin North Am 71(2):243–258, 1987

Massie MJ, Holland JC: Depression and the cancer patient. J Clin Psychiatry 51:12–17; discussion 18–19, 1990

Maunsell E, Brisson J, Desehenes L, et al: Psychological distress after initial treatment of breast cancer. Assessment of potential risk factors. Cancer 70(1):120–125, 1992

Maunsell E, Brisson MJ, Deschenes ML: Social support and survival among women with breast cancer. Cancer 76(4):631–637, 1993

McNair DM, Lorr M, Droppleman LF: EdITS Manual for the Profile of Mood States. San Diego, CA, Educational and Industrial Testing Service, 1971

Mermelstein HT, Lesko L: Depression in patients with cancer. Psychooncology 1:199–225, 1992

Moos RH, Schaefer JA: The crisis of physical illness: an overview and conceptual approach, in Coping With Physical Illness 2: New Perspectives. Edited by Moos RH. New York, Plenum, 1984, pp 3–25

Morris T, Greer HS: Psychological characteristics of women electing to attend a breast screening clinic. Clin Oncol 8(2):113–119, 1982

Morris T, Greer HS, White P: Psychological and social adjustment to mastectomy: a two-year follow-up study. Cancer 40(5):2381–2387, 1977

Morrow GR, Morrell C: Behavioral treatment for the anticipatory nausea and vomiting induced by cancer chemotherapy. N Engl J Med 307(24):1476–1480, 1982

Mulder C, van der Pompe G, Spiegel D, et al: Do psychosocial factors influence the course of breast cancer? A review of recent literature methodological problems and future directions. Psychooncology 1:155–167, 1992

Myers JK, Weissman MM, Tischler GL, et al: Six-month prevalence of psychiatric disorders in three communities 1980 to 1982. Arch Gen Psychiatry 41(10):959–967, 1984

Neale AV: Racial and marital status influences on 10 year survival from breast cancer. J Clin Epidemiol 47(5):475–483, 1994

Nelson DV, Friedman LC, Bear PE, et al: Subtypes of psychosocial adjustment to breast cancer. J Behav Med 17(2):127–141, 1994

Northouse LL, Swain MA: Adjustment of patients and husbands to the initial impact of breast cancer. Nurs Res 36(4):221–225, 1987

Omne-Ponten M, Holmberg L, Burns T, et al: Determinants of the psychosocial outcome after operation for breast cancer. Results of a prospective comparative interview study following mastectomy and breast conservation. Eur J Cancer 28A(6–7):1062–1067, 1992

Omne-Ponten M, Holmberg L, Sjoden PO, et al: Psychosocial adjustment among women with breast cancer stages I and II: six-year follow-up of consecutive patients. J Clin Oncol 12(9):1778–1782, 1994

Pettingale KW: Coping and cancer prognosis. J Psychosom Res 28(5):363–364, 1984

Plumb MM, Holland J: Comparative studies of psychological function in patients with advanced cancer, I: self-reported depressive symptoms. Psychosom Med 39(4):264–276, 1977

Psychological response to mastectomy: A prospective comparison study. Psychological aspects of Breast Cancer Study Group. Cancer 59(1):189–196, 1987

Quigley KM: The adult cancer survivor: Psychosocial consequences of cure. Semin Oncol Nurs 5(1):63–69, 1989

Reynolds P, Kaplan GA: Social connections and risk for cancer: prospective evidence from the Alameda County Study. Behav Med 16(3):101–110, 1990

Richardson JL, Shelton DR, Krailo M, et al: The effect of compliance with treatment on survival among patients with hematologic malignancies. J Clin Oncol 8(2):356–364, 1990

Rieker PP, Edbril SD, Garnick MB: Curative testis cancer therapy: psychosocial sequelae. J Clin Oncol 3(8):1117–1126, 1985

Rodin G, Voshart K: Depression in the medically ill: an overview. Am J Psychiatry 143(6):696–705, 1986

Rose RM: Overview of endocrinology of stress, in Neuroendocrinology and Psychiatric Disorder. Edited by Brown GM. New York, Raven, 1984, pp 95–122

Schottenfeld D, Robbins GF: Quality of survival among patients who have had radical mastectomy. Cancer 26(3):650–655, 1970

Spiegel D: Facilitating emotional coping during treatment. Cancer 66(suppl 6):1422–1426, 1990

Spiegel D: Mind matters: effects of group support on cancer patients. Journal NIH Research 3:61–63, 1991

Spiegel D: Living Beyond Limits: New Help and Hope for Facing Life-Threatening Illness. New York, Times Books/Random House, 1993

Spiegel D, Bloom JR: Group therapy and hypnosis reduce metastatic breast carcinoma pain. Psychosom Med 45(4):333–339, 1983a

Spiegel D, Bloom JR: Pain in metastatic breast cancer. Cancer 52(2):341–345, 1983b

Spiegel D, Bloom JR, Yalom I: Group support for patients with metastatic cancer. A randomized outcome study. Arch Gen Psychiatry 38(5):527–533, 1981

Spiegel D, Bloom J, Gottheil E, et al: Family environment of patients with metastatic carcinoma. Journal of Psychosocial Oncology 1:33–44, 1983

Spiegel D, Bloom JR, Kraemer HC, et al: Effect of psychosocial treatment on survival of patients with metastatic breast cancer. Lancet 2(8668):888–891, 1989

Stavraky KM, Donner AP, Kincade JE, et al: The effect of psychosocial factors on lung cancer mortality at one year. J Clin Epidemiol 41(1):75–82, 1988

Steckel S: Predicting, measuring, implementing and following up on patient compliance. Nurs Clin North Am 17(3):491–498, 1982

Stewart MA, Drake F, Winokur G, et al: Depression among medically ill patients. Dis Nerv Syst 26:479–485, 1965

Temoshok L: Biopsychosocial studies on cutaneous malignant melanoma:

psychosocial factors associated with prognostic indicators, progression, psychophysiology and tumor-host response. Soc Sci Med 20(8):833–840, 1985

Timko C, Janoff-Bulman R: Attributions, vulnerability, and psychological adjustment: the case of breast cancer. Health Psychol 4(6):521–544, 1985

Turns DM: Psychosocial factors, in Cancer of the Breast. Edited by Donegan WL, Spratt JS. Philadelphia, PA, WB Saunders, 1988, pp 728–738

Vinokur AD, Threatt BA, Caplan RD, et al: Physical and psychosocial functioning and adjustment to breast cancer. Long-term follow-up of a screening population. Cancer 63(2):394–405, 1989

Vinokur AD, Threatt BA, Vinokur-Kaplan D, et al: The process of recovery from breast cancer for younger and older patients. Changes during the first year. Cancer 65(5):1242–1254, 1990

Watson M, Greer S, Young J, et al: Development of a questionnaire measure of adjustment to cancer: the MAC scale. Psychol Med 18(1):203–209, 1988

Watson M, Pruyn J, Greer S, et al: Locus of control and adjustment to cancer. Psychol Rep 66(1):39–48, 1990

Watson M, Greer S, Rowden L, et al: Relationships between emotional control, adjustment to cancer and depression and anxiety in breast cancer patients. Psychol Med 21(1):51–57, 1991

Waxler-Morrison N, Hislop TG, Mears B, et al: Effects of social relationships on survival for women with breast cancer: a prospective study. Soc Sci Med 33(2):177–183, 1991

Wood PE, Milligan M, Christ D, et al: Group counseling for cancer patients in a community hospital. Psychosomatics 19(9):555–561, 1978

Yalom I: Theory and Practice of Group Psychotherapy. New York, Basic Books, 1995

Zeltzer L, LeBaron S: Hypnosis and nonhypnotic techniques for reduction of pain and anxiety during painful procedures in children and adolescents with cancer. J Pediatr 101(6):1032–1035, 1982

PART VI

Family Therapies

13

Family Therapies

Efficacy, Indications, and Treatment Outcomes

Ira D. Glick, M.D.

Strong pressures to cut costs, in the context of two decades of accumulated research on treatment efficacy and outcomes, have provided an opportunity to update the indications for family therapy. The message to both clinical researchers and clinicians is that family therapy does work, but we are still not clear for whom, or for what. Given that introduction, in this chapter I review the literature on the indications and efficacy of family therapy and also cover, by way of background, the history of family therapy, its definition, goals, mechanisms, and techniques.

Research on efficacy and treatment outcomes has produced significant data on treatment of families with such Axis I diagnoses as mood disorders and schizophrenia, as well as other marital and family problems and dysfunctions. It would be well to review the pitfalls and limitations in interpreting these results, critique the data, and attempt to formulate critical issues.

When, if ever, is marital or family therapy indicated? Using the four steps of a family decision tree (Glick et al., in press) developed from a critical review of the literature, we can aid in both clear-cut and complicated decision making. The theory and practice of how one combines family therapy and medication is also discussed.

Given the implications of the new economic realities, can family therapy survive in the future? More research on process and outcome, better therapists, and what I consider to be a quality treatment equation will help to assure the future of family therapy.

Background, Definition, Goals, and Models

Compared with individual or group psychotherapy formats, marital and family therapy is the newest of the psychotherapies. Nevertheless, many would agree that family therapy has a better early (i.e., its first two decades) history of controlled research on both its process and its outcomes than any of the other psychotherapies. *Marital and family therapy* can be defined as a professionally organized attempt to produce beneficial changes in a disturbed marital or family unit essentially through interactional, nonpharmacological methods. Its aim is the establishment of a more satisfying way of living for the entire family. There is a continuum between the intrapsychic system, the interactional family system, and the sociocultural system, but the major uniqueness of family therapy is that the emphasis is put on the family.

The goals of family therapy are based on a thorough evaluation of the strengths and weaknesses of each family member and of the family as a group. Ideally, the entire family should function more satisfactorily and each family member should derive personal benefit from the experience and results of family therapy. Goals must be in some way congruent with what the family members seem to want, and what they are realistically capable of achieving at any particular point in time. Families enter therapy either because of gross symptomatic difficulty in one member or general family system problem issues, such as marital troubles (most commonly) or family unhappiness. Goals should be based not only on the specific problems of the family (i.e., a problem-oriented approach to each family), but also on the following general goals: 1) to facilitate communication of thoughts and feelings among family members, 2) to shift disturbed, inflexible roles and coalitions in the family, and 3) to increase options and demythologize dysfunctional family myths. Of course the therapist must differentiate short-term goals from long-term goals.

As to mechanisms and techniques, family therapy uses all the general elements of the psychotherapies (e.g., a good patient-therapist relationship, release of emotional tension, cognitive learning). However, objectives are all set with the goal of improving the overall functioning of the entire family, and the specific mix of the elements varies. Family therapists place their emphasis on such different dimensions as 1) the present (versus the past), 2) action techniques (versus interpretation), 3) the presenting problem (versus "growth"), 4) developing a special plan for each problem (versus a general method for all problems), and 5) keeping a therapeutic focus on two or more individuals (versus a focus on one patient).

Therapists have adopted treatment techniques from different schools of family therapy as described in Table 13–1. To summarize this material most simply: 1) with the insight-awareness approach, observation, clarification, and interpretations are used to foster understanding and presumably change; 2) in the systemic-structural approach, manipulations are devised to alter family structures and conduct; 3) in the cognitive-behavioral approach, family members learn to eliminate dysfunctional behaviors and use new and more effective interpersonal behaviors; 4) in the experiential-existential approach, emotional experience is designed to change the way family members see, and presumably react to, one another; and 5) in the narrative approach, a new reality is constructed. We emphasize in this chapter three major therapeutic strategies to achieve these goals: 1) strategies that facilitate communication of thoughts and feelings; 2) strategies that shift disturbed, inflexible roles and coalitions; and 3) strategies that aid family role assumption, education, and demythologizing.

Efficacy, Indications, and Treatment Outcomes

The latest reviews concerning family therapy fall into two groups. The first are those of Pinsof and Wynne (1995) and Lebow and Gurman

TABLE 13–1

Models of family treatment

Treatment approach (school)	Major proponents	Strategies and techniques	Therapist role	Therapeutic goals	Data base
1. Insight-awareness (aka historical, psychodynamic, or psychoanalytic)	Ackerman Nagy and Spark Paul Nadelson Bowen	1. Observation 2. Clarification 3. Interpretation	1. Listener 2. "Therapeutic distance" 3. Therapeutic stance of technical neutrality	Foster understanding and insight in effecting change	1. History 2. Unconscious derivatives 3. Transference
2. Systemic-structural (aka systems, communications, or structural)	Palo Alto Group (Jackson, Bateson, Haley, Satir) Sluzki Dowen Minuchin M. Erickson	1. Strategies to alter family structure and behavior 2. Observe and transform using directives	Therapist observes and moves in and out of process	Change structure, communications, pattern, and roles, which change perception and behavior	1. Sequences 2. Communication 3. Rules 4. History
3. Cognitive-behavioral	Weiss Jacobson Patterson Falloon	1. Communication teaching 2. Problem-solving skills 3. Contingency contracting	Therapist is collaborator in the development of interpersonal skills	Eliminate dysfunctional behaviors and learn to use new and more effective interpersonal behaviors	1. Observation of overt behaviors 2. Functional analysis of problematic behavioral sequences

Continued on next page

TABLE 13–1 (*continued*)

Treatment approach (school)	Major proponents	Strategies and techniques	Therapist role	Therapeutic goals	Data base
4. Experiential-existential	Whitaker Bowen Nagy	1. Therapist designs and/or participates with family in the emotional experience	Therapist offers self for interaction to minimize distance between family members	1. Change ways family members experience (and presumably react to) each other 2. Growth and differentiation	1. Observed verbal and nonverbal behavior 2. Shared feelings (including the therapist's feelings)
5. Narrative	White Epson	1. Externalizing the problem 2. Mapping influence of problem over family and influence of family over the problem	Therapist collaborates with family on a therapeutic conversation	1. Develop an alternative narrative story about the problem 2. Liberate the family from being controlled by the problem toward authoring their own study	Linguistic behavior

Source. Reprinted from Click ID, Berman E, Clarkin JF, et al: Marital and Family Therapy, 4th Edition. Washington, DC, American Psychiatric Press, in press. Used with permission.

(1995), which are overviews of outcome data summarized in the October 1995 issue of the *Journal of Marital and Family Therapy* (Table 13–2). The second is the Shadish et al. (1993) meta-analysis.

These reviews suggest that the strongest indication for family therapy is for the treatment of schizophrenia. Figure 14–5 outlines the well-developed literature and findings supporting this therapeutic indication. The type of family therapy used for treating schizophrenia most commonly is *psychoeducational*, a therapy that emphasizes teaching about the details of schizophrenia as well as working on decreasing expressed emotion and increasing both compliance and the ability of the family to cope with life stress. Needless to say, this family therapy must be combined with medication to obtain the most efficacious outcomes for both patient and family.

A second indication for family therapy is for mood disorder in women who also have couple or marital problems. Prince and Jacobson's (1995) review suggests that medication plus marital therapy is more efficacious than individual therapy alone. In these situations, individual therapy alone is often inefficient and ineffective for moderate to severe depressive symptoms. Likewise, drugs alone are ineffective for the marital disorder part of the equation. In addition, Clarkin et al. (1998) have reported that marital therapy in addition to medication is more effective than medication alone for bipolar disorder.

A third indication for family therapy is for what is described as "out-of-control children and adolescents." The disorders studied are 1) child and adolescent conduct disorder, 2) adolescent drug abuse, 3) aggression and noncompliance in children diagnosed with attention deficit hyperactivity disorder (ADHD), and 4) childhood autism. Here, the use of three specific family treatments is advocated: 1) a type of social learning applied to family therapy, 2) structural family therapy, and 3) an ecological approach (i.e., involving the larger family system of counselors, teachers, etc.) targeting treatment in multiple relevant systems.

A fourth area of application is the treatment of couples or marital distress and/or conflict. The data from more than three decades suggest that couples therapy is superior to individual therapy for most of these situations, but the effects wash out over time, working for only about 40% of couples. The strongest effects are for increasing marital satis-

TABLE 13-2

Adult, adolescent, and childhood disorders or problems for which marital (MT) and family (FT) therapy have significant effects

Patient age	FT > no treatment controls	FT > standard or individual treatment	MT > no treatment controls	MT > standard or individual treatment
Adult	Schizophrenia[a] Alcoholism[a] Drug abuse Dementia Cardiovascular risk factors	Schizophrenia[a] Alcoholism[a] Drug abuse Dementia Cardiovascular risk factors	Depressed women in distressed marriages Marital distress or conflict Obesity Hypertension	Women with unipolar depression in distressed marriages, treated as outpatients Marital distress or conflict
Adolescent	Conduct disorders[a] Drug abuse[a] Obesity Younger adolescents with anorexia of <3 years	Conduct disorders[a] Drug abuse[a]		
Child	Conduct disorders[a] Aggression and non-compliance in ADHD Autism[a] Chronic physical illnesses Obesity	Autism[a] Aggression and non-compliance in ADHD		

Note. Significant effects meaning that there are at least two published, controlled studies with significant results supporting the efficacy of marital and family therapy.

[a] Indicates multicomponent packages with at least one marital and family therapy component.

Source. Reprinted from Pinsof WM, Wynne LC: The efficacy of marital and family therapy. Journal of Marital and Family Therapy 21:586–613, 1995. Used with permission.

faction and reducing conflict. Thus, the therapy helps to decrease the risk of divorce.

A fifth indication for family therapy is to induce difficult-to-engage patients and family units to enter therapy (e.g., individuals who abuse substances, patients with schizophrenia, and children or adolescents who are delinquent).

Most researchers in this area have agreed that for Axis I disorders, the duration of the treatment effect for family therapy dissipates rapidly after the family therapy is terminated. This, of course, should be no surprise to anyone who treats chronic medical illness. Like hypertension and diabetes, these illnesses need continual boosters to maintain the progress resulting from effective intervention in the acute phase. In summary, combining or integrating family therapy with drug therapy for most Axis I disorders may be an effective strategy.

Lebow and Gurman (1995) discuss a number of methodological issues, pointing out many areas where knowledge is scant. First, we do not know whether a number of the well-known types of family therapy work differentially. Second, we do not know whether such common clinical indications as treatment of the family of origin or of intergenerational conflict are effective. Second, how the marital process relates to outcome still needs to be studied. Third, we do not understand the influence, or effect, of gender and cultural issues on outcome. Finally, very little work has been done on the use of family therapy with such child and adolescent problems as anxiety and depression.

The other major review to be considered is Shadish et al. (1993). This study was a meta-analysis of 163 randomized trials focusing on 1) theoretical orientation effects, 2) family and marital therapy versus individual therapy, 3) outcomes, 4) clinical significance versus statistical significance of the marital therapy, 5) mediating variables, and 6) family therapy versus alternative therapies. The main issue here is that unlike some meta-analyses, there was no quality control of the studies. That is, the studies were not rated as to their quality, using only the best ones, so many poorly designed studies were included in this review.

Given that limitation, Shadish's review suggested that two-thirds of families receiving treatment versus one-third of the control families benefited. This assertion is consistent with previous literature. Shadish et al. (1993) found only minimal negative effects when they looked at the effect of the different types of family therapy. Most seemed better than the control situations. As to effect sizes, Shadish et al. (1993) found that marital therapy was more effective than family therapy for certain problems. Marital therapy was effective for conduct disorders, phobias, schizophrenia and "global psychiatric disorders" (p. 994) including depression in females and communication problems with couples. Marital and family therapy seemed better than individual and conjoint therapy. Finally, all types seemed to work, except for what has been labeled *humanistic therapy*. As to the issue of clinical versus statistical significance, Shadish and colleagues (1993) judged that the effects *were* clinically significant.

As to methodological issues, Shadish et al. (1993) felt that generally the quality of the studies was "good" (p. 1000), I assume compared with other psychotherapy studies and not with psychopharmacological studies. The authors wisely pointed out that several areas needed strengthening, including: 1) internal validity (i.e., although the cases were randomly assigned, the studies had high attrition), 2) statistical conclusion validity (the authors pointed out that these studies had very low power), 3) construct validity (very little exploration of the process of therapy was done, perhaps an appropriate omission given the uncertainty about outcome) and, 4) external validity (the sample was mostly obtained from university settings and was experimenter-solicited, rather than drawn from cases being treated in clinical practice. This led to high exclusion rates, therefore limiting generalizability).

In 1987, Glick et al. summarized the available literature using a series of rhetorical questions. More recent data suggest some new answers.

What percentage of families receiving family therapy improve?
Roughly two-thirds improve: 40%–60% of marital cases and 70% of family cases.

Does the developmental level of the identified patient help to predict outcome?
If a child or an adolescent is the identified patient, there may be a slightly better outcome than if the patient is an adult.

What percentage of patients or families get worse during (if not because of) therapy?

We think the answer is about 5%–10%, although Pinsof and Wynne (1995) believe that the rate is lower, and describe family therapy as "not harmful" (p. 604).

What therapist characteristics are associated with poor outcome?

If the therapist has poor relationship skills and attacks frontally too early, or provides no structure for the session or support for the family, this is associated with poor outcome.

Which family therapies are not effective?

We found conjoint (same therapist with one couple) to be the best of the marital (nonbehavioral) therapies; that is, it is better than collaborative (two therapists each treating a spouse) or concurrent (same therapist treating both partners) therapy.

Which is better, individual therapy or marital therapy, for marital problems?

Marital therapy has a better improvement rate and about half the rate of deterioration.

What are the best "ingredients?"

Increasing communication is a necessary but not a sufficient ingredient.

What length of treatment works best?

Brief treatment (defined as up to 20 sessions) has been found equal to long treatment. (With the arrival of managed care, most therapy *is* now brief.)

Whose participation betters the outcome of family therapy?

A better outcome occurs if the father is included. Likewise, a better outcome occurs if both parents are included.

Do other variables affect outcome?

No evidence exists that the use of a cotherapist, a team, or videotape improves outcome.

The Decision Tree

We have recently (Glick et al., in press) reviewed the available research literature on the indications for family therapy to construct a decision tree for use in deciding whether to use marital or family treatment. We propose four steps:

Step I: Evaluation

We defined the family evaluation as one or more family interviews designed to assess the structure and process of family interaction to discover how this phenomenon is related to the behavior and symptoms of individual members. We concluded that situations in which family or marital evaluation is usually essential include 1) when a child or adolescent is the presenting patient; 2) when the presenting problem is sexual difficulty or dissatisfaction; 3) when the presenting problem is a serious family or marital problem, especially when the future of the marital relationship, the adequate care of the children in the family, or family members' vocational stability or health is at stake; 4) when a recent stress or emotional disruption in the family, caused by such family crises as serious illness, injury, loss of job, death, birth, or the departure from the home of a family member has occurred; 5) when the family or the marital pair, or an individual within the group, defines the problem as a family issue and family evaluation is sought.

In addition, we consider that family evaluation is usually indicated when referral of a family member for hospitalization or acute psychiatric treatment is being considered. In such circumstances, family evaluation is of value for history-gathering, to clarify the relationship between family interaction patterns and the course of the identified patient's illness, and to negotiate a treatment plan with the whole family. Other less powerful indications for family evaluation include 1) situations where more than one family member is simultaneously in psychiatric treatment (this is especially true when both members of a couple are in individual treatment); 2) when improvement in a patient coincides with the development of symptoms in another such as the spouse, or a deterioration in their relationship; 3) when individual or group therapy is failing or has failed, and the patient is very involved with family problems, has difficulty dealing with family issues or shows evidence of too intense transference to the therapist, or when family cooperation appears necessary so the individual can change; and 4) when during individual evaluation it appears that the advantages to the family of the patient's symptoms can be understood in the light of the psychological functioning of the family.

Step II: Differential Diagnosis and Therapy

Making a differential diagnosis and conducting therapy involves deciding whether family or marital treatment is required, as opposed to individual treatment, sex therapy, or treatment in hospital. We suggest that family or marital therapy may be indicated 1) when couples or marital distress problems are a presenting complaint, without an identifying patient; 2) when a family presents with current problems in the relationships between family members; 3) where problems in perception and communication are chronic and severe, such as in projective identification, in which members blame each other for problems and disclaim their own parts in them, or there is paranoid-schizoid functioning, or various severely disturbed forms of communication such as are seen in schizophrenia and mood disorder; 4) in the presence of such adolescent antisocial behavior as drug abuse, delinquency, or violence; 5) when problems involve adolescent separation; 6) when control or manipulation of the parent by the child is found; 7) following the failure of other treatment, for example when individual therapy sessions have been used mainly to discuss family problems; 8) when the family group is motivated to accept treatment but an individual is not; 9) where improvement in one family member leads to symptoms or deterioration in another; and finally, 10) when more than one person needs treatment, and resources are available for only one treatment.

The next choice is to decide between administering family or marital therapy. In making this choice, the therapist must consider whether the main problems are in the spouse subsystem or in the family as a whole and the motivation of the different family members to become involved in one or another type of therapy. If marital therapy is selected, the decision has then to be made whether or not to include sex therapy as a part or the major component of the intervention. This decision depends upon 1) whether sexual problems are present, 2) how severe they are, and 3) whether the marital problem is clearly centered about the sexual difficulties. In addition, 4) the couple must be motivated to have sex therapy and be willing and able to carry out the appropriate tasks.

Step III: Duration and Intensity of Therapy

The choice here is among using family crises therapy, brief family therapy, or long-term family therapy. Of course, financial support for greater than six sessions must be available to choose long-term treatment. Family crises therapy (up to six sessions) is most likely to be indicated when the problems with which the family presents are associated with a developmental or other crisis, and particularly, when the problems are acute and urgent. Brief family therapy, defined as more than six sessions, but lasting less than six months and consisting of sessions no more often than once a week, is indicated for less urgent problems. These include the following situations: 1) when there is a focal symptom or conflict involving a child, adolescent, or marital pair, and the family is highly motivated to change; 2) when family involvement is necessary to support another method of treatment, such as regular attendance at a day hospital; 3) when a couple presents seeking help in deciding whether to separate; and 4) in family situations too complex to be understood in a brief evaluation. In this situation, brief family therapy may enable the therapist to learn more about the situation and test the response to treatment. Long-term therapy (greater than 20 sessions) may be indicated for more complex and chronic problems, especially where a family's motivation to change is strong and in instances where the family has failed to respond to family crisis therapy or brief treatment.

Step IV: Choosing the Type of Therapy

Considering which brand or type to use consists of determining which family therapy approach is likely to be most useful in a particular case. Currently, little scientifically acceptable information on this subject is available, and few controlled trials in which two or more different methods of family therapy have been tried using matched or randomly allocated cases. Lebow and Gurman (1995) have suggested that the 1) cognitive-behavioral, 2) structural, 3) psychoeducational, and 4) problem-oriented approaches are those with demonstrated effectiveness.

The decision tree described previously is a recent development, and its value is still not certain. Although it is derived from an extensive review of the literature, this in turn has many limitations because it consists largely of personal views resulting from therapists' own experiences, rather than being based on scientifically sound studies. Nevertheless, the principle of using a decision tree of this type, considering first the circumstance in which family or marital evaluation is indicated and then considering a number of steps before deciding what treatment to use (if any is required) seems a useful one.

Combining Family Interventions With Medication

For the first time in the last three decades, new medications for the treatment of psychoses — namely, clozapine, anticonvulsants, and new atypical antipsychotics — have created the opportunity to improve the prognosis for patients with major psychoses. Two major treatment questions have arisen: What else is useful? How can compliance be increased? An important part of the answer is to combine psychotherapy or rehabilitation strategies, especially family intervention ones, with newer medication strategies.

What are the objectives of combining medications with psychotherapy? Simply put, the objective is to treat not only the symptoms of the identified patient, but also the associated family problems (i.e., the effects of the symptoms on the family). Most clinicians know that combining medication with psychotherapy is necessary and indicated for several reasons:

1. Patients value psychotherapy, and often value it more than do their nonpsychiatric physicians.
2. Patients may not be on medications at different points in the course

of an illness for a variety of reasons and thus may need to be carried by psychotherapy.

3. Although the etiology of these illnesses are biological, stress may precipitate an episode.

4. Although the pathogenesis does not lie with the family, symptoms of the patient's illness affect the family, and the family's response can make the symptoms better or worse.

5. Psychotherapy is advisable to increase medication compliance. Even after successful acute therapy, patients often do not want to give up certain behaviors: for example, the perception of increased sexual intensity, productivity, and creativity associated with a manic mood disorder for the treatment effects of drugs.

Controlled Clinical Research Studies of Combined Medication and Family Therapy

A modest body of controlled studies suggests that medication and family interventions are synergistic. Each covers different domains: medication is useful for certain symptom clusters (e.g., hallucinations and delusions), and family intervention is useful for improving interpersonal skills and relationships. By extension, an assumption to be made is that both treatments improve compliance. The rationale is that, given the cognitive disorder inherent in the major psychosis, family intervention with a heavy psychoeducational focus is believed to be necessary to increase the effectiveness of medication. By way of example, in our Inpatient Family Intervention study (Glick et al. 1991a), family intervention improved compliance among those who were noncompliant prior to hospitalization. The obvious next questions are which diagnoses need which combination of therapies, in which sequence, and at what doses?

General and Specific Guidelines for Combining Treatments

We use a model that assumes that biological and psychological factors interact to produce most Axis I disorders. Using this model, we (Glick .

et al. 1991b, 1994) have developed the following Quality Care Equation:

Effective treatment of major psychoses =
Medication + Family intervention + Individual intervention +
Consumer group support

With respect to practical guidelines, first, making both a DSM-IV (American Psychiatric Association 1994) and a family systems diagnosis is important. Next, having specific goals for each modality is necessary. Third, one should be aware not only of target symptoms, but the side effects of both the drug therapy and the family psychotherapy, as well as their interaction. Finally, determining for whom combined treatment is not indicated is important.

The next issue is effectively and efficiently to sequence the modalities. As a first step, a working therapeutic-alliance must be established. Only after that should medication be prescribed. Simultaneously, referral of the family to the appropriate consumer group (i.e., National Alliance for the Mentally Ill, National Depressive and Manic-Depressive Association, Alcoholics Anonymous) is recommended. Next, provide psychoeducation for the family and the patient, but only if both are cognitively able to hear the information, as a crucial early step. *Psychoeducation* is defined as the systematic administration over time of information about symptoms and signs, diagnosis, treatment, and prognosis. Later, individual supportive therapy and/or family supportive interventions are made, and only still later are dynamic individual psychotherapy or systemic family models used. Much later (months or even years), rehabilitation is added to the equation, at a point when the patient can cognitively or behaviorally benefit.

Psychiatric Management

The term *psychiatric management* refers to a whole range of psychiatric services, including medical, supportive, psychosocial, and rehabilitation strategies. The rationale of psychiatric management is that no psychosocial strategy by itself can change the life course for either schizophrenia or mood disorder. The question arises as to which type and in which phase management should occur. I suggest family intervention (rather than individual treatment) in acute phases, and family therapy combined with individual therapy in the maintenance phases. The model is the psychoeducational one (rather than a psychodynamic or cognitive family therapy model). The psychotherapeutic alliance is characterized by a more receptive, less judgmental stance than the pharmacotherapeutic alliance. Finally, and most important, the patient as well as the family is viewed as partners on the treatment team.

Family Intervention

Data from our inpatient study (Glick et al. 1990) and from five outpatient studies have lent strong support for the concept that combining family intervention with medication is effective in treating schizophrenia. Lam (1991) has described seven components of effective family approaches to schizophrenia. Each of these can be adapted to most Axis I and II disorders. They include 1) a positive approach and genuine working relationship between the therapist and family; 2) the provision of family therapy in a stable, structured format with the availability of additional contacts with therapists if necessary; 3) a focus on improving stress and coping in the here and now, rather than dwelling on the past; 4) encouragement of and respect for interpersonal boundaries within the family; 5) the provision of information about the biological nature of schizophrenia in order to reduce blaming of the patient and family guilt; 6) use of behavioral techniques, such as breaking down goals into manageable steps; and 7) improving communication among family members.

Saying it another way, the family intervention may educate, improve communication skills, improve problem-solving skills, and resolve dynamic and systems issues. The pharmacological intervention may normalize the illness and suppress symptoms.

Summary

As to *survivability* of this modality, first, given the economic realities, more research on process and outcome is needed. Second, given the economic realities of our times, a better quality of therapist is going to be demanded by those providing the money to pay for it. Third, the field should move out of its marginalized place and back into the mainstream of the mental health field (Shields et al. 1994).

As to the future, I am suggesting that quality care in terms of full resolution requires the following equation:

Episode resolution =
Diagnosis + Treatment + Patient and family compliance

To achieve the best quality of care, the appropriate diagnosis must be made followed by the appropriate treatment, with the patient and family as full, active members of the treatment team. I am advocating an interactive process among patients, family, and treatment team. Thus, I am suggesting that treatment for most Axis I disorders should be a medication or medications, family intervention plus a supportive individual intervention, psychoeducation for both patient and family, and a link between the family and consumer organizations. For family problems and dysfunction, marital and family therapy will play an increasingly important role as the data on its efficacy accumulates in a variety of clinical situations.

References

American Psychiatric Association: Diagnostic and Statistical Manual of Mental Disorders, 4th Edition. Washington, DC, American Psychiatric Association, 1994

Clarkin JF, Carpenter D, Hull J, et al: Effects of psychoeducational intervention for married bipolar patients and their spouses. Psychiatr Serv 49:531–533, 1998

Glick ID, Clarken JF, Kessler DR: Marital and Family Therapy, 3rd Edition. Washington, DC, American Psychiatric Press, 1987, pp 393–417

Glick ID, Spencer JH, Clarkin JF, et al: A randomized clinical trial of inpatient family intervention, IV: followup results for subjects with schizophrenia. Schizophr Res 3:187–200, 1990

Glick ID, Clarkin JF, Haas G, et al: A randomized clinical trial of inpatient family intervention, VI: mediating variables and outcome. Fam Process 30:85–99, 1991a

Glick ID, Burti L, Suzuki K, et al: Effectiveness in psychiatric care: I. A cross-national study of the process of treatment and outcomes of major depressive disorder. J Nerv Ment Dis 179:55–63, 1991b

Glick ID, Burti L, Okonogi K, et al: Effectiveness in psychiatric care: III. Psychoeducation and outcome for patients with major affective disorder and their families. Br J Psychiatry 164:104–106, 1994

Glick ID, Berman E, Clarkin JF, et al: Marital and Family Therapy, 4th Edition. Washington, DC, American Psychiatric Press, in press

Lam DH: Psychosocial family intervention in schizophrenia: a review of empirical studies. Psychol Med 21:423–441, 1991

Lebow J, Gurman AS: Making a difference. Annual Review of Psychiatry 46:27–57, 1995

Pinsof WM, Wynne LC: The efficacy of marital and family therapy: an empirical overview, conclusions, and recommendations. J Marital Fam Ther 21:585–613, 1995

Prince SE, Jacobson NS: A review and evaluation of marital and family therapies for affective disorders. J Marital Fam Ther 21:377–401, 1995

Shadish WR, Montgomery LM, Wilson P, et al: Effects of family and marital psychotherapies: a meta-analysis. J Consult Clin Psychol 61:992–1002, 1993

Shields CG, McDaniel SH, Wynne LC, et al: The marginalizaton of family therapy: a historical and continuing problem. J Marital Fam Ther 20:117–138, 1994

14

New Directions in Family Intervention Programs for Psychotic Patients

Implications From Expressed Emotion Research

Michael J. Goldstein, Ph.D.[†]

Radical changes in the pattern of treatment for psychotic patients occurring over the last 15 years have focused attention on the application of appropriate models for community-based care. As hospitalizations are measured in days rather than in weeks or months, a three-phase model has emerged, consisting of inpatient resolution of the most acute positive symptoms, stabilization of the patient in the postdischarge period, and a maintenance phase in which the gains of the stabilization period are continued and enhanced. Clearly, family-focused psychoeducational programs initiated during the immediate postdischarge period can substantially decrease the risk of a psychotic disorder relapse during the first year following an index episode (Goldstein and Miklowitz 1995). Many of these programs have been inspired and guided by research on the concept of expressed emotion (EE; Kavanagh 1992).

The concept of EE refers to specific attitudes and behaviors, manifested by relatives of psychotic patients during a semistructured inter-

---

[†]Dr Goldstein died in 1998.

view, the Camberwell Family Interview (CFI; Vaughn and Leff 1976). The repeated observation has been made that patients returning to live, or remain in substantial contact with, relatives that rated as having high EE on excessive criticism and/or emotional overinvolvement are at substantially higher risk for relapse than patients whose relatives do not express these attitudes. Many early psychoeducational family programs followed an epidemiological perspective and were designed to modify risk factors, and indeed, the goal of these programs was often to reduce high EE attitudes.

A number of implicit assumptions were inherent in the EE hypothesis. For example, high EE behaviors observed in the laboratory were presumed likely to be manifested in day-to-day family interactions once the patient returned home, and variance in EE attitudes was thought to be reasonably independent of the attributes of the patient as such, which possessed prognostic value in their own right. Our research group at UCLA has been investigating these assumptions using in vivo observations of the interactions of recently discharged psychotic patients diagnosed with schizophrenia and bipolar-manic disorder. In this chapter we describe some of our findings from these studies and relate them to the literature on the efficacy of psychoeducational programs.

The Family Assessment Procedure

To appreciate the findings of these studies, it may be helpful for the reader to understand the exact procedures used by our group to elicit interactional behavior between a recently discharged psychotic patient and certain close relatives. The CFI was administered by members of one research team. In addition, a number of measures were administered in the following order: 1) a 7-card version of the Thematic Apperception Test (Jones 1977) designed to provide a communication sample scorable by the communication deviance system; 2) a Five Minute Speech Sample (FMSS-EE) (Magana et al. 1986) designed to assess EE in a brief period; 3) an Adjective Rating Scale (Friedman and Goldstein 1994) that asked relatives to rate their typical interactional behaviors over the previous 3 months by checking applicable positive and negative adjectives, as well as their patient-relatives' typical behavior toward them over the same period.

Following this, the patient and relative(s) were interviewed in an interaction assessment in separate rooms. They were interviewed by another research team that was blind to the observed EE status concerning typical problems that can arise in a family, which can be particularly acute when a psychiatric patient returns home or is in very close contact with relatives. This interview was designed to identify problems that were particularly significant for the person being interviewed. When such a problem was identified, the interviewer asked the respondent to imagine that some instance of the problem was occurring at that moment, and to role-play, in their natural tone of voice, what they would say to the other person (patient to relative or vice versa) if that person were present in the room. Generally, two such vignettes were identified, and role-played statements were audiotaped for each one. These audiotapes were then taken to the room where the target of the comment was located, and the individual's audiotaped segments were played for that person. The target's response was recorded on the same tape, forming a simulated interactional segment for each of the two identified problem areas.

Of the various problems discussed, two were selected for a discussion in person, one generated initially by the patient and the other by a relative. If two relatives participated in the discussion, statements were used from only one of them that had sufficiently broad applicability for the three-person group (patient and two relatives).

The next phase of the assessment involved two 10-minute interactions, in which relatives and patients were brought together in the same room, played one of the simulated interactions, and instructed to tell each other why they said what they did on the tape, how they felt about the issue, and to attempt to resolve the issue in the next 10 minutes. The interviewer then left the family alone for 10 minutes. After 10 minutes, the interviewer returned and repeated the procedure for the second identified problem discussion. Across families, the order of the presentation was counterbalanced, with half starting with a patient-generated problem and the other half with a problem initiated by a relative.

Because we select only two from a larger set of problems, the question often arises as to how we select the two problems used. In general, our criteria have been that the problem is of a level of generality such that it could involve all family members, that it is a problem of family life that would be true of most families, and that the problem is not related to the obvious symptoms of the patient's disorder. For example, a problem that referred to a specific incident (i.e., the patient had not cut the lawn 2 days previously) was considered a poor stimulus for discussion because it could be dismissed as an irrelevant one-time issue. If the problem only involved the mother and the patient, and the father was not relevant, it was considered less useful. If the problem focused on the patient's delusions or hallucinations, it was also considered less useful than if it referred to some interactional behavior that was difficult to deal with (e.g., consistently playing the hi-fi too loudly at night).

Do Family Members Classified by Test Procedure as High or Low EE Interact With Their Schizophrenic Patient-Relatives in a Manner That Parallels Their Attitudes?

To answer this question, we used a comparison of the CFI-based status of relatives with relatives' verbal behavior during the direct interaction task. The direct interaction data were coded using a system developed by Jeri Doane, termed affective style (AS) (Doane et al. 1981). The AS system is applied to verbatim transcripts of relatives' remarks during the two 10-minute interactions and identifies the following behaviors: 1) support statements; 2) benign criticisms that refer to specific behaviors; 3) personal or harsh criticisms that refer to general traits or motives of the other; 4) guilt-inducing statements; and 5) intrusions that refer to statements about the patient's needs, motives, or desires, and imply a special knowledge by the relative not completely justified by the patient's own remarks. Category 5 is considered one potential manifestation of the high EE category of emotional overinvolvement, whereas categories 2, 3, and 4 are hypothesized to parallel the criticism component of the EE system.

The AS system was applied to three family samples in which relatives were classified by their EE status prior to the interactional measurement described earlier (Miklowitz et al. 1984, 1989; Strachan et al. 1986). Two of these studies were done in Los Angeles and one in London by Angus Strachan, a postdoctoral fellow working on our project, with the kind cooperation of Julian Leff at the Maudsley Hospital. The results of the first two studies supported a direct relationship between relatives' CFI status and their AS patterns. Figure 14–1 presents the rationale of the AS scores (sum of criticisms, guilt-inducing remarks, and intrusions) and relatives' EE status from these two studies.

However, in our more recent study (Miklowitz et al. 1989), we failed to find such a clear relationship between AS and CFI, although the interval between the CFI and the interactional assessment was longer than was the case in the first two studies. This may have played a role in the failure to find a correlation between AS and the CFI-EE status of the relatives. Also, the patient sample in the third study was much less chronic than the earlier two, being composed of two-thirds recent onset, first episode cases.

Fortunately, we did introduce the FMSS-EE procedure (as opposed to the CFI evaluation) in the third study, giving it on the same

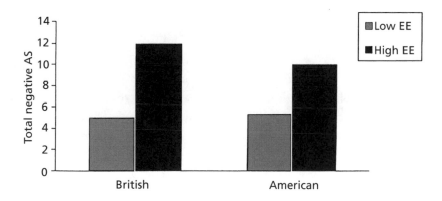

FIGURE 14–1. *Total number of negative AS statements made by British (Strachan et al. 1986) and American (Miklowitz et al. 1984) high and low EE relatives of schizophrenic patients.*

day as the family assessment. Relatives' FMSS-EE status was highly predictive of their AS pattern. Further, when we compared relatives with respect to the stability of their EE status from the original CFI to the FMSS-EE procedure, only those relatives who were classified as high EE on both indices were discriminable from low EE relatives (Fig. 14–2).

Of course, based on these observations, we cannot say whether the discrepancy we noted across time speaks to a distinction between relatives with stable or unstable EE attitudes, respectively, or to something about the potential of the two methods (CFT or FMSS) for eliciting high EE attitudes. It is also intriguing to consider the possibility that there are two types of high EE relatives, one type whose attitudes are transitory and related to the stresses associated with having a patient-relative with an acute episode of psychosis, and a second type, whose EE attitudes and negative AS behaviors persist into the postdischarge period. It is interesting to note that in the Goldstein et al. (1989) sample we found that those relatives whose EE ratings were high on the original CFI *and* on the subsequent FMSS (and who, in turn, were likely to express negative AS behaviors in direct interactions with the patient) were much more likely than other relatives to have a lifetime history of major and severe mental disorder. This would suggest that these relatives, based on their own vulnerability, may have had fewer resources to cope with the stresses posed by the existence of schizophrenia in a close family member.

Although the CFI did not predict the subsequent verbal behavior of relatives in the direct interaction task in the third study (Goldstein et al. 1989), as reflected in the AS coding, we were surprised to find that it was highly predictive of the patient's verbal behavior directed toward his or her relatives. The patient's behavior was coded using another system, called patient coping style (CS; Strachan et al. 1989). The pattern of patient CS codes was reliably predicted from the relative's CFI, and in particular, one code reflecting the patient's tendency to be critical of the relative was closely related to the family status being defined as high EE-critical type. Thus, we found that relatives' affective attitudes from the inpatient to the immediate posthospitalization period could vary considerably, but that the original attitudinal assessment predicted the patient's behavior, independent of whether the

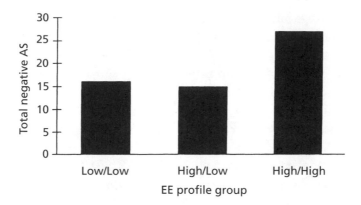

FIGURE 14–2. *Association between EE patterns (CFI and FMSS) and family AS scores.*

relatives' attitude is modulated over time. Stated otherwise, relatives behaved toward patients more or less in keeping with their *current* affective attitude, but patients reacted to relatives according to the relative's *prior* affective attitudes. At the time, we did not fully appreciate the implications of these findings.

Are Relatives' Affective Attitudes Independent of Patient Behavior?

In general, the data from numerous studies supported Vaughn's (Vaughn 1989) conclusion that there was no correlation between the form and severity of patient symptoms and relative or family EE status. However, frequent observations of the videotapes of our direct inter- action task indicated that there was a variety of what might be termed *subclinical* or *subsyndromal* behaviors, manifested by patients while interacting with other family members. Possibly, we reasoned, high or low EE family attitudes were related in some way to these more subtle manifestations of psychopathology of the patients that would not reach the level of clinical significance on standard rating scales. Also, we wondered whether these patterns of subclinical psychopathology could be seen as triggers of high or low EE attitudes.

Two investigators from our group, Irwin Rosenfarb (Rosenfarb et al. 1995) and Stephanie Woo (Woo et al., 1997) approached this problem from different perspectives. Rosenfarb looked at the verbal behavior of patients from transcripts, and Woo examined nonverbal and paraverbal behavior observable on videotapes. Both developed coding systems based on scales from the expanded version of the Brief Psychiatric Rating Scale (BPRS; Lukoff et al. 1986). Both also carried out factor analyses of their multiple codes. They found that the verbal codes yielded two factors, and the nonverbal or paraverbal codes yielded three factors. One factor from each domain was very similar, and was termed *odd or disruptive behavior* for the verbal behavior, and *hostile-unusual behavior* from Woo's system. This factor had two major components in both systems: odd thought patterns (or behavior) and hostile behavior, verbally or nonverbally assessed. The EE status of relatives was highly related to patient scores on this factor, with patients from high EE homes showing significantly greater amounts on the total factor, and on each of its two components (odd behavior and hostility). For the nonverbal behavior only, Woo found that nonverbal codes akin to negative symptoms in the patients were connected to the relatives EE status, despite some earlier suggestions (Hooley et al. 1987) that negative symptoms might be more distressing for high EE relatives (Figs. 14–3 and 14–4).

To this point, the data on patient subclinical psychopathology were obtained roughly 5 weeks after hospital discharge, when the family assessments were conducted. It is possible that over extended periods, symptoms fade and negative-type symptoms become more pronounced as sources of frustration to relatives, particularly those with high EE proclivities.

Differences in patient subclinical psychopathology as related to relatives' EE status are open to a number of interpretations or hypotheses:

1. Patients from high EE homes may recover more slowly after an index episode of schizophrenia and therefore show more residual symptoms when interacting with relatives.
2. Patients from high EE homes may have persistent differences in odd and hostile behavior that exist in either premorbid or inter-

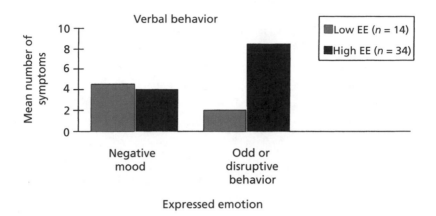

FIGURE **14-3.** *Mean number of negative mood statements and odd or disruptive symptoms displayed by patients from high and low EE families.* Source. *Reprinted from Rosenfarb I, Goldstein MJ, Mintz J, et al: Expressed emotion and subclinical psychopathology observable within the transactions between schizophrenic patients and their family members. J Abnorm Psychol 104:259–267, 1995. Used with permission.*

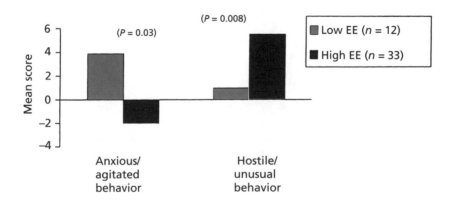

FIGURE **14-4.** *Mean scores for two BPRS symptom factors by family EE status.* Source. *Reprinted from Woo SM, Goldstein MJ, Neuchterlein KH: Relatives' expressed emotion and non-verbal signs of subclinical psychopathology in schizophrenic patients. Br J Psychiatry, in press. Used with permission.*

morbid periods. This hypothesis would be in keeping with George Brown's (Brown et al. 1962) original finding that notable behavioral disturbance was more prominent in patients from high EE families. This interpretation is also consistent with relatives' reports of the typical behavior of the patient toward them over the prior 3 months (Friedman and Goldstein 1994).

3. Subclinical psychopathology may represent specific stress responses to being in direct contact with high EE relatives.

Rosenfarb (Rosenfarb et al. 1995) attempted to examine these different interpretations by studying significant patterns in the interactions, focusing on patient subclinical behaviors and relatives' AS criticism, expressed to the patient in the direct interactions. He focused on a high frequency code in the odd-disruptive cluster, termed unusual thought expression, one more commonly — but not exclusively — seen in patients from high EE families. He found that most often these unusual thoughts were expressed early in the interactions by patients from high EE families, prior to the expression of a critical comment by the relative. (Recall that the expressions of critical comments are much more likely in high than low EE families.) Rosenfarb found the probability that another unusual thought would be expressed in a later section of a 10-minute interaction depended on whether a critical remark by a relative appeared subsequent to the odd thought.

These findings strongly support Hypotheses 2 and 3 listed earlier, and may also be congruent with Hypothesis 1. Unusual thoughts are more likely to occur in patients from high, as compared with low, EE homes, and to occur before relatives respond with criticism to their behavior. However, if criticism is expressed, then it appears that the greater base rate of unusual thoughts may represent a stress response to criticism. Put in colloquial terms, patients from high EE homes are different from those in low EE homes. High and low EE relatives respond differently to these differences in their patient-relative's behavior. Finally, these differences in relatives' responses further augment the distinctiveness of patients from high and low EE homes. If any data support a family system view of relative-patient interaction, they are these data.

Findings From the First and Second Generation of Family Intervention Programs

As indicated in our prior review (Goldstein and Miklowitz 1995) and in the review by Glick in Chapter 13 of this volume, the first generation of psychoeducationally oriented family programs has been found to reduce relapse over the short-to-intermediate term. These studies all used an add-on design in which some form of family intervention was added to standard medication management. As indicated in a review of these first generation studies, they all engaged the individual family unit (Goldstein 1996) (Fig. 14–5).

Since this first generation of studies appeared, other studies have been reported that have addressed more refined research questions. We refer to the studies in Amsterdam with young, largely first episode patients (Linszen et al. 1996), the NIMH Treatment Strategies Study

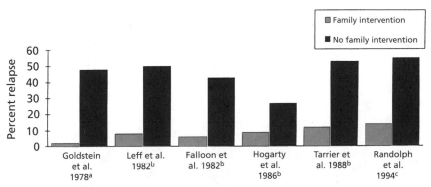

FIGURE 14–5. *Relapse rates from the six first generation studies, contrasting a family intervention program with the absence of such a program (schizophrenic patients on continuous medication).*
[a]*6-month follow-up*
[b]*9-month follow-up*
[c]*12-month follow-up*
Source. *Reprinted from Goldstein MJ, Miklowitz DJ: The effectiveness of psychoeducational family therapy in the treatment of schizophrenic disorders. Journal of Marital and Family Therapy 21:361–376, 1995. Used with permission.*

(TSS; Keith et al. 1989), a multisite study within the United States and the McFarlane et al. study (1995), which tested variations in the modality of family treatment. All three studies build on the first generation of studies by assuming that some degree of family involvement is a necessary condition for effective community treatment of psychotic patients.

In the Amsterdam study, relatives received psychoeducation shortly after the patient was admitted to the inpatient unit for an extended period of care (average 3 months of inpatient care, 3 months of day hospital care, and 9 months of sustained outpatient care, carried out by the same clinical team throughout). Linszen et al. (1996) tested whether a psychoeducational family program added on during the 9-month outpatient program could add anything to this rich program of psychosocial and pharmacological treatment. They found that it did not do so, and in fact the relapse rates for the sample as a whole were strikingly low. However, they did find that despite the attempt to lower EE, those patients from families originally categorized as high EE still had a higher relapse rate at the end of the trial.

The TSS represents a far more complex research design than those described already, in which two forms of family involvement were added onto a variant of pharmacological treatment consisting of either standard dose, low dose, or intermittent dose antipsychotic medication for the patient. The two psychosocial treatments applied were termed *supportive* (SFM) and *applied* family management (AFM). The SFM referred to use of groups offered on a monthly basis for relatives and patients, but largely attended by relatives. The AFM involved in-home family treatment sessions that closely followed the Falloon et al. model (1982). All those assigned to the AFM condition also were offered the SFM group as well and in fact used the SFM to the same extent as did the SFM group. No group was treated by medication management alone in the TSS study, so all families had some degree of involvement in the patient's treatment. The contrast studied involved whether the more intensive family management was more effective in reducing relapse than was the less intense one. The results of this study suggest that it was not.

Unfortunately, the TSS study, unlike the Linszen et al. (1996) study, did not stratify the families on the EE factor, so it is difficult to know whether high EE families responded differentially to the different dosages of family treatment. Also, the absence of a no-family treatment group limits any conclusion about whether either SFM or AFM was effective. We can conclude, however, that SFM and AFM did not interact systematically with the three variations in pharmacotherapy.

The McFarlane et al. study (1995) also began with the assumption that some form of psychoeducational family program was necessary for the most effective community treatment of schizophrenic patients. This study considered whether one method for delivering this treatment, which involved multiple family groups (MF), was as effective as working with single family units alone (SF). In both the SF and MF groups, patients were present in the treatment sessions, which contrasted with the SFM condition in the TSS study, which largely involved relatives only and few patients. Entry into the MF condition was preceded by 3–4 individual family sessions, found necessary to engage the family in treatment. These investigators found an advantage for MF or SF in relapse reduction, and particularly for patients who left the hospital with notable persisting systems.

Implications of These Second Generation Studies for Future Treatment Development

These second generation studies raise a number of important questions concerning what the optimum model is for designing and delivering a psychoeducational family program. First, whether programs that involve relatives primarily are as effective as those that engage the patients as well is a relevant question. Programs for relatives only are consonant with the original interpretations of the EE literature, which emphasized relatives' affective attitudes as the major risk factor for relapse. Yet the research summarized in the earlier part of this chapter suggests that such a model may be incomplete because it ignores the patient's contribution to the affective quality of the family environment. How and in what ways relatives' groups affect the odd and unusual behavior of patient-relatives identified in our interactional studies is another important question. Are these behaviors best addressed in social skills programs, as was part of the Hogarty et al. study (1986), or are these more complex transactional processes best addressed when family members meet together, either singly or in multiple family groups? Relevant to this question, the one study that contrasted relatives-only groups with in-home family treatment (Leff et al. 1989) revealed a disappointing attrition rate in the relative-only condition, so it is not clear how effective relatives-only groups are for most of families of the severely mentally ill.

In a previous review (Goldstein 1996), we considered whether some forms of family intervention are more relevant than others at different phases of a patient's psychotic disorder. Although the evidence here is circumstantial rather than direct, it appeared that for first episode or recent onset patients, very favorable results in terms of relapse reduction were found when patients and relatives were seen as individual family units. In contrast, and here the evidence is much less solid, it appears that some type of group format is most effective with very chronic patients, particularly those with persisting symptoms at the time of hospital discharge. Although highly speculative, these data suggest that early in the stages of a patient's illness, the potential exists to modify the kind of negative transactional cycle identified in our family interaction research. However, as the illness becomes more chronic and recurrent, family programs primarily provide support for relatives and serve as a vehicle for limiting persisting high EE attitudes in daily interactions with patient-relatives.

Adaptation of Psychoeducational Programs for Other Psychotic Disorders

The focus of research on psychoeducational family programs has been on patients with schizophrenia. Yet nothing is so specific to these programs that would prevent their adaptation to patients with bipolar disorder or schizoaffective disorder. Studies have found that the EE status of relatives is also a powerful predictor of relapse in bipolar patients (Miklowitz et al. 1988). Furthermore, the earlier study by Glick et al. (1985), which involved an eight-session program of inpatient psychoeducational family therapy, found more positive results for affectively disordered patients than for schizophrenic patients. We are currently engaged in a randomized controlled trial of patients with bipolar manic disorder, testing the relative efficacy of family versus individual patient management programs, added to standard maintenance pharmacotherapy (Goldstein and Miklowitz 1990). Although this study is still ongoing, it is clear that a program adapted for patients with bipolar disorder and their relatives has high consumer acceptance and very low rates of attrition. Similar family-focused programs are currently underway at Brown, Cornell, and the University of Colorado.

Conclusion

Both social forces and research on EE have stimulated the development and testing of community-based, psychoeducational, family-focused treatment programs. The first generation of family programs relied on a narrow view of the direction of causality implied by the EE index. More recent family interaction research has suggested that a more complex bidirectional model of EE is more appropriate. Future development of family-focused programs for patients with severe mental illness could profit from considering the patient's contribution to the family environment. Further consideration of this issue can clarify programmatic design features related to the optimum format of the next generation of family-focused programs for psychotic patients and how these design features relate to the phase of a patient's disorder.

References

Brown GW, Monck EM, Carstairs GM, et al: Influences of family life on the course of schizophrenic illness. British Journal of Preventive Social Medicine 16:55–68, 1962

Doane JA, West KL, Goldstein MJ, et al: Parental communication deviance and affective style. Arch Gen Psychiatry 38:679–685, 1981

Falloon IRH, Boyd JL, McGill CW: Family management in the prevention of exacerbations of schizophrenia: a controlled study. N Engl J Med 306:1437, 1982

Friedman MS, Goldstein MJ: Relatives' perceptions of their interactional behavior with a schizophrenic family member. Fam Process 33:377, 1994

Glick ID, Clarkin JF, Spencer JH, et al: A controlled evaluation of inpatient family intervention. Arch Gen Psychiatry 42:882–886, 1985

Goldstein MJ: Psycho-education and family treatment related to the phase of a psychotic disorder. Int Clin Psychopharmacol 11:77–83, 1996

Goldstein MJ, Miklowitz DJ: Behavioral family treatment for patients with bipolar affective disorder. Behav Modif 14:457–489, 1990

Goldstein MJ, Miklowitz DJ: The effectiveness of psychoeducational family therapy in the treatment of schizophrenic disorders. J Marital Fam Ther 21:361–376, 1995

Goldstein MJ, Miklowitz DJ: Family intervention for persons with bipolar disorder, in Family Intervention in Mental Illness. Edited by Hatfield AB. San Francisco, CA, Jossey-Bass, 1994, pp 23–35

Goldstein MJ, Miklowitz DJ, Strachan AS, et al: Patterns of expressed emotion and patient coping styles that characterize the families of recent-onset schizophrenics. Br J Psychiatry 155:107–111, 1989

Hogarty GE, Anderson CM, Reiss DJ, et al: Family education, social skills training, and maintenance chemotherapy in the aftercare of schizophrenia. Arch Gen Psychiatry 43:633–642, 1986

Hooley JM, Richters JE, Weintraub S, et al: Psychopathology and marital distress: the positive side of positive symptoms. J Abnorm Psychol 96:27–33, 1987

Jones JE: Patterns of transactional style deviance in the TAT's of parents of schizophrenics. Fam Process 16(3):327–338, 1977

Kavanagh DJ: Recent developments in expressed emotion and schizophrenia. Br J Psychiatry 160:601–620, 1992

Keith S, Schooler N, Bellack A, et al: The influence of family management on patient stabilization. Schizophr Res 2:224–227, 1989

Leff J, Kulpers L, Berkowitz R, et al: A controlled trial of social intervention in the families of schizophrenia patients. Br J Psychiatry 141:121–134, 1982

Leff J, Gerkowitz R, Shavit N, et al: A trial of family therapy, V: a relatives group for schizophrenia. Br J Psychiatry 154:58–66, 1989

Linszen D, Dingemans P, Van der Does JW, et al: Treatment, expressed emotion and psychotic relapse in recent-onset schizophrenic disorders. Psychol Med 26:333–342, 1996

Lukoff D, Neuchterlein KH, Ventura J: Appendix A: manual for expanded Brief Psychiatric Rating Scale. Schizophr Bull 12:594–602, 1986

Magana AB, Goldstein MJ, Karno M, et al: A brief method for assessing expressed emotion in relatives of psychiatric patients. Psychiatry Res 17:203–212, 1986

McFarlane WR, Lukens E, Link B, et al: Multiple-family groups and psychoeducation in the treatment of schizophrenia. Arch Gen Psychiatry 52:679–687, 1995

Miklowitz DJ, Goldstein MJ, Falloon IRH, et al: Interactional correlates of expressed emotion in the families of schizophrenics. Br J Psychiatry 144:482–487, 1984

Miklowitz DJ, Goldstein MJ, Nuechterlein KH, et al: Family factors and the course of bipolar affective disorder. Arch Gen Psychiatry 45:225–231, 1988

Miklowitz DJ, Goldstein MJ, Doane JA, et al: Is expressed emotion an index of transactional process? I: relative's affective style. Fam Process 28:153–167, 1989

Randolph ET, Eth S, Glynn SM, et al: Behavioural family management in schizophrenia. Outcome of a clinic-based intervention. Br J Psychiatry 164:501–506, 1994

Rosenfarb I, Goldstein MJ, Mintz J, et al: Expressed emotion and subclinical psychopathology observable within the transactions between schizophrenic patients and their family members. J Abnorm Psychol 104:259–267, 1995

Strachan AM, Leff JP, Goldstein MJ, et al: Emotional attitudes and direct communication in the families of schizophrenics: a cross-national replication. Br J Psychiatry 149:279–287, 1986

Strachan AM, Feingold D, Goldstein MJ, et al: Is expressed emotion an index of transactional process? II: patient's coping style. Fam Process 28:169–181, 1989

Tarrier N, Barrowclough C, Porceddu K: The community management of schizophrenia: a controlled trial of behavioral intervention with families to reduce relapse. Br. J Psychiatry 153:532–542, 1988

Vaughn CE: Expressed emotion in family relationships. J Child Psychol Psychiatry 30:13–22, 1989

Vaughn CE, Leff JP: The influence of family and social factors on the course of psychiatric illness: a comparison of schizophrenic and depressed neurotic patients. Br J Psychiatry 129:125–137, 1976

Woo SM, Goldstein MJ, Neuchterlein KH: Relatives' expressed emotion and non-verbal signs of subclinical psychopathology in schizophrenic patients. Br J Psychiatry, 170:58–61, 1997

PART VII

Methodological Considerations in Psychotherapy Research

CHAPTER 15

The Relative Efficacy of Drugs and Psychotherapy

Methodological Considerations

Steven D. Hollon, Ph.D.

Drugs and psychotherapy are both widely used in the treatment of mental and emotional disorders. Although each has often been effective, comparisons between the two modalities (and their combination) have been fraught with interpretative difficulties. This has been true especially when one modality has already been established as the standard of treatment for a particular disorder, as in the treatment of depression.

This chapter examines the nature of the controls required for adequate interpretation of drug-psychotherapy comparisons and the related issue of allegiance effects. If the two modalities are to be compared in a meaningful way, it is essential that both are implemented in a competent and representative fashion. Studies often disagree with respect to the relative efficacy of the two modalities, and some of this variability may reflect differences in the implementation of the respective modalities across the various trials. The chapter also examines

Preparation of this chapter was supported by Grant R10MH55875 from the National Institute of Mental Health.

the problems inherent in testing the long-standing claim that psychotherapy can produce broader and more enduring effects than drugs. Although widely believed and quite possibly true, it has been surprisingly hard to document in any scientifically acceptable fashion. Finally, the chapter concludes by considering the utility of drug-psychotherapy comparisons for testing the role of causal mediators associated with each of the single modalities. Such comparisons offer a unique opportunity for testing theories of change, if they incorporate the necessary controls and avoid certain high-probability errors in interpretation.

Pill-Placebo Controls and the Role of Allegiance Effects

In an exchange that began over the Internet and continued in a major journal, Klein (1996) argued that comparisons between drugs and psychotherapy that did not also include pill-placebo controls were essentially uninterpretable. According to Klein, in the absence of such controls, telling whether pharmacotherapy was adequately implemented would be impossible, as would whether the sample selected was actually drug-responsive. Drugs are often included as a known standard in such trials precisely because they have already been shown to be more effective than pill-placebo controls. However, because different groups may differ in their capacity to execute pharmacotherapy in a competent fashion, and because heterogeneity typically exists within a population with respect to likely response to any given treatment, there is no guarantee that pharmacotherapy will be adequately implemented or that the particular patients selected in any given study will be responsive to medications. Thus, according to Klein, any drug-psychotherapy comparison that fails to include a pill-placebo control could well fail to detect a bias against pharmacotherapy and thereby falsely overestimate the efficacy of psychotherapy.

In a companion piece, Neil Jacobson and I agreed with Klein that the inclusion of pill-placebo controls in such comparisons represents a desirable methodological feature, but disagreed that it was either necessary or sufficient for an appropriate interpretation of study findings (Jacobson and Hollon 1996a). In that article, we argued that making an informed judgment regarding the quality of execution of the respective modalities should be possible (and the nature of the sample) regardless of whether such controls were included or not. Moreover, we further argued that finding drugs superior to pill-placebo controls would still not guarantee that pharmacotherapy was adequately implemented, because even mediocre execution might produce a significant advantage in a large enough sample. Inclusion of a pill-placebo control and the detection of a *true* drug effect would increase our confidence that pharmacotherapy was adequately implemented, but it is neither necessary nor sufficient for such a judgment to be made.

Allegiance Effects and the Adequacy of Pharmacotherapy

In this regard, early studies that found cognitive therapy (CT) superior to drugs in the treatment of depression have been criticized by myself and others for failing adequately to implement pharmacotherapy (Hollon et al. 1991; Meterissian and Bradwejn 1989). In the first of these studies, Rush and colleagues found CT superior to imipramine pharmacotherapy in terms of acute response (Rush et al. 1977). However, in that study, pharmacotherapy was provided by inexperienced psychiatric residents, medication doses were less than optimal (no more than 250 mg/day), no plasma monitoring was conducted to check on compliance and absorption, and drug withdrawal was begun two weeks before the end of treatment. This was hardly adequate pharmacotherapy. Similarly, in another early study, Blackburn and colleagues found CT superior to drugs (typically either amitriptyline or clomipramine) in a general practice setting (Blackburn et al. 1981). However, drug dosage levels were again low (no more than 150 mg/day) and plasma medication levels were again not monitored. Moreover, drugs in that setting were managed by general practitioners, who are notorious for failing to implement adequate pharmacotherapy. (In that study, only 14% of the general practice sample responded to medications.) No differences were evident in a psychiatric outpatient sample when pharmacotherapy was provided by experienced research psychiatrists.

Even to an advocate like myself, it is obvious that neither of these studies appeared to provide consistently adequate pharmacotherapy, something that was evident despite the fact that neither incorporated a pill-placebo control. Reviews of the outcome literature have suggested that differences between treatments are most likely to be found when the group conducting the study has a vested interest in one of the interventions (Luborsky et al. 1975; Robinson et al. 1990; Smith and Glass 1977). Such allegiance effects require no intent to bias the results; frequently, they reflect nothing more than different levels of competence with (or interest in) the respective interventions. For example, the study by Rush and colleagues (1977) was conducted at the center at which CT was developed by people (including me) who had a vested interest in that modality's success; it is likely that more effort went into assuring that the psychosocial intervention was adequately implemented than was the case for pharmacotherapy. In particular, our decision to begin medication withdrawal prior to treatment termination was clearly misguided, but it was made in good faith (we were trying to ensure that patients were "done" with treatment by the time of the termination interview and thought that we needed to begin withdrawal early to compensate for the half-life of the medication).

Similarly, the decision by Blackburn and colleagues (1981) to rely on less experienced nonpsychiatric personnel to provide the pharmacotherapy in their general practice setting was doubtless driven by expediency; that is, who was already treating patients in that setting. By way of contrast, the same experienced cognitive therapists (two of the authors) provided CT in both the relevant settings in that study. Looking at these two studies, it seems likely that pharmacotherapy was less than adequately implemented in each (at least in the general practice setting in Blackburn et al. [1981]). Thus, the two studies suggesting that CT is superior to drugs in the treatment of depression appeared to be biased against pharmacotherapy, and this bias was apparent despite the absence of pill-placebo controls.

Comparable Efficacy When Allegiance Effects Are Balanced

Those studies that have done an adequate job of implementing pharmacotherapy have typically found little evidence of any advantage for CT over drugs, at least with respect to acute response. As already mentioned, Blackburn and colleagues (1981) found little difference between CT and drugs when both were implemented by experienced practitioners in a psychiatric outpatient setting. Similarly, Murphy and colleagues (1984) found few differences between nortriptyline pharmacotherapy versus CT in a separate sample of outpatients who were depressed and diagnosed with unipolar illness. Although the authors of this latter study did rely on inexperienced psychiatric residents to provide the pharmacotherapy, they went to considerable trouble to ensure that both modalities were adequately implemented, including monitoring plasma medication levels (nortriptyline has a therapeutic window for optimal response) and providing ongoing supervision for therapists in both modalities throughout the study. Given that the study was conducted at the psychiatry outpatient clinic at the Washington University in St. Louis, long a bastion of biological psychiatry, it is likely that these efforts were most necessary to ensure that CT was adequately implemented.

Our own group found virtually identical response to imipramine pharmacotherapy versus CT in a similar sample of outpatients who were depressed and diagnosed with unipolar illness in a project we called the cognitive-pharmacotherapy (CPT) project (Hollon et al. 1992). As did Murphy and colleagues (1984), we also went to considerable trouble to ensure that both modalities were adequately implemented. In particular, we tried to offset my own considerable identification with, and allegiance to, CT by making common cause with an experienced group of psychopharmacology researchers (headed by V. B. Tuason, M.D., a research psychiatrist trained at Washington University in St. Louis) and conducting the study at their treatment site (the St. Paul-Ramsey Medical Center in St. Paul, Minnesota), a setting best known for its biological orientation. Not only did the research group consist of strong advocates for each approach, but imipramine dosage levels were pursued aggressively (up to 450 mg/day) and monitored with plasma medication checks, whereas treatment was provided by experienced practitioners in both modalities who were provided with ongoing on-site supervision throughout the study.

I have trouble finding fault with the quality of execution of pharmacotherapy in these latter two studies, because both were overseen by experienced research pharmacotherapists and monitored with plasma medication checks to ensure that patients received adequate dosage levels. Nonetheless, neither included a pill-placebo control. Therefore, there is no guarantee that the medications produced a *true* drug effect in either. Klein (1996) would dismiss these studies; Jacobson and Hollon (1996a) would not. Although we agree with Klein that it would have been better if both studies had included pill-placebo controls, we think that the quality of implementation of the respective modalities can be ascertained with reasonable certainty by a consideration of the methods actually employed. Clearly, pharmacotherapy was more adequately implemented in these latter two studies than it was in the earlier studies conducted by Rush and colleagues and Blackburn and colleagues (1981) (at least in the general practice sample). My sense is that neither the study conducted by Murphy and colleagues (1984) nor the study conducted by our own group (Hollon et al. 1992) was biased by differences in the quality of execution between the respective interventions. Nonetheless, that is a matter of opinion about which reasonable people can disagree. I think Klein (1996) goes too far in dismissing these studies out of hand, but I think he is correct when he suggests that inclusion of pill-placebo controls would have made their findings far easier to interpret.

Was CT Adequately Implemented in the NIMH Collaborative Program?

Some in the field, including myself, have raised questions about the adequate implementation of CT in the NIMH Treatment of Depression Collaborative Research Program (TDCRP), the one study that found pharmacotherapy superior to CT in the treatment of depression (Jacobson and Hollon 1996a; Thase 1994). Whether these questions are fair or reflect the biases of the persons raising those issues (including me) remains an ongoing source of controversy (Elkin et al. 1996). Because the TDCRP did incorporate a pill-placebo condition, such controls clearly do not resolve all interpretative ambiguity, but they do clarify the issue to a considerable extent, at least with respect to the adequacy of the pharmacotherapy provided.

In the TDCRP, 250 outpatients who were depressed and diagnosed with unipolar illness were randomly assigned to 16 weeks of treatment with either CT, interpersonal psychotherapy (IPT), imipramine pharmacotherapy (up to 300 mg/day), or a pill-placebo control (Elkin et al. 1989). Although few differences were observed among the treatments in the full sample, there were indications of a treatment-by-severity interaction favoring drugs over psychotherapy (particularly CT) among the patients who were more severely depressed and functionally impaired. These differences were even more pronounced (and robust across measures) when the data were reanalyzed using random regression techniques and other strategies that better handled heterogeneity of regression and missing data; CT was consistently outperformed by drugs and sometimes by IPT and was often no better than the pill-placebo among the patients who were more severely depressed and functionally impaired (Elkin et al. 1995; Klein and Ross 1993). These findings have raised questions about the relative (and absolute) efficacy of CT in the treatment of depression in outpatients and have been translated into specific treatment guidelines that suggest that psychotherapy not be used as the sole treatment for patients who are more severely depressed (American Psychiatric Association 1993; Depression Guideline Panel 1993).

The problem I have with basing such conclusions on the TDCRP is that it is not clear to me that those findings were either robust across sites or consistent with earlier studies. In their original report of the TDCRP data, the authors noted that ". . . patients receiving CBT at one site did extremely well and had mean scores very similar to those for patients receiving imipramine-CM. The same was true for patients receiving IPT at another site . . ." (Elkin et al. 1989, p. 980). This suggested to me that the quality with which CT was implemented may

have varied across sites in the TDCRP, and that it was this variability
in implementation (and not any inherent limitation in the psychosocial intervention itself) that led it to perform with less effectiveness
than pharmacotherapy with the patients who were more severely depressed and functionally impaired.

Although the original article did not report actual posttreatment
scores as a function of site, the subsequent publication of the TDCRP
data set did make it possible to pursue this question. Figure 15–1
presents, as a function of treatment condition, the TDCRP posttreatment Hamilton Rating Scale for Depression (HRSD; Hamilton 1960)
scores at 16 weeks for the patients completing treatment who were
more severely depressed (Jacobson and Hollon 1996b). Scores for the
CT condition are further broken down by site. As can be seen, CT
performed quite poorly at two of the sites (being no more effective

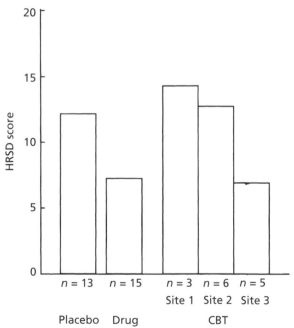

FIGURE 15–1. *Site differences in the TDCRP for high severity patients
completing treatment (N = 42). Source. Reprinted from Jacobson NJ,
Hollon SD: Prospects for future comparisons between psychotropic drugs
and psychotherapy: lessons from the CBT vs. pharmacotherapy exchange. J Consult Clin Psychol 64:74–80, 1996. Copyright © 1996,
American Psychological Association. Reprinted with permission.*

than pill-placebo), but performed quite well at a third (doing about as well as pharmacotherapy). In fact, the magnitude of the difference between the effect of CT at the third site versus the effect of CT at the other two sites combined was about as large as the magnitude of the difference between drugs versus pill-placebo (the *true* drug effect) across the full subsample. As shown in Figure 15–2, these differences were attenuated somewhat on the HRSD in the intent-to-treat sample (suggesting that some portion of the difference between the sites may have been due to differences in keeping patients who were nonresponsive in treatment). Nevertheless, the magnitude of this effect was relatively robust regardless of how outcome was measured or whether dropouts were included in the analyses (Jacobson and Hollon 1996b).

Does this mean that CT was differentially effective across the sites? I think it probably does, but, as someone with a vested interest in CT, my judgment must be suspect in this matter. Elkin and colleagues (1996) did respond to this issue by calculating Bayesian estimates of

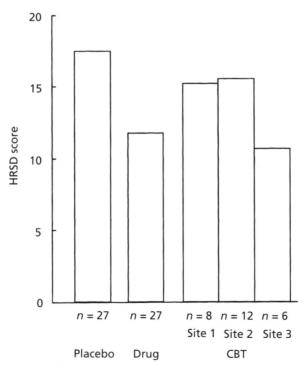

FIGURE 15–2. *Site differences in the TDCRP for all assigned high severity subjects (N = 106).*

individual response based on random regression models that suggested little differentiation between the sites. One advantage of their method is that it generates estimates of endpoint scores for treatment dropouts that take into account their individual trajectory of response, clearly a better procedure than relying on the last available score at the time of attrition. However, the disadvantage of this method is that it also estimates posttreatment scores for subjects for whom the actual data are available; that is, two patients with identical scores at termination receive different estimated scores in this analysis if they showed different rates of improvement across the preceding treatment interval. In fact, 4 of the 6 patients treated with CT at Site 3 in the TDCRP had scores of 7 or less on the HRSD at week 16 (more than at any other site), yet the Bayesian estimates provided in Elkin and colleagues' article (1996, Figure 1) showed only one patient from the third site in that range and several patients from the other sites. I do not object to estimating scores for patients when the actual data are missing (in fact, I rather like the notion), and I do not mind adjusting data for individual differences that were present prior to randomization, but I am nervous about estimating data for patients for whom it already exists, especially when the conclusions that one would draw from those estimates are different from what might be drawn from the actual data. Thus, although I find the Bayesian estimates interesting, I do not think they necessarily resolve the issue of differences between the sites.

Given that we (Hollon et al. 1992) found no indication that CT was less effective than drugs with patients who were more severely depressed (or that severity predicted response within CT), it was of interest how the two modalities compared with one another across the two studies. Figure 15–3 compares response with treatment in the TDCRP versus that observed by our CPT project among subjects of comparable severity who completed treatment. As can be seen, patients treated with CT in the TDCRP were doing considerably worse at 12 weeks (the end of treatment in Hollon et al. [1992]) and were still lagging behind 4 weeks later. Comparing Figure 15–1 with Figure 15–3 indicates that patients treated with CT at the third site in the TDCRP did about as well as they did in the study by Hollon and colleagues (1992), but that patients treated with CT at the other two sites did considerably worse. Again, this is consistent with the notion

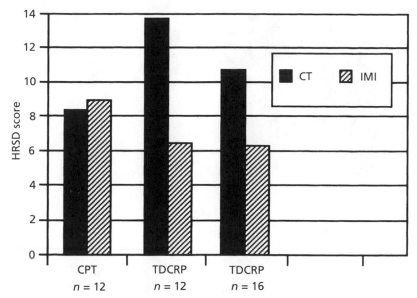

FIGURE 15–3. *HRSD scores among subjects with initial high severity who completed treatment, after 12 weeks in CPT and TDCRP, and after 16 weeks in TDCRP.*

that CT may have been less than adequately implemented at two of the sites in the TDCRP.

In all fairness, it should be pointed out that the picture is not so clear if subjects who did not complete treatment are taken into consideration. As shown in Figure 15–4, differences favoring CT in our CPT project over CT in the TDCRP are no longer so pronounced and are no greater than those favoring imipramine in the TDCRP over that provided in our CPT study. This suggests that the studies may have differed in terms of those they kept in treatment and raises the possibility that pharmacotherapy was less than adequately done in our CPT trial. Although seeing what more we could have done with respect to the implementation of pharmacotherapy in CPT is hard for me, I cannot dismiss the possibility that apparent differences between the two studies had as much to do with the lesser effectiveness of drugs in CPT as it did with any purported problems in the implementation of CT in the TDCRP.

Direct comparisons between different studies are always treacherous. In particular, at least two differences in the actual protocols

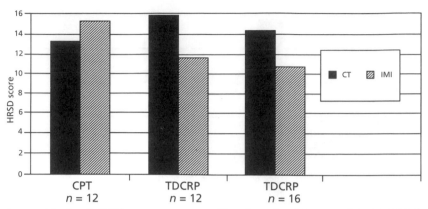

FIGURE 15–4. *HRSD scores among all assigned subjects with initial high severity, after 12 weeks in CPT and TDCRP, and after 16 weeks in TDCRP.*

followed might have contributed to differences in the findings. First, protocol in the TDCRP called for less intensive treatment than protocol in the CPT project; patients in both studies received a maximum of 20 sessions, but patients in the TDCRP did so across 16 weeks whereas patients in CPT had only 12 weeks to do so. This means that patients in the TDCRP received less frequent sessions during the first half of treatment (typically dropping back to once-weekly sessions after week 4, whereas patients in CPT could continue twice-weekly sessions through week 8). This may have contributed to a lesser efficacy for CT in the TDCRP for the patients who were more severely depressed and functionally impaired. Second, patients in the TDCRP had to sustain minimum levels of symptomatology over a 1-week washout period prior to qualifying for admission to the study, whereas patients in the CPT project did not. This suggests that patients in the TDCRP may have been more stable in their symptomatology than patients in the CPT trial, even when selected for comparable levels of severity.

Thus, although a variance exists between the trials, it is not clear whether the problem lies with the quality of implementation of CT in the TDCRP or the quality of implementation of pharmacotherapy in the CPT study (or the other studies already described). If the problem lies with the implementation of CT in the TDCRP, how could that have happened? Training in that study was quite intensive and conducted by Dr. Brian Shaw, a recognized expert in the modality (and one of the people most important in my own training). All therapists conducted a number of pilot cases under ongoing supervision, and none were admitted to the study proper until they were deemed ready by a committee of independent experts in the modality (including Drs. Rush, Kovacs, Emery, and Young). Judgments were made from actual videotapes of therapist performance and ongoing quality of execution ensured by a red-line technique that reinstituted intensive supervision whenever a therapist's performance fell below a predefined minimum level of acceptance. This is a very comprehensive regime, one designed to ensure that each of the respective modalities was adequately implemented. If something went wrong, what could that have been?

My own sense is that the training regime, rich though it was, was not sufficient to ensure the adequate implementation of CT. In particular, I was concerned when I learned (before the publication of the initial findings) that the frequency of supervision was going to be cut back to only once a month during the study proper. Most of the therapists selected were experienced psychotherapists, but few had any formal training in CT prior to their participation in the project. My sense is that recently trained cognitive therapists require continued ongoing supervision to maintain adequate levels of competent performance; in my own studies I typically like to meet with therapists seeing active study cases at least once (and preferably twice) weekly. This is a much higher frequency of ongoing supervision than was maintained in the TDCRP. Moreover, supervision was provided off-site, which may have further impeded ready access of the therapist to a supervisor. Again, my own experience when doing controlled trials is that being able to talk over tough aspects of ongoing cases regularly is helpful for therapists to alter what they are doing by the next treatment session. That has typically been possible in the single-site studies already described, but may have been harder to obtain in the multisite TDCRP.

If there were problems with the amount of ongoing supervision provided, why should it have affected some sites more than others? Although the authors of the TDCRP have been reluctant to link outcome to site, I have long presumed that CT might fare better at the Oklahoma site than at either Pittsburgh or George Washington (Hollon et al. 1991; Jacobson and Hollon 1996a). Oklahoma had an independent history of participation in studies of CT and seemed to have a general cognitive-behavioral orientation that predated its involvement in the TDCRP (that is where John Rush went after he left Philadelphia and where site principal investigator Watkins had a cognitive orientation). Similarly, Pittsburgh had a history of participation in studies of dynamic-eclectic psychotherapy and principal investigators on site with a strong interest in that modality. It is less clear that the George Washington site had an a priori orientation, but it did have several experienced dynamic-eclectic therapists available for participation in the study. If Oklahoma was site 3 (and Pittsburgh site 2), then I think it is possible that the findings from the TDCRP with respect to the relative efficacy of the two psychotherapies may reflect the operation of differential allegiance effects (Jacobson and Hollon 1996a). At the same time, neither John Rush nor site principal investigator John Watkins were directly involved in the training of the therapists who took part in the TDCRP at the Oklahoma site. Nonetheless, my sense is that the general ambience of the setting was more conducive to a cognitive approach in Oklahoma than at the other two sites, and I stand by my prediction that cognitive therapists at that site produced better results than did therapists at the other two sites.

The TDCRP investigators clearly went to great lengths to forestall the operation of allegiance effects. Nonetheless, I suspect this may not have been sufficient and that the quality of the CT practiced at the other two sites (especially Pittsburgh) may not have represented what has been done in other comparable studies. The authors of the TDCRP have argued that their findings may represent what is likely to happen when experienced practitioners try to use a novel approach (Elkin et al. 1996). That may be true, but I question whether their findings represent what can be done by practitioners who are fully competent with the intervention they are being asked to provide.

In short, I question the representativeness of the findings from the TDCRP with respect to CT so long as they are averaged across sites; that is, I suspect that CT is about as effective as drugs for outpatients who were more severely depressed and functionally impaired, as it was at the third site in the TDCRP and as it has been in other non–placebo-controlled comparisons. Nonetheless, I am aware that the existing data are open to multiple interpretations, and I recognize that my own biases are likely to color my perceptions in this regard. I appreciate the fact that the TDCRP included a pill-placebo control and can only wish that we had done so as well in our own design (or that Murphy [Murphy et al. 1984] had in his). However, I also recognize that the inclusion of such a control can only serve as a manipulation check for the adequacy of pharmacotherapy. Ensuring that psychosocial interventions like CT are adequately implemented may require that not only that therapists are adequately trained (as I believe they were in the TDCRP), but also that they are adequately supervised across the duration of the study proper (as I believe they were not in the TDCRP).

Placebo Controls and the Prevention of Allegiance Effects

Klein was clearly correct when he argued that inclusion of pill-placebo controls makes comparisons between drugs and psychotherapy more readily interpretable, but such controls may be neither necessary nor sufficient. Studies that do an inadequate job of operationalizing pharmacotherapy can often be seen for what they are, even in the absence of pill-placebo controls, and the inclusion of such controls does not guarantee pharmacotherapy will be adequately implemented. Nonetheless, such controls are a desirable design feature and comparisons between drugs and psychotherapy are stronger for their inclusion.

Ensuring that psychotherapy is adequately implemented and detecting when it is not may be even more complicated than is the case for pharmacotherapy. Psychotherapy is inherently more complex and depends to a greater extent on the skill of the practitioner for its effects. This makes it more susceptible to the influence of allegiance by the clinician. Few pharmacotherapists have a strong attachment to any single medication, but most experienced psychotherapists have a strong investment in a particular type of treatment. Training to the point of competence takes time, and there is reason to think that therapists become technically proficient before the underlying essence of the therapy becomes second nature to them.

Determining whether the treatment was competently implemented can also be problematic. Rating scales exist, but they essentially depend upon the expertise of the judges. In that regard, the TDCRP did use independent experts to rate the therapy sessions (Elkin et al. 1996). This is a desirable design feature that other investigators would do well to emulate. However, they failed to include samples of tapes generated by acknowledged experts in the respective modalities; thus, they had to rely on an arbitrary criterion for determining whether implementation was adequate. We made the same mistake with respect to our pharmacotherapy condition in our CPT trial (Hollon et al 1992). In essence, we not only need to rate tapes on measures of competence and adherence, we also need to calibrate those ratings against tapes of known quality for each of the respective modalities.

Inclusion of attention-placebo controls for the psychotherapy conditions does not solve the problem of detection, because there are still major questions regarding whether such conditions can be made sufficiently credible to serve their intended purpose or even whether psychotherapy needs to have a specific effect to be of value clinically (Parloff 1986). Similarly, including multiple sites that provide a separate expertise in the respective interventions to be compared is not sufficient; steps must be taken to ensure that each site can competently implement each intervention (Jacobson and Hollon 1996a). A recent trial in the treatment of social phobias provides an example of how that can be done. In that study, the principal investigators at each of the respective sites provided intensive supervision of the implementation of their preferred treatment at the other site (listening to every minute of every session and providing ongoing supervision in a timely fashion) with no apparent indication of any site-by-treatment interaction (R. G. Heimberg, personal communication, November 1995).

In short, the issue of allegiance effects in comparisons between drugs and psychotherapy has no easy solution. At the very least, allegiance effects should be balanced at each participating site. Protocols should be designed with input from advocates of each approach, and therapists should be selected who are (or can become) competent to deliver the respective interventions. Treatment should be followed on an ongoing basis by supervisory personnel who can provide feedback in sufficient time that problems can be corrected, and implementation should be monitored by independent experts who can pass judgment on its competence. (My sense is that the TDCRP did the latter, but not the former.) Ideally, these judges should also be asked to rate sessions conducted by therapists acknowledged to be experts with the interventions to provide an internal calibration for therapy execution.

These procedures are complex and time-consuming, but they should enhance the quality of the inferences that can be drawn from the outcome literature. Even a casual perusal of the depression literature suggests that differences in the quality of implementation may account for a considerable portion of the variability among the treatment trials. My sense is that studies that have implemented either modality inadequately are the ones that have found differences, whereas studies that have implemented both modalities adequately have tended not to find differences between them, at least with respect to acute response. Yet, it is possible that subsequent studies will show that it is the TDCRP that has done the most evenhanded job, and that drugs are truly superior to CT in the treatment of outpatients who are more severely depressed and functionally impaired. Nonetheless, despite what future studies tell us, quality of implementation is clearly a major concern, one that may go a long way to explaining apparent allegiance effects in the comparative literature.

Does CT Have an Enduring Effect?

In our earlier paper, Jacobson and I speculated that variability in the quality of execution across sites may have obscured evidence for an enduring effect for CT in the TDCRP (Jacobson and Hollon 1996a). Most of the earlier studies already cited, comparing CT and drugs in the treatment of depression, found evidence that patients treated to remission pharmacologically were at twice the risk for symptom return following treatment termination as were patients treated to remission with CT (Blackburn et al. 1986; Evans et al. 1992; Kovacs et al. 1981; Simons et al. 1986). Although none of these studies was conclusive (samples were small and definitions of remission and relapse varied from study to study), overall, they suggested that CT had an enduring effect that survived the termination of treatment and that reduced risk by 50% relative to prior pharmacotherapy; a reduction in risk comparable in size to the magnitude of the effect associated with continuation medication (Hollon et al. 1991).

It is not clear that this was the case in the TDCRP. In that study, patients treated with CT faired better than patients treated with pharmacotherapy over an 18-month posttreatment follow-up (more patients got better and stayed better in CT than in the other conditions), although it was somewhat less effective than drugs during the acute treatment phase (Shea et al. 1992). Nonetheless, differences between the modalities in rates of relapse may not be as large as they were in the earlier studies already cited. Elkin and colleagues (1996) have argued that their absolute rates of relapse are not that different from what has been observed in some other studies. However, our concern is less with absolute rates than with relative ones, because absolute rates can vary from study to study as a function of definitions of response and relapse and the nature of the sample. Rates of relapse reported in the TDCRP were 36% for prior CT versus 50% for prior drug therapy (a reduction of 28% for prior CT relative to prior pharmacotherapy), as opposed to 21% for prior CT versus 50% for prior drug therapy in our CPT trial (for reduction of risk of 58% for prior CT vs. prior pharmacotherapy). It is this reduction in relative risk that I think is most important, and I note with some interest that the magnitude of this differential reduction in risk was somewhat greater in the TDCRP (and consistent with earlier studies) over the first year of the 18-month follow-up.

The fact that those earlier trials did not include pill-placebo controls is not relevant to the current discussion, but concerns about the quality of implementation of CT in the TDCRP are germane. If CT was less than adequately implemented at one or more of the TDCRP sites, then estimates of its effects based on data averaged across the whole study may underestimate its capacity to prevent subsequent relapses (Jacobson and Hollon 1996a). As with the acute treatment data, it would be of real interest to know if site 3 (presumably Oklahoma) produced a lower rate of relapse that the other two sites, and, if so, whether this lower rate approximated that observed in the other earlier studies. In a footnote in their paper, Elkin and colleagues (1996) declined to present the relapse data broken down by treatment, severity, and site because they did not see how meaningful conclusions could be drawn given the large number of cells and the small number of relapses. They did indicate that an examination of the data did not suggest any site differences. I would still like to see the actual rates of relapse for patients treated with CT as a function of site, so that I could draw my own conclusions.

Placebo Controls and the Detection of Mediation

Pill-placebo controls not only facilitate the interpretation of drug and psychotherapy comparisons, they can also play a role in detecting causal mediation. Drug-psychotherapy comparisons provide a unique opportunity for such tests, because it is likely that the respective approaches produce their effects through maximally dissimilar mechanisms. In essence, each modality can serve as a control for the other; change in purported mediators cannot be dismissed as a simple epiphenomenal consequence of change in depression (reverse causality) if that change is specific to one or the other modality and change in depression is not. That does not mean that a construct must change differentially to be a mediator, but if it does, then reverse causality can be ruled out (Hollon et al. 1987).

At the same time, inclusion of a less effective control condition (for example, a pill-placebo control) increases the likelihood of a sufficient variance in outcome to support sophisticated causal modeling strategies designed to rule out third variable causality. Simply comparing two or more active treatments may not provide sufficient variability, because both are likely to produce comparable levels of response. For example, in our CPT trial, we tested for causal mediation with respect to the prevention of relapse (and found that change in attributional style was specific to CT and appeared to have mediated its enduring effect) because prior CT reduced risk for symptom return relative to prior pharmacotherapy (Hollon et al. 1990). However, we were not able to conduct comparable tests for mediation with respect to response to treatment, because both CT and drugs produced nearly comparable change. Had we included a pill-placebo control in the original design, we could have conducted far more powerful tests of causal mediation of acute response (DeRubeis et al. 1990).

This is all to say that the inclusion of pill-placebo controls (or their logical equivalents) may be at least as important to the detection of causal mediation as they are to the ascription of causal efficacy to a particular treatment. Determining whether a treatment works is quite straightforward logically; determining how it works is inevitably more complex, largely because the purported mediators are not under direct experimental control. Treatment outcome studies are essentially two variable designs; some treatment variable is manipulated and its differential effects are observed. Tests for mediation essentially involve at least three variable causal chains; some treatment variable is manipulated and its effects on both purported mediator and outcome are observed and (hopefully) related to one another. Because the purported mediator is not itself directly manipulated (unlike the treatment itself), covariation between it and the outcome is always subject to multiple interpretations, including that it itself was influenced by change in the outcome (reverse causality) or another third variable (epiphenomenality). As already discussed, inclusion of the appropriate control conditions can help rule out these alternative explanations for covariation (if it is observed) and increase confidence in the inferences that can be drawn regarding the process of causal mediation.

Conclusion

Klein (1996) was right when he argued that the inclusion of pill-placebo controls can facilitate the interpretation of comparisons between drugs and psychotherapy. Such controls are useful in that they can help determine whether pharmacotherapy was adequately implemented (and whether the sample was pharmacologically responsive). At the same time, they are nothing more than a useful manipulation check; inferences can sometimes be drawn in their absence regarding the quality of the pharmacotherapy provided, and they do nothing to guarantee that either treatment was adequately implemented. I would be reluctant to design another comparison of drugs and psychotherapy that was not placebo controlled, but I would not dismiss entirely the findings from earlier studies that failed to include such controls.

I suspect that much of the variance in outcome literature can be explained in terms of allegiance effects, and that allegiance effects largely operated through differing levels of competence; neither modality fares particularly well compared with the other when it is implemented by people who are not expert in its delivery. Those studies that have suggested that CT is superior to drugs have generally done a poor job of implementing pharmacotherapy, and the one study that has suggested that drugs are superior to CT may have had the opposite problem with respect to CT at some of its sites. Given the indications that CT may have enduring effects not found with medications, it seems important to ensure that both modalities are adequately implemented in any study that tries to compare the two. The best way to do this is to be sure that knowledgeable advocates oversee the execution of each modality at each participating site (rather than depending on off-site supervision), and that implementation is monitored and compared with known standards and feedback provided to the therapists regularly throughout the life of the project.

References

American Psychiatric Association: Practice guideline for major depressive disorder in adults. Am J Psychiatry 150(No 4, suppl):1–26, 1993

Blackburn IM, Bishop S, Glen AIM, et al: The efficacy of cognitive therapy in depression: a treatment trial using cognitive therapy and pharmacotherapy, each alone and in combination. Br J Psychiatry 139:181–189, 1981

Blackburn IM, Eunson KM, Bishop S: A two-year naturalistic follow-up of depressed patients treated with cognitive therapy, pharmacotherapy and a combination of both. J Affective Disord 10:67–75, 1986

Depression Guideline Panel: Clinical Practice Guideline: Depression in Primary Care, Vol 2: Treatment of Major Depression. Agency for Health Care Policy and Research Publication No. 93–0551. Rockville, MD, U.S. Department of Health and Human Services, 1993

DeRubeis RJ, Evans MD, Hollon SD, et al: How does cognitive therapy work? Cognitive change and symptom change in cognitive therapy and pharmacotherapy for depression. J Consult Clin Psychol 58:862–869, 1990

Elkin I, Shea MT, Watkins JT, et al: NIMH Treatment of Depression Collaborative Research Program, I: general effectiveness of treatments. Arch Gen Psychiatry 46:971–982, 1989

Elkin I, Gibbons RD, Shea MT, et al: Initial severity and differential treatment outcome in the National Institute of Mental Health Treatment of Depression Collaborative Research Program. J Consult Clin Psychol 63:841–847, 1995

Elkin I, Gibbons RD, Shea MT, et al: Science is not a trial (but it can sometimes be a tribulation). J Consult Clin Psychol 64:92–103, 1996

Evans MD, Hollon SD, DeRubeis RJ, et al: Differential relapse following cognitive therapy and pharmacotherapy for depression. Arch Gen Psychiatry 49:802–808, 1992

Hamilton M: A rating scale for depression. J Neurol Neurosurg Psychiatry 23:5652, 1960

Hollon SD, DeRubeis RJ, Evans MD: Causal mediation of change in treatment for depression: discriminating between nonspecificity and noncausality. Psychol Bull 102:139–149, 1987

Hollon SD, Evans MD, DeRubeis RJ: Cognitive mediation of relapse prevention following treatment for depression: implications of differential risk, in Psychological Aspects of Depression. Edited by Ingram RE. New York, Plenum, 1990, pp 117–136

Hollon SD, Shelton RC, Loosen PT: Cognitive therapy and pharmacotherapy for depression. J Consult Clin Psychol 59:88–99, 1991

Hollon SD, DeRubeis RJ, Evans MD, et al: Cognitive therapy and pharmacotherapy for depression: singly and in combination. Arch Gen Psychiatry 49:802–808, 1992

Jacobson NJ, Hollon SD: Cognitive behavior therapy vs. pharmacotherapy: now that the jury's returned its verdict, its time to present the rest of the evidence. J Consult Clin Psychol 64:74–80, 1996a

Jacobson NJ, Hollon SD: Prospects for future comparisons between psychotropic drugs and psychotherapy: lessons from the CBT vs. pharmacotherapy exchange. J Consult Clin Psychol 64:104–108, 1996b

Klein DF: Preventing hung juries about therapy studies. J Consult Clin Psychol 64:81–87, 1996

Klein DF, Ross DC: Reanalysis of the National Institute of Mental Health Treatment of Depression Collaborative Research Program general effectiveness report. Neuropsychopharmacology 8:241–251, 1993

Kovacs M, Rush AJ, Beck AT, et al: Depressed outpatients treated with cognitive therapy or pharmacotherapy. Arch Gen Psychiatry 38:33–39, 1981

Luborsky L, Singer B, Luborsky L: Comparative studies of psychotherapies: is it true that "everyone has won and all must have prizes"? Arch Gen Psychiatry 32:995–1008, 1975

Meterissian GB, Bradwejn J: Comparative studies on the efficacy of psychotherapy, pharmacotherapy, and their combination in depression: was adequate pharmacotherapy provided? J Clin Psychopharmacol 9:334–339, 1989

Murphy GE, Simons AD, Wetzel RD, et al: Cognitive therapy and pharmacotherapy, singly and together in the treatment of depression. Arch Gen Psychiatry 41:33–41, 1984

Parloff MB: Placebo controls in psychotherapy research: a *sine qua non* or a placebo for research problems? J Consult Clin Psychol 54:79–87, 1986

Robinson LA, Berman JS, Neimeyer RA: Psychotherapy for the treatment of depression: a comprehensive review of controlled outcome research. Psychol Bull 108:30–49, 1990

Rush AJ, Beck AT, Kovacs M, et al: Comparative efficacy of cognitive therapy and pharmacotherapy in the treatment of depressed outpatients. Cognitive Therapy and Research 1:17–38, 1977

Shea M, Elkin I, Imber S, et al: Course of depressive symptoms over follow-up: findings from the National Institute of Mental Health Treatment of Depression Collaborative Research Program. Arch Gen Psychiatry 49:782–787, 1992

Simons AD, Murphy GE, Levine JL, et al: Cognitive therapy and pharmacotherapy for depression: sustained improvement over one year. Arch Gen Psychiatry 43:43–48, 1986

Smith ML, Glass GV: Meta-analysis of psychotherapy outcome studies. Am Psychol 32:752–760, 1977

Thase MF: After the fall: cognitive behavior therapy in depression in the "post-collaborative" era. The Behavior Therapist 17:48–52, 1994

CHAPTER 16

A Checklist for Developing and Reviewing Comparative Treatment Evaluations in the Areas of Psychotherapy and Pharmacotherapy

Donald F. Klein, M.D.

That the randomized, controlled, comparative, double-blind, or independently measured treatment trial is the gold standard for treatment evaluation is generally accepted. However, controversies occur despite several supposedly adequate trials in a fairly well-defined subject area. This chapter argues that there are many features of supervision, measurement, design, and analysis that must be considered in evaluating the probative value of a psychopharmacology or psychotherapy study (American Psychological Association Task Force on Psychological Intervention Guidelines 1995; Baar and Tannock 1989; Begg et al. 1996; Kazdin and Wilson 1978; Laupacis et al. 1992; Luborsky et al. 1993; Maher 1978; Sackett and Gent 1979; Simon and Wittes 1985; The Standard of Reporting Trial Group 1994).

These issues are partially enumerated as a checklist. The complexities of comparative pharmacotherapy and psychotherapy studies

This chapter was supported in part by PHS Grant MH-30906, MHCRC-New York State Psychiatric Institute.

The author wishes to acknowledge the editorial assistance of Lauren Smith.

are particularly addressed. Ideally, this checklist should guide protocol production as well as facilitate report analysis. I critique the irrationality of most meta-analyses elsewhere (D. F. Klein, unpublished manuscript), and do not address that here, but rather focus on design and analysis of individual studies. The topics are ordered with regard to nodal points in protocol production.

Kazdin (1998) has clearly spoken to the issues of internal, external, construct, and statistical validity. His summary appears in Table 16–1.

I do not cross-reference my concerns to these rubrics, because many are not subsumed or are multiply relevant to these categories. However, the reader can see that many concerns affect multiple aspects of validity. I have become particularly concerned with what I call procedural validity. This stems from the well-established allegiance effect (Robinson et al. 1990), whereby the best outcomes are achieved by those invested in a method's success, particularly those with parental interests. This disconcerting fact may be due to at least two factors:

TABLE 16–1

Types of experimental validity and the questions they address

Type of validity	Questions addressed
Internal validity	To what extent can the intervention, rather than extraneous influences, be considered to account for the results, changes, or group differences?
External validity	To what extent can the results be generalized or extended to people, settings, times, measures, and characteristics other than those in this particular experimental arrangement?
Construct validity	Given that the intervention was responsible for change, what specific aspects of the intervention or arrangement was the causal agent, that is, what is the conceptual basis (construct) underlying the effect?
Statistical conclusion validity	To what extent is a relation shown, demonstrated, or evident, and how well can the investigation detect effects if they exist?

Source. *Reprinted from Kazdin AE: Research Design in Clinical Psychology, 3rd Edition. Needham Heights, MA, Allyn & Bacon, 1998, p. 16. Copyright © 1998. All rights reserved. Reprinted with permission of Allyn & Bacon.*

1) those invested in a method do it particularly well, or 2) those invested in a method induce subtle biases in subject allocation, differential attrition, treatment and measurement validity, or statistical analyses that sabotage unbiased treatment estimates. Further, these biases usually cannot be detected from published reports. This last hypothesis (which has much support) makes suspect even apparently excellent, but unreplicated, experimental studies if they are conducted by advocates. Thus, we are left with the uncomfortable conclusion that our gold standard may be producing promissory notes without a drawing account.

The only solution to this problem is independent replication and critical collaboration, not by unbiased scientists, because they are hard to find, but by scientists with declared antithetic views willing to put them to the test of conducting mutually monitored, joint studies that they agree would be of probative value. Further, the statisticians involved in a given study should be blinded to treatment identities. This should be promulgated as a new design and funding standard. The feasibility of this more objective approach has been demonstrated, as in the joint studies of Heimberg and Liebowitz (Heimberg et al. 1995).

As a concrete example, let us say we wish to study the effects of therapist training on treatment outcome. Would the reader's convictions differ if the study were conducted by a training enthusiast, a training skeptic, or by a mutually monitoring joint collaboration? The answer seems clear to me. Does anyone disagree? If not, why not call for this as a general principle? Such a criterion would call for a level of scientific collaboration that has been sorely missing in the evaluation of therapeutics. In the following pages I have outlined a checklist relevant to these issues. It is assumed that the subjects are real patients, because analog studies are regularly more misleading than useful.

I.   Hypothesis and Background Regarding Treatment
    A.   How firm are the historic data supporting the proposed treatment?
        1.   Have there been detailed reports of a consecutive series of longitudinally treated cases, independently assessed for dropout, termination, and change in clinical status prior to embarking on this comparative trial?

2. Have there been adequate dose ranging trials?
3. Have side effect management procedures been developed?
4. Is the outcome known following treatment discontinuation?
5. How have the patients been followed up, and have longitudinal change patterns been assessed?
6. Was a double-blind, randomized, placebo substitution and withdrawal trial attempted in putative medication responders? with what results?
7. What length of acute treatment appears necessary for specific clinical benefit?
8. Did preliminary experience yield an estimate of proportions markedly benefited, somewhat benefited, or not helped?
9. Are there published data contradictory to the hypothesis?
B. Is the goal of the trial pragmatic? That is, is an attempt made to comparatively evaluate the net result of the total treatment program, including its dropouts and nontreated patients?
C. Is the goal explanatory, attempting to demonstrate the reality of a specific treatment effect?
D. What is the hypothesis regarding magnitude and direction of each pairwise treatment contrast for each measure over time?
E. Are proposed mechanisms of specific therapeutic action stipulated for each treatment?
1. Is each outcome hypothesis stipulated in advance?
2. Does this lead to specific process hypotheses (e.g., does cognitive improvement or interpersonal process amelioration necessarily antecede affective change)?
3. Are there stipulated process tests to determine if any benefits may not be attributable to proposed specific mechanisms, but rather to nonspecific common process (e.g., demoralization relief)?
F. In comparative, multitreatment trial, is the clinical meaningfulness of each pairwise treatment contrast stated? This allows per comparison hypothesis testing appropriate for meaningful pairwise treatment contrasts without concern for multiple group contrasts and per family error rates, thus obviating coun-

terproductive conservative adjustments such as the Bonferroni correction.

G. Are hypothetical biological or other moderating variables measured?

H. Is there a prior definition of the magnitude of change considered clinically significant for each measure?
   1. How is this determined?
   2. Are there normative standards (derived how?) for each measure, allowing an estimate of degree of clinical normalization?

I. What primary reference groups allow estimation of the magnitude of differential therapeutic activity?
   1. Pill placebo-case management?
      a. Placebo-active (side effect producing)
      b. Placebo-inactive
   2. Psychological placebos (e.g., attention controls)?
   3. Standard accepted treatments?
   4. Alternative putative treatments?
   5. Waiting lists? (Such lists do not control for expectancy or treatment setting, may be toxic, and do not estimate specific treatment effect. Waiting lists only estimate the course of the illness under the stressful condition of deferred treatment and should be avoided.)

J. Do any contrasts estimate the magnitude of nonspecific therapeutic activity?
   1. Waiting lists versus pill placebo?
   2. Can the natural history of the illness be estimated?

K. What are the qualifications, special training, motivation, attitudes toward treatment, affective and cognitive abilities of the therapists?
   1. Are nonprofessionals or paraprofessionals included?
   2. Is a preliminary, as well as longitudinally checked, standard of demonstrated proficiency in carrying out the prescribed treatment required?
   3. Do therapists deliver all treatments or are they nested within treatments?

L. If the treatment fails, what happens to the patients?
   1. How is failure determined?

    2. Can patients be switched to another protocol after a period of poor progress while remaining within the study?

    3. Are they discharged from the study?

    4. Is poststudy treatment offered to the patients, free of cost?

    5. Are there referrals to community resources?

    6. Are dropouts followed up for the study period and evaluated?

  M. What are the investigators' attitudes toward each treatment?

  N. Is there joint mutual supervision by investigators with opposing beliefs?

  O. Is treatment credibility assessed?

II. Design

  A. Sample definition: Is the sample to be representative of clinical practice, is it narrowly defined to rule out confounding variables, or is it simply a sample of convenience?

    1. Inclusion and Exclusion

      a. How are inclusion and exclusion criteria specified?

      b. How are subjects recruited?

      c. Is there a standardized registration system?

      d. Is there a required diagnosis with specified inclusion and exclusion criteria?

    2. Psychiatric History

      a. Are the amount of previous treatment and previous treatment outcomes recorded?

      b. How are suicidal tendencies and attempts measured and what is the effect on eligibility?

      c. How are previous hospitalizations and outcomes measured?

    3. How is chronicity determined?

    4. Are symptomatic minima and maxima for specified historic periods stipulated?

    5. Are impairment minima and maxima for specified historical periods stipulated?

    6. Is there a priori treatment referent substratification or covariate identification?

    7. Is there a measure of intelligence?

    8. Medical evaluation

      a. Is there a preliminary medical evaluation?

        b. Is there a preliminary clinical laboratory screening?

        c. Is there an examination for neurological difficulty (e.g., soft signs)?

    9. How are psychiatric and medical comorbidity dealt with?

  10. How are patients' social and economic competence measured?

  11. What demographics indices are measured?

        a. Age

        b. Sex

        c. Social class

        d. Income

        e. Other

B. Site specification

    1. What is the history of site experience?

    2. What is the history of site treatment allegiance?

    3. Is there provision of supervision across sites by alternative treatment experts?

C. Treatment definition

    1. Is there a period of treatment washout or initial placebo treatment to remove rapid responders?

        a. Length of trial

        b. Number of treatment sessions

    2. How are psychotherapies defined?

        a. Manuals

        b. Narratively

    3. How are medications applied?

        a. Fixed dose

        b. Fixed-flexible dose

        c. Possible modifications and sequences of treatments given initial failure

    4. Are patients afforded equal time and an equivalent caring environment?

    5. Are combined treatments assessed?

    6. How are adjunctive, ad hoc, prescribed, or self-administered agents administered?

    7. Is there standardization of postacute trial treatment and follow up?

D. Are criteria for initial clinically useful change as well as positive marked response stipulated, allowing estimates of rapidity of onset?

E. Is an a priori sample size determined, and what are the power implications?
   1. For trial termination
   2. Sequential analysis
   3. Adaptive assignment

F. Is an a priori maximum percent of nonevaluable patients stipulated for study validity?

G. How is informed consent defined and carried out?

H. Randomization
   1. How is randomization accomplished?
      a. Is it done in terms of individuals or larger groups?
      b. How is the method of allocation concealed?
   2. Are nonrandomized comparisons stipulated?

III. Measures

A. Are measures normatively standardized?

B. Blinding
   1. How is blinding accomplished?
      a. If a pill placebo is used, is it credible?
         (i) Does it look like the active treatment?
         (ii) Does it taste like the active treatment?
   2. Are there measures of blinding effectiveness?
   3. Can piercing the blind be attributed to therapeutic improvement or side effects?
   4. In case of emergency how can blind be broken?

C. Rationale and design
   1. How are the measures, occasions of measurement, and means of measurement justified?
   2. Are primary measures of importance stipulated?
   3. How was measurement reliability established?
      a. Historical
      b. Concurrent
      c. Details of training and longitudinal checking
   4. Are multiple measures counterbalanced?
   5. Are measurements obtained by therapist evaluation, patient self-evaluation, knowledgeable informant, objective measures, or blind independent evaluators?

      6.   Are there categorical scales of clinically relevant outcome?

      7.   Are process measures taken by recordings during treatment?

      8.   What is the timing of the outcome assessment?

  D. Types of measures

      1.   Are continuous or dichotomous measures of change used?

      2.   Are objective measures of functioning, such as work, income, staying out of trouble with the law, graduation from approved training programs, cessation of positive urine tests, used?

      3.   Are initial and repeated measures of treatment acceptability, credibility, and guessed treatment identification obtained from patients? Note initial credibility may be gullibility and terminal credibility is confounded with success.

      4.   How is treatment compliance measured?

        a.   Diaries?

        b.   Informants?

        c.   Pill counts?

        d.   Blood and urine tests?

      5.   Is there urine or blood screening or self-screening for self-administered psychotropic agents?

      6.   How are adverse events defined and evaluated?

      7.   Are there measures of quality of life?

      8.   How is the integrity of the treatment process established?

        a.   By recorded comparison with a manual?

        b.   By narrative notes or tapes of a therapist, independent evaluator, patient?

        c.   Measures of treatment compliance (e.g. urine, blood tests)?

  E. Are dropouts followed, assessed, and incorporated into the analytical model?

  F. Are costs of care estimated?

  G. Do individual therapists provide sufficient data to allow estimation of their specific effects?

IV. Statistical Analysis

  A. Is an intention to treat model used? If not, how is it justified?

B. Is a minimum period of actual treatment required to be included in the data base?

C. Is a last observation carried forward approach used?

D. Is a random regression or repeated measures approach used?

E. Can completer analysis be justified?

F. Are statistical analysts blind to treatment objective?

G. What alpha level is selected? One-tailed or two-tailed?

H. Is a target sample size stipulated in advance?

I. Is each stipulated hypothesis tied to a specified analysis?

J. Are data distributions presented?

K. If complex analyses are performed, are sufficient summary data presented to allow independent reanalysis?

L. Are baseline scores of randomized treatment groups comparable? If not, how is this addressed?

M. Are analytical models for treatment contrasts stipulated and justified with special reference to covariates and treatment relevant subgroups (e.g., has there been stratification for diagnostic heterogeneity related to outcome or is this approached by analysis of covariance)?

N. Are a priori analyses clearly distinguished from post hoc analyses?

O. Are order analyses appropriate and conducted?

P. Are requirements for pairwise contrast of homogeneity of slope in the analysis of covariance model met at appropriate nonstringent levels?

Q. If the analysis of covariance model is questionable, is a Johnson-Neyman or analogous resampling analysis performed, rather than simply dropping the initial value covariate?

R. How are site interactions analyzed?

S. How are power analyses calculated? In particular, what is the power with regard to clinically significant contrasts?

T. If "null hypotheses" cannot be invalidated, what is the power with regard to clinically significant contrasts?

U. Dropouts

    1. Is there any differential dropout number or type of patient?

    2. Do dropouts and completers differ by treatment?

3. Can the dropout process be modeled and included in the efficacy analysis?

V. What are the confidence limits on all treatment outcomes and contrasts?

W. Are there implicit or explicit affirmations of the null hypotheses, especially in the contrasts of two active treatments?

X. Are effect size measures presented?

Y. Are actual probability values presented?

Z. Are there analyses for relative speed of onset and costs of specific treatment effects?

AA. Are there analyses for individual therapist effects?

BB. Is there any relationship between deviation from manuals and outcome?

CC. Do deviations from a manual occur differentially before or after lack of improvement?

DD. Are there analyses in terms of clinically relevant, treatment specific, longitudinal patterns (e.g., very quick onset of improvement, maintaining major improvement, delayed improvement with maintenance gains versus fluctuating course)?

EE. If combined treatments are assessed in a factorial design, are individual cell contrasts evaluated?

V. Results

A. Has the trial completed its intended course or been terminated early or late and why?

B. In carrying out the trial, are deviations from the protocol noted, explained, and dealt with in the analysis?

C. Sample composition

1. What proportion of trial applicants are considered eligible? What are the reasons for ineligibility and relevant Ns?

2. What proportion of suitable patients accepted the proposed study?

3. What proportion of study entrants actually failed study criteria?

4. What proportion of study-accepting subjects do not ac-

cept their treatment assignment or drop out after a few sessions?

5. What are the reasons for dropouts?
6. What is the status of the dropouts at drop out and after a period equivalent to the treatment course?
7. What treatment did the dropouts receive after the study but during the period of the trial?

D. Is evidence of integrity of treatment provision satisfactory?

1. Are there analyses regarding medication and psychotherapeutic administration, compliance, and informed supervision?
2. Are there analyses of biological evidence that putatively unmedicated patients are actually unmedicated?
3. Is use of ad hoc self-administered adjunctive agents detected? How is this handled?
4. Are there analyses regarding process monitoring?
5. Did outcome relate to antecedent or subsequent process variations?

E. Are there analyses of site treatment interactions?

F. What are the measures of comparative benefit?

1. Relative risk reduction
2. Absolute risk reduction
3. Categorical
4. Endpoint
5. Trend over time
6. Adjusted or raw means
7. How are these related to clinical significance?

G. What is the evidence for benefit?

1. If dichotomous variables were used, are the results presented as proportions?
2. Does it only consist of showing within treatment or after contrasts?
3. Is this explained as a change during treatment or as due to treatment?
4. Does it consist of statistical superiority to waiting lists, which lack expectancy of help, hope, and therapeutic al-

liance? Is this explained as insufficient for estimating specific treatment efficacy?

5. Does it consist of statistical superiority to other credible therapies?

6. Does it consist of superiority to putatively inactive psychotherapy placebo, pill placebo-case management, or both?

7. Has the psychotherapy placebo been calibrated against pill placebo? (In the Liebowitz and Heimberg trial, in subjects with social phobia the psychological placebo was significantly inferior on two assessor-rated measures to pill placebo. Therefore, it does not suffice to stipulate by fiat that a psychological procedure is a placebo because it may contain a beneficial or toxic specific ingredient.)

8. Is equivalent efficacy demonstrated by affirming the hypothesis of no clinical differences between putative and standard treatment, using confidence limit analyses and a priori standards?

9. Has the benefit been shown in studies by therapists without strong allegiance to the treatment?

10. Are there individual therapist or site effects?

11. Is there evidence of a dose-response relationship?

12. Is comparative speed of improvement addressed?

13. Are comparative costs of treatment addressed?

14. Are hypothesized moderating variables demonstrated?

15. Can improvement or toxicity be modeled in terms of baseline or process variables?

16. What is the level of patient satisfaction?

H. Has it been demonstrated in the trial that the medication is superior to pill placebo, thus calibrating the putatively medication responsive sample as actually medication responsive?

I. What is the evidence that the proposed mechanism of action is the actual mechanism?

1. Does it antecede the development of benefit?

2. If inadequately effectuated, is there less benefit?

3. Is degree of therapist training or professional experience correlated with the amount of benefit produced?

4. Can it be shown that the treatment actually affects the target illness or whether it only affects demoralization?

J. Do the survival curves over each treatment course differ?

K. Is there comparative, prospective evidence for posttreatment maintained or prophylactic benefit?

L. Is there an analysis in terms of the intent to treat sample, extending through follow up, thus allowing a pragmatic programmatic evaluation?

M. Are statistically significant effects translatable into clinically meaningful effects as calibrated against a priori standards or normative samples?

N. Has the study been replicated?

O. Have the findings been replicated?

P. When does unblinding occur, and can this information be kept from the study team?

Q. Are the raw data supporting a publication available in analyzable form, at the point of publication or shortly after data collection completion, for independent analysis? (The investigators should, of course, have a reasonable period to complete and report their analyses.)

R. Overall assessment of the study in the context of the literature
  1. Is the effect size of the medication-placebo contrast consonant with the literature?
  2. Do the results match those previously found, and how are the differences explained?
  3. What are the practical and theoretical implications of the findings?
  4. What are the weaknesses of this study?
  5. What are the implications for future studies?

References

American Psychological Association Task Force on Psychological Intervention Guidelines: Template for Developing Guidelines: Interventions for Mental Disorders and Psychosocial Aspects of Physical Disorders. Washington, DC, American Psychological Association, February, 1995

Baar J, Tannock I: Analyzing the same data in two ways: a demonstration model to illustrate the reporting and misreporting of clinical trials. J Clin Oncol 7:969–978, 1989

Begg C, Cho M, Eastwood S, et al: Improving the quality of reporting of randomized controlled trials. JAMA 276:637–639, 1996

Heimberg RG, Liebowitz MR, Hope DA, et al (eds): Social Phobia: Diagnosis, Assessment and Treatment. New York, Guilford, 1995

Kazdin AE: Research Design in Clinical Psychology, 3rd Edition. Needham Heights, MA, Allyn & Bacon, 1998

Kazdin AE, Wilson GT: Criteria for evaluating psychotherapy. Arch Gen Psychiatry 35:407–416, 1978

Laupacis A, Naylor CD, Sackett DL: How should the results of clinical trials be presented to clinicians? ACP J Club A12–A14, 1992

Luborsky L, Diguer L, Luborsky E, et al: The efficacy of dynamic psychotherapies: is it true that "everyone has won and all must have prizes"? in Psychodynamic Treatment Research: A Handbook for Clinical Practice. Edited by Miller NE, Luborsky L, Barber JP, et al. New York, Basic Books, 1993, pp 497–516

Maher BA: A reader's, writer's, and reviewer's guide to assessing research reports in clinical psychology. J Consult Clin Psychol 46:835–838, 1978

Robinson LA, Berman JS, Neimeyer RA: Psychotherapy for the treatment of depression: a comprehensive review of controlled outcome research. Psychol Bull 108:30–49, 1990

Sackett DL, Gent M: Controversy in counting and attributing events in clinical trials. N Engl J Med 301:1410–1412, 1979

Simon R, Wittes RE: Methodologic guidelines for reports of clinical trials. Cancer Treat Rep 69:1–3, 1985

The Standard of Reporting Trial Group: A proposal for structured reporting of randomized control trials. JAMA 272:1926–1931, 1994

PART VIII

Psychotherapy in the Era of Managed Care

17

Psychotherapy and Managed Care

Compatible or Incompatible?

Steven S. Sharfstein, M.D.

Great economic and social pressures are bearing down on the practice of psychotherapy, and the future of psychotherapy as a valued treatment is uncertain. This topic is an emotional issue, engendering much anger, sadness, and anxiety between psychiatrists and other psychotherapists across the country. As the market for psychotherapeutic services shrinks, competition for patients among therapists intensifies and, as hours open up, demoralization takes hold. Fees and therapists are depressed simultaneously. Of course there is a causal association between the shrinking of the market for psychotherapy and the ever-expanding number of helpers who hang out the shingle of psychotherapist. Supply and demand are important influences on the psychotherapy market today in the United States that remains mostly an unregulated industry for which the rules of supply and demand have always applied. Now, with managed care and cost containment as the current major thrust for all of health care, extra scrutiny of psychotherapy takes on an added and ominous significance.

Psychiatry is being depleted of its future as potential medical students, observing the narrowing of opportunity to practice psychotherapy, choose primary care specialties or alternative graduate education opportunities. Psychiatrists are upset about their loss of autonomy and their inability to practice their science and art as they have for many decades. Other mental health professionals as well have expressed concern about the viability of psychotherapy as a career choice, including psychologists, social workers, nurses, and family and marriage counselors (Goleman 1996).

Let me state my biases about psychotherapy up front. Psychotherapy is very much a part of my identity as a psychiatrist and as a mental health professional, and it was the bedrock of my experience in residency training. Like many medical students trained in the 1960s, the excitement over psychoanalysis was a main motivation for me to pick psychiatry as a specialty. I have always had a psychotherapy practice. For eight years I ran a group for 8–12 patients with severe mental illness. Today, along with my rather demanding administrative and management role, I continue to treat patients with short- and long-term dynamic psychotherapy and to supervise residents in our excellent residency training program at Sheppard Pratt that teaches psychotherapy so superbly.

I am not trained as a psychoanalyst, but I have had personal psychoanalysis, and a number of years ago I was made an honorary member of the Washington Psychoanalytic Society. My bias is that psychotherapy is more than an effective treatment; it is an overall social good and, in many respects, it represents the antidote in the 20th century to anomie, mass culture, and the bureaucratized and mechanized suppression of the individual. I strongly agree with Freud's statement, made in 1919 in the famous Copper and Gold speech, that "one may reasonably expect that at some time or other the conscience of the community will awaken and admonish it that the poor man has just as much right to health for his mind as he now has for the surgeon's means of saving his life" (Freud 1919/1966, p. 157–158. Thus, these are the biases to which I subscribe, and my own research into psychotherapy and its cost effectiveness have always been informed by these values.

In this chapter I make a stab at defining psychotherapy and review the abundant evidence showing that psychotherapy is effective, both as a treatment and in the marketplace. Under current health insurance practices, some obstacles to adequate coverage of psychotherapy and specific economic problems do exist in that competitive marketplace today. Finally, I discuss managed care with respect to its current role in containing costs through controlling the use of psychotherapy and point to some options for harnessing this approach to provide more, not fewer, opportunities for appropriate and effective psychotherapy to more patients in the future.

Defining Psychotherapy

Psychotherapy is the systematic use of an interpersonal relationship designed to treat symptoms, alleviate pain, and cure disease. This treatment is in contrast to pharmacologic, procedural, or social methods of treatment. Today, psychotherapy is often provided in combination with other methods of care. The goal of any psychotherapy is to produce change in behavior, cognition, and feelings. The goals of some psychotherapies may transcend symptomatic relief and include individual enhancement, the obtainment of personal autonomy, and improved self-esteem. This gives psychotherapy a strong preventive focus in that the more personal autonomy and self-esteem a patient retains throughout life, the more that patient will be able to deal with life's future difficulties and vicissitudes.

For psychotherapy to succeed it needs structure and space. Structure means a regular time and place that are secure and safe enough so that the patient can explore thoughts and feelings in a controlled way, and where the normal consequences of verbalizing these thoughts and feelings do not apply. Space implies a situation facilitative of the necessary development of dependency, some regression, and a capacity to explore the transferential feelings of the patient toward the therapist in the longer term dynamic forms of psychotherapy. The structure of psychotherapy is a *holding environment*, and financial security is a part of that environment. If psychotherapy threatens the economic security of the individual, sustaining it is difficult, and this is true for either long-term or short-term psychotherapy.

Psychotherapy is costly and requires the skills of professionals who have trained for many years in the theoretical and practical aspects of the science and art of it. It is not, and will never be, a free good. Psychotherapists need to be commensurately paid for their work; that is, to be able to earn a living and pay their bills. If these payments are not forthcoming, psychotherapy will be difficult to sustain in the future.

Is Psychotherapy an Effective and Cost-Effective Treatment?

In a meta-analysis of several hundred placebo-controlled psychotherapy experiments, Smith and colleagues answered the question "Is psychotherapy effective?" decidedly in the affirmative (Smith et al. 1980). The average effect size, as these authors define it, of psychotherapy was approximately one standard deviation. This means that the average psychotherapy patient did better than 85% of control subjects. Another way the authors put it is that 70% of the psychotherapy patients evaluated improved, whereas 30% did not. Conversely, 30% of the controls improved, whereas 70% did not. In these various studies, placebo groups included nonspecific chats and unfocused discussion groups.

The effectiveness of psychotherapy is also attested to by medical cost offset data. Seventy studies have now looked at the impact on medical costs of the provision of psychotherapy. These studies demonstrate a decrease in medical costs when psychotherapy is accessible, and this decrease is due to a decrease in the number of hospitalizations and hospital days, the number of consultations with physicians, and a decrease in the use of expensive medications (Jones and Vischi 1979; Sharfstein et al. 1994).

The offset issue is important from a health policy perspective, because our society has determined to do what it can to control total medical costs. Forty years ago in what was then West Germany, a major study took place that led to a very broad expansion of national health insurance benefits for psychotherapy (Duhrssen 1957, 1972). This West German follow-up study evaluated patients' health and mental health status at the onset and at the end of psychotherapy treatment, and then at follow-up after 5 years. Of the 1,000 patients who underwent individual psychotherapy, the average number of treatment hours was 100; 12% ended treatment prematurely, 12% continued privately after their limit of 200 treatments ran out, 10% wanted further treatment after 200 treatments, but could not afford it.

At 5-year follow-up, 845 of the 1000 patients were evaluated. It was estimated that approximately 13% of the patients had experienced one relapse in their mental condition during this 5-year follow-up period. The number of hospital stays per year for the follow-up group was .78, which compared with a pretreatment average of 5.3 days per year and a general average for the insured population matched by age and sex of 2.5 hospital days per year, and these were hospital days for any illness, not just mental illness.

Although this pioneering study has several methodological problems, it was persuasive enough, along with several confirmatory studies on the cost offset of psychotherapy, to expand the health insurance benefit for mental illness in Germany to 250 lifetime psychotherapy visits, as long as the care is preapproved using prognostic factors and periodically evaluated by a peer review committee.

There are, in addition, many studies that examine the outcome of psychotherapy for specific conditions such as acute depression. Many of these studies show psychotherapy to be as effective as pharmacotherapy and the combination of psychotherapy and pharmacotherapy to be even more effective for specific conditions. Other studies demonstrate that the number of hospital days for a given psychiatric illness is decreased when access to intensive psychotherapeutic care is provided. Many of these studies were quoted in that important journal of our times, *The Wall Street Journal* (Pollack 1995).

In 1995 *Consumer Reports* conducted a major study using a sample of their subscribers and reported in an article entitled "Mental Health: Does Therapy Help?" that consumers felt greatly helped by psychotherapy. More than 80% felt that they had been helped a lot or helped somewhat, and most interestingly and significantly, those who saw a "mental health specialist" for more than six months did better than those who received shorter term care. The best outcomes were reported by individuals who stayed in treatment for more than two years (Seligman 1995).

To summarize then, psychotherapy is an effective treatment for a broad range of conditions, and there are cost offsets caused by it in general medical care, as well as in expensive psychiatric care. Patients are satisfied, and the outcomes are excellent. So what is the problem? As a society, why do we not pay for it like we pay for cancer treatment, organ transplantations, or cardiac care?

Psychotherapy and Health Insurance: Some Basic Incompatibilities

Despite the arguments already elucidated, at this time virtually all health insurance programs, either public or private, severely limit psychotherapy. In contrast to other effective and appropriate treatments, and even treatments that have dubious effectiveness and high costs, where full coverage is provided under health insurance, psychotherapy is universally limited through limitations in annual number of visits, caps on the amount of lifetime or annual dollars that can be spent, on the fees that can be charged, and by requiring copayments, paid out-of-pocket by patients. The Clinton Health Security Act is a typical example of this situation, with a benefit of 30 psychotherapy visits and requirement of a 50% copay. This bill, however, did provide an interesting tradeoff, allowing for more visits if it could be demonstrated that inpatient psychiatric days could be saved. Medicare limits psychotherapy through its fee schedule and via copayments. The current fee schedule for psychotherapy of 50% of a national average of approximately $80 per hour is now a baseline for most private insurance plans, which underscores the unwillingness of the insurance industry to pay adequately for psychotherapy. In a recent survey, only 6% of all private health insurance companies provided psychotherapy on the same basis as other medical treatments (Scheidemandel 1993).

Stigma and stereotyping obviously play a role in shaping these restrictive policy decisions, but rather than focus on this traditional lament, there are some serious and concrete economic problems for psychotherapy under current health insurance practices deserving of our attention. These realities make the politics of psychotherapy coverage under managed care more complex and uncertain.

Health insurance has several conceptual underpinnings that compromise its appropriateness as the principal payment method for psychotherapy. Health insurance, in many ways, is like other insurance because it is primarily a method designed to pay for unforeseen financial losses of some magnitude that the few endure unexpectedly, while the many contribute a small amount to a large risk pool. Health insurance implies the spreading of risk and the ability of the many who are well to pay for the few who are sick. As such, three important principles are necessary for the treatment of any medical condition to be covered.

First, the illness must have definable epidemiology. Diseases and disorders must be defined discretely and distinctly, with a special focus on being able to define the moment of onset and conclusion of a condition. Epidemiology is an essential medical science that helps determine whether health insurance can pay for the economic loss implied by a countable, discrete disease.

Second, in addition to a definable epidemiology, there is the need to have a definable treatment (that is, an appropriate and necessary treatment), an understanding about who can provide it, a knowledge of the technical skills required and other technologies appropriately applied to relieve symptoms effectively and care well for patients or even effect a cure. A definable treatment with the definable epidemiology defines the loss to be covered. These concepts in health insurance are primary aspects of underwriting an insurance company's assessment of the potential payout of certain coverages for specific populations. It is important that both the treatment and the condition are not discretionary, and that people cannot not easily forego the treatment if they need it. Third, and finally, under health insurance accountability is necessary, and utilization review is the main method for accountability, with outcome studies beginning to emerge on the horizon as the preferred method for accountability. Utilization review implies a model of diminishing marginal returns. That is, with each treatment a definable improvement is occurring to the point where those improvements begin to diminish and plateau, and at that point treatment should cease.

From these principles, one can see that the current health insurance model, more accurately called acute illness insurance, is most compatible with coverage for infectious disease, acute surgical conditions, and short-term medical events.

Does psychotherapy conform to these basic tenets of health insurance? Many believe that almost everyone with developmental issues and life crises could benefit from psychotherapy, and if a nearly 100% epidemiology or prevalence exists, psychotherapy is not an insurable good. Even with the more narrow epidemiologic focus of DSM-III-R and DSM-IV (American Psychiatric Association 1987, 1994), studies that show 30% of the American population with a psychiatric disorder and only 20% of that 30% in treatment, gives any payer a basis for concern about generous insurance coverage and a need to add limits to coverage for psychotherapy (Regier et al. 1993). If the epidemiologic catchment area data is correct, and I have no reason to doubt these data, approximately 50 million Americans can benefit from psychotherapy, but as *Consumer Reports* mentions, fewer than 10% of these individuals are actually in treatment ("Mental health: does therapy help?"). The second issue to consider is whether psychotherapy is a definable treatment. Hundreds of psychotherapies are practiced in the United States, and although the studies are many, no one major type of psychotherapy as such can be consistently demonstrated to be more effective than any other (Banta and Saxe 1983). This truism includes individual or group therapy, short-term or long-term therapy, cognitive-behavioral therapy, and psychoanalysis. Obviously these treatments vary considerably on the matter of cost. Second, effectiveness may have more to do with the therapist than with the therapy per se. I am not aware of any study that consistently shows that those with an M.D. degree are superior to those with any other degree from the point of view of effectiveness or outcome. *Consumer Reports* showed that people were just as satisfied with treatment they received from a psychiatrist, a psychologist or a social worker, but less likely to feel they had been helped by a marriage or family counselor; and they were more satisfied with mental health specialists than family practitioners ("Mental health: does therapy help?").

Third, there is a notable lack of specificity in many studies on treatment; that is, the specificity of a particular psychotherapy for specific patients and conditions. Psychotherapy remains a very individualized treatment approach, with a lack of clear practice guidelines or protocols. The therapy being received generally depends on the type or theoretical orientation of the therapist and not on the patient's particular problem. Economists called this *the matching problem*; that is, how do the right people get the right treatment? Given the number of providers and the number of therapies, the matching of patients, therapists, and therapies leads to economic consequences that undermine the compatibility of health insurance as the main way to pay for care.

Finally, can utilization review of psychotherapy demonstrate incremental improvements with sessions over time? We all know as practicing psychotherapists that patients experience resistance and regression, and that learning is complicated; it is not a smooth marginal curve but a wavy one, often with improvements in the first 10 sessions followed by some decrement, and, perhaps much more significant, improvement occurring in sessions much later in the overall treatment. Thus, each psychotherapy session is not a discrete treatment on which one scrutinizes with utilization review!

We must ask how discretionary psychotherapy is compared with other medical treatments. The price sensitivity of psychotherapy has been studied in more than 20 well-designed experiments (Frank and McGuire 1986). It has been observed that the demand responsiveness of ambulatory mental health and medical care is different, and that psychotherapy is more responsive to price than is general medical care. The Rand Health Insurance Experiment, a study having one of the best prospective randomized designs, showed that as coinsurance rates increased for patients, medical care decreased 50% and psychotherapy decreased 75%. Patients more willingly forego psychotherapy if a third party was not willing to pay (Wills and Manning 1989). One study, however, showed that those patients who reduced visits for psychotherapy because of lack of insurance had the most need in terms of their Axis I, DSM-III-R diagnosis (Landerman et al. 1994).

Therefore, the very broad epidemiology of mental disorders, the many psychotherapies and psychotherapists, the difficulties inherent in reviewing psychotherapy, and psychotherapy's price sensitivity undermine the compatibility of psychotherapy with health insurance, and lead the actuaries and other policy makers to act on their ingrained prejudice against psychotherapy by limiting coverage. The actuarial literature is replete with statements of the inability effectively to offer coverage for psychotherapy for a variety of the reasons as discussed already, and based on statements concerning overutilization, unnecessary care, providers openly marketing to consumers, and the like.

Despite these limitations, insurance coverage for psychotherapy has grown in recent years, and the costs for treatment have also grown. From 1955 to 1985, outpatient mental health costs increased 77 times, most being for psychotherapy. This contrasts with an increase in the gross national product of 10 times national health expenditures, 24 times during the same period (Taube and Barrett 1985). The need for psychotherapy care is compelling. The consumers want it. We need to find a method that works for paying for it adequately.

Managed Care and Psychotherapy

If the epidemiology for the appropriate provision of psychotherapy can be more narrowly defined, if practice guidelines and clinical models for appropriate and necessary care are developed, and if the group of competent licensed practitioners is limited, I believe we can provide for a reasonable and predictable state of affairs and develop not only indications for psychotherapy, but methods for utilization review. This is essentially what was done in Germany 35 years ago.

Managed care in America, however, has been introduced primarily as a means for limiting costs. Utilization review under managed care has been used to interrupt psychotherapy, create chaos for the therapist and the patient, and to cut costs through the denial of care.

The first phase of managed care in the early 1990s has been managed costs and mangled care, and there are many examples of managed care that have just been another chapter of discrimination against mental illness under health insurance (Sharfstein 1994).

Managed care has invaded the psychotherapist's office, compromised the confidentiality of the patient-therapist relationship, and may be one of the best examples of what has been called "rationing by harassment" (Grumet 1989). But counterintuitively and perhaps with some undue optimism, I would like to suggest that with managed care there may be the opportunity to preserve and expand psychotherapy in the face of the cost containment imperatives of the 21st century. The techniques of managed care include prior, concurrent, and retrospective review of medical necessity and appropriateness of services, the application of financial incentives or disincentives related to the use of specific providers or services, controlled access to and coordination of services by a case manager, and efforts to identify treatment alternatives and modify benefits so that high-cost patients can be treated efficiently and effectively. These techniques could be harnessed to lead to a cost-controllable expansion of psychotherapy for many individuals who could greatly benefit from the treatment.

What I am suggesting is that managed care could be an effective method to deal with the problems of uncertain epidemiology, many competing treatments and providers, utilization review issues, price sensitivity problems, the matching problem, the overall issue of cost effectiveness.

If I were the president of a large HMO, I would put together systems of care with psychotherapy as a key element integral to the efficiency of my medical care system by users the cost offset of the high users of medical care with psychotherapy. I would develop criteria for clinicians, including psychiatrists, directly to provide more psychotherapy rather than less. I would aim for having many of my enrollees in short-term psychotherapy, and then having a number of those at risk for chronic illness in long-term psychotherapy. Those patients who are at risk for medical or psychiatric hospitalizations are prime candidates for this approach. Their numbers are large. I would aim for 30% of my covered population being evaluated for psychotherapy, and between 10% and 15% of my overall costs being devoted to it. Obviously, I would want good outcome data and high patient satisfaction, and all this has to work within an overall budget and a competitive marketplace. Given these restrictions, I believe we could achieve a broad expansion for psychotherapy in the context of an organized system of care. I am suggesting nothing less than a revaluing of psychotherapy and its expansion within the broad medical marketplace, a change that should be possible and desirable as we move toward population-based health reform.

Opportunities Today for Contracting With Managed Care for Psychotherapy

What is the private practicing clinician to do today in the face of the incursions of managed care? In contracting with managed care and becoming part of networks, the clinician in private practice has the opportunity not only to continue his or her psychotherapy practice, but to make the case to the managed care system that psychotherapy is cost effective and necessary. To do this, I would offer the following suggestions to the psychotherapist.

First, use a case's medical offset potential to justify treatment. Describe your patient's history of use of medical and surgical care, as well as inpatient psychiatric care, and show how the psychotherapy proposed may be expected to reduce these expenses. This makes the idea of *medical necessity of psychotherapy* more directly apparent to reviewers and the medical directors of managed care companies.

Second, be clear as to the specific objectives of the psychotherapy being offered, and the progress being made toward accomplishing these objectives. Focused short-term objectives are important to clarify and be specific about up front, and if extended psychotherapy is needed, justifying it again from the point of view of specifiable and achievable objectives is important.

Third, not exaggerating symptoms is important in the process of utilization review, such as making the patient seem excessively suicidal, to gain permission for more sessions. Honesty is always the best policy.

Even with these suggestions, it may be that managed care organizations will only allow for a few visits to deal with the most acute and intensive symptoms. At that point, working with the patient in justifying the costs and benefits of more extended treatment is important. Many patients avail themselves of the opportunity and pay out of pocket. Some patients from the beginning prefer not to use their insurance and be subjected to managed care review because of confidentiality breaches and lack of privacy in the communication of sensitive information from therapist to reviewer. To some extent, managed care has brought psychotherapy back into the era of out-of-pocket payment. Many Americans have disposable incomes between $2,000 and

$10,000 a year, and via these individuals, psychotherapy will continue to flourish outside the mainstreams of third party financing.

The final decision on the role of and reimbursement for psychotherapy will take place in the political and economic marketplace. It is important to not be too pessimistic nor too optimistic. It is important that we shape the future and manage it as best we can, and continue to be good psychotherapists.

References

American Psychiatric Association: Diagnostic and Statistical manual of Mental Disorders, 3rd Edition, Revised. Washington, DC, American Psychiatric Association, 1987

American Psychiatric Association: Diagnostic and Statistical manual of Mental Disorders, 4th Edition. Washington, DC, American Psychiatric Association, 1994

Banta DH, Saxe L: Reimbursement for psychotherapy: linking efficacy research and public policymaking. Am Psychol 38(8):918–923, 1983

Duhrssen A: Die beurteilung des behandlungserfolges in der psychotherapie. Z Psychosom Med 3:3, 1957

Duhrssen A: Katamnestische ergebnisse bei 1004 patienten nach analytischer psychotherapie. Z Psychosom Med 7:2, 1972

Frank RG, McGuire TG: A review of studies of the impact of insurance on the demand and utilization of specialty mental health services. Health Serv Res 21:241–265, 1986

Freud S: Lines of advance in psychoanalytic therapy (1919), in The Standard Edition of the Complete Psychological Works of Sigmund Freud, Vol 17. Translated and edited by Strachey J. London, Hogarth Press, 1966, pp 157–168

Goleman D: Critics say managed-care savings are eroding mental care. New York Times, January 24, 1996, p 1

Grumet GW: Health care rationing through inconvenience. N Engl J Med 321:609–611, 1989

Jones KR, Vischi TR: Impact of alcohol, drug abuse and mental health treatment on medical care utilization: a review of the research literature. Medical Care 17:12, 1979

Landerman LR, Burns BJ, Swartz MS, et al: The relationship between insurance coverage and psychiatric disorder in predicting use of mental health services. Am J Psychiatry 151(12):1785–1790, 1994

Mental health: does therapy help? Consumer Reports, November 1995, pp 734–739

Pollack EJ: Managed care's focus on psychiatric drugs alarms many doctors. Wall Street Journal, December 1, 1995, p 1

Regier DA, Narrow WE, Rae DS, et al: The de facto US mental and addictive disorders service system: epidemiologic catchment area perspective 1-year prevalence rates of disorders and services. Arch Gen Psychiatry 50:85–94, 1993

Scheidemandel P: The Coverage Catalog, 3rd Edition. Washington, DC, American Psychiatric Association 1993

Seligman ME: The effectiveness of psychotherapy. The *Consumer Reports* study. Am Psychol 50(12):965–974, 1995

Sharfstein SS: Economics redefining the practice of psychiatry. Bull Menninger Clin 58(4):647–653, 1994

Smith ML, Glass GV, Miller TI: The Benefits of Psychotherapy. Baltimore, MD, Johns Hopkins University Press, 1980

Taube CA, Barrett SA (eds.): Mental Health, United States, 1985 (DHHS Pub. No. ADM 85–1378). Washington, DC, U.S. Government Printing Office, 1985

Wills KB, Manning WH: The effects of insurance generosity on the psychological distress and psychological well-being of a general population. Arch Gen Psychiatry 46(4):315–320, 1989

Index

Note: *Page numbers printed in **boldface** type refer to tables or figures.*